with contributions by

CYNTHIA L. BECKER, R.N., B.S.N.

Formerly Staff Nurse, Combined MICU-CCU,
Veterans Administration Hospital, San Francisco

CAROL A. CARROLL, R.N., B.S.N.

Formerly Head Nurse, Combined MICU-CCU,
Veterans Administration Hospital, San Francisco

THOMAS P. FORDE, M.D.

Clinical Instructor in Medicine,
University of California School of Medicine,
San Francisco; Courtesy Staff, Samuel Merritt,
Providence and Peralta Hospitals, Oakland

MERVIN J. GOLDMAN, M.D.

Professor of Medicine,
University of California School of Medicine;
Assistant Chief, Medical Service, Veterans
Administration Hospital, San Francisco

ALBERT D. HALL, M.D.

Vice Chairman and Associate Professor of Surgery,
University of California School of Medicine;
Chief, Surgical Service,
Veterans Administration Hospital, San Francisco

STEPHANIE A. SEDLOCK, R.N., M.S.

Lecturer in Nursing,
University of California School of Nursing,
Regional Medical Program, Area I, San Francisco

ARTHUR N. THOMAS, M.D.

Assistant Professor of Surgery,
University of California Medical Center;
Chief, Thoracic Surgery,
San Francisco General Hospital, San Francisco

THE CARDIAC PATIENT

A Comprehensive Approach

RICHARD G. SANDERSON, M.D.

Associate in Surgery, University of Arizona
College of Medicine, Tucson; Formerly Chief,
Cardiac Surgery, Veterans Administration
Hospital, San Francisco

Saunders Monographs in Clinical Nursing—2

W. B. SAUNDERS COMPANY
Philadelphia, London, Toronto

W. B. Saunders Company: West Washington Square
Philadelphia, Pa. 19105

1 St. Anne's Road
Eastbourne, East Sussex BN21 3UN, England

833 Oxford Street
Toronto, M8Z 5T9, Canada

The Cardiac Patient: A Comprehensive Approach   ISBN 0-7216-7095-6

Print No.:   9   8   7   6

Preface

The concepts and contents presented in this book are the direct result of the challenging interplay between the cardiac nurses and their attending physicians. The cardiac nurse, with her medical training, clinical judgment and underlying experience, plays a very direct role in the formulation of the patient's medical regimen as well as in his actual nursing care. Her intellect should be stimulated as her opinions are actively solicited; she is asked to personally evaluate clinical situations and take independent action rather than to blindly follow a prescribed ritual of patient care. In this individualized approach, she plays a very integral part in every phase in the interplay with her patients, from the diagnostic inquiries to the therapeutic formulations and actual patient care.

In a sense, the cardiac nurse is expected to play a new and expanded role in comprehensive patient care. The cardiac nurse should have an in-depth knowledge about the underlying disease processes, the diagnostic and therapeutic maneuvers used to treat cardiac disease, and the techniques of meticulous care of these critically ill patients. It is the purpose of this book to give the cardiac nurse a comprehensive understanding of each of these aspects.

The first three chapters of the book lay the foundations for understanding the basic problems—the underlying anatomy and pathology of cardiac disease and the concepts of medical and surgical treatment. The next six chapters describe the "tools" that are used in cardiac care—electrocardiography, diagnostic techniques, respiratory care, cardiac drugs, specialized equipment and cardiopulmonary resuscitation. The final two chapters, intentionally saved to serve as a conclusion and a summary of the preceding chapters, are written by medical and surgical cardiac nursing specialists and embody their application of these basic concepts to direct nursing care.

v

   Although the book is intended for cardiac nursing specialists of varying degrees of experience, it is intentionally written at a relatively advanced nursing level. It is our hope that the advanced cardiac nurse will find the text adequately stimulating, particularly if supplemented with additional reading from the selected bibliographies at the conclusion of each chapter, and that the beginning nurse specialist can "reach out" to the text as a reference source. Hopefully, the many illustrations and drawings will enhance the understanding of both the beginner and the expert.

RICHARD G. SANDERSON, M.D.

Acknowledgments

The acknowledgments involved in such a collaborative effort are legion and my thanks are extended to many people. Primary recognition is given to the inquisitive intellect and dedicated care of the cardiac nursing specialists who stimulated the writing of the book; they are too numerous to name. To Dr. J. Englebert Dunphy and Dr. Albert Starr go my thanks for their role in providing me not only with my basic training, but also with whatever understanding, clinical judgment and teaching attitudes form the undercurrent of this book. The hard work and expertise of the other collaborators will hopefully be recognized by the readers' understanding of cardiac care that their chapters have provided.

Every author or editor has a great debt of gratitude for the secretarial and technical assistance that he has received. The untold hours of work in rough drafts and manuscript preparation by Mrs. Dorothy Archbold, Mrs. Ada Glen and Mrs. Helen Hafner are gratefully recognized and appreciated. Mrs. Lou Scanlon and Mrs. Rae Brooks have been equally helpful in the preparation of the galley proofs. The superlative medical illustrations provided by Mary Anne Olson, Nancy Morris, Jean Koelling and Laurel Schaubert are highlights of the book, as are the works of the medical photographers, Henry Raphael and Charles Francis; their help is also greatly appreciated. To the staff of W. B. Saunders Company, particularly to Robert Wright, Helen Dietz, George Laurie and Jane Kelsey, go my thanks for their encouragement, support and patience during the formulation and production phases of the book.

Finally, I should like to give very special recognition to my family. My wife Paula has been a paragon of helpful support and patient understanding during all phases of preparation of the book;

without her help, little would have been accomplished. I hope my four children will forgive me the hours that my work on the book has kept me from them.

RICHARD G. SANDERSON, M.D.

Contents

SECTION I

The Problem

CHAPTER 1

Anatomy, Embryology, Physiology, and Pathology

By RICHARD G. SANDERSON, M.D.

In order to lay a firm foundation for the succeeding chapters, basic concepts of anatomy, embryology, physiology, and pathology of the heart will be discussed in the first chapter.

The heart is unique among the body's vital organs (liver, kidney, lung, brain, and other organs) because its function is purely mechanical—it pumps blood. It does not excrete fluid, filter blood, exchange oxygen, or synthesize proteins; but it does propel blood to the body's tissues by a most amazing and complex series of events.

The heart is also a remarkably durable organ. It beats 60 times a minute, 3600 times an hour, 86,400 times a day, and so on, but normally it never tires. It can be cut wide open, and yet when sewn back together it continues to beat and resumes near-normal function. Its extrinsic nerve supply can be severed (as in cardiac transplantation), yet it will continue to beat by virtue of its own intrinsic rhythm. The pumping walls of the heart comprise the body's most concentrated mass of muscular tissue, yet the heart also contains some very delicate tissues, the cardiac valves. When the heart is damaged by a variety of diseases it compensates remarkably. Only in the later stages of these diseases does it fail and cause symptoms.

Anatomy

The heart is a hollow muscular pump which lies in the middle portion of the chest slightly to the left side. It is flanked by the right and left lungs. It is protected anteriorly by the sternum and attached ribs, and posteriorly by the vertebral column and the other ends of the ribs. It lies in close proximity not only to the lungs, but also to the esophagus and descending thoracic aorta posteriorly and to the diaphragm below.

The heart is contained within a fibrous sac, the pericardium, whose serous inner layer normally allows free cardiac motion. The pericardium forms a barrier through which infections from the lung and mediastinum seldom pass. Moreover, the pericardial fluid prevents external trauma from being transmitted directly to the heart. The limiting perimeters of the pericardium are shown in Figure 1–1. Note the sites of entry and exit of the great vessels, the prominence of the esophagus posteriorly, and the lungs flanking the pericardium on either side. All the heart lies within the pericardium, but only short segments of the attached vessels (aorta, pulmonary artery, venae cavae, pulmonary veins) reside within the pericardial cavity.

The heart itself is composed of three separate layers—the epicardium, the myocardium, and the endocardium. The outermost layer, the epicardium, covers the surface of the heart, extends onto

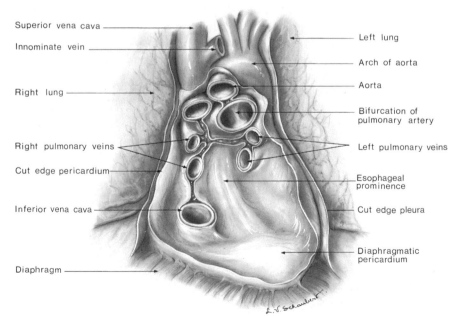

Superior vena cava

Innominate vein

Right lung

Right pulmonary veins

Cut edge pericardium

Inferior vena cava

Diaphragm

Left lung

Arch of aorta

Aorta

Bifurcation of pulmonary artery

Left pulmonary veins

Esophageal prominence

Cut edge pleura

Diaphragmatic pericardium

Figure 1–1. Drawing of the pericardial cavity with the heart removed.

the great vessels and there becomes continuous with the inner lining of the pericardium. The muscular portion of the heart is called the myocardium. The innermost layer, the endocardium, is a thin, delicate layer of tissue which lines the inside of the cardiac chambers and covers the surfaces of the cardiac valves.

CARDIAC CHAMBERS

Although the cardiac chambers are named "right" and "left," these determinations are embryologic rather than positional. The most posterior cardiac chamber is the left atrium, while the right ventricle lies anteriorly, just underneath the sternum. The left ventricle is situated laterally on the left side (and slightly posteriorly), and the right atrium lies laterally on the right side. These positions are shown diagrammatically in Figure 5–6. The following discussion of the cardiac chambers will be presented in the same sequence as the flow of blood—right atrium, right ventricle (pulmonary artery, lungs, pulmonary veins), left atrium, and left ventricle.

Right Atrium (RA)

The right atrium is the receiving chamber for venous (unoxygenated) blood from the systemic circuit—from the arms, head, abdomen, and legs. It normally has a pressure of 2 to 7 mm Hg, which varies with respiration. During inspiration, as the chest expands and the diaphragm descends, the pressure inside the chest cavity falls, causing the RA pressure to similarly decrease. The pressure in the venous system outside the chest changes only slightly with respiration. Therefore, with inspiration, the RA pressure will be lower than the pressure in the veins outside the chest. Blood will then flow from the area of higher pressure to the area of lower pressure. It is this difference in pressure which causes blood to flow into the right atrium.

Portals of entry into the right atrium include the superior vena cava (draining blood from the head and upper extremities), the inferior vena cava (bringing blood from the abdominal viscera and the lower extremities), the coronary sinus (draining blood from the circulation of the heart), and the many tiny Thebesian veins (draining small amounts of blood directly from the atrial wall itself). Blood from the inferior vena cava has a slightly higher oxygen concentration (80 per cent saturated), as compared with blood draining from the superior vena cava (70 per cent saturated). As cardiac muscle has a tremendous capability of extracting oxygen from blood from the coronary arteries, the blood draining from the coronary sinus is very dark and desaturated—about 30 per cent oxygen saturation. A sample of mixed venous blood (combining all these entry sites) has an oxygen saturation of about 75 per cent or a P_{O_2} of 40 mm Hg (see Chapter 6 for discussion of oxygen saturation and gas tensions).

The right atrium is separated from the left atrium by the interatrial septum, a dividing wall which lies medially (to the left) and posteriorly. During embryologic life, this dividing wall is perforated by a large hole, allowing right atrial blood to shunt to the left atrium. Soon after the child is born a flap of tissue covers this hole, eliminating the right-to-left shunt and leaving a slight depression called the fossa ovalis (Fig. 1–2). There is a small outpocketing of the right atrium, projecting anteriorly, which is called the right atrial appendage.

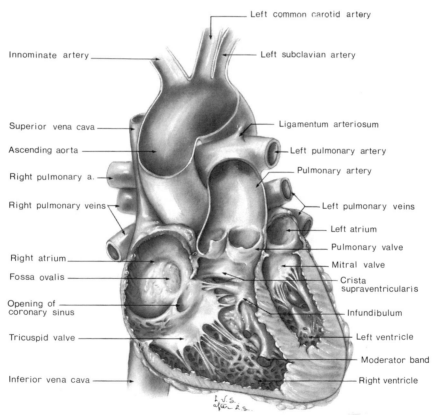

Figure 1–2. Drawing of the heart with some of the anterior structures removed to allow illustration of the underlying anatomy. The labeled structures are described in the text.

Right Ventricle (RV)

The right ventricle is a flat muscular pump which lies on the most anterior surface of the heart. It is divided into two parts—the inflow (or body of the RV) near to the tricuspid valve and the outflow (also called the infundibulum). The inner surface of both these parts is composed of crisscrossing bands of muscular tissue called trabeculations, the most prominent of which is called the moderator band (see Fig. 1–2). The papillary muscles which form the support to the tricuspid valve also take origin from these muscular walls (see discussion of cardiac valves).

The entrance to the right ventricle from the right atrium is guarded by the tricuspid valve and the exit by the pulmonary valve. Normally, the right ventricular wall is about 0.5 cm thick, but may become much thicker in lesions which obstruct its outflow (see later under discussion of pathology of pulmonary outflow obstructions). As the pulmonary circuit has a relatively low resistance, high pressures are not required to pump blood into the lungs. Normal right ventricular pressure is 20/0–5 mm Hg. Right ventricular blood has the same oxygen concentration as the blood in the right atrium.

Left Atrium (LA)

The left atrium is the receiving chamber for oxygenated blood draining from the lungs. Its portals of entry are the superior and inferior pulmonary veins draining the right lung and a similar pair draining the left lung. Normal left atrial pressure is 5 to 10 mm Hg and changes only slightly with respiration, since both the lungs and the left atrium are subjected to the same intrathoracic pressures. The oxygen saturation of left atrial blood is 96 to 98 per cent (a P_{O_2} of 95 mm Hg), assuming normal oxygen exchange in the lungs.

The left atrium lies on the posterior surface of the heart, where it rests on the esophagus. The proximity of these two structures becomes important when the left atrium enlarges; it then displaces the esophagus posteriorly, allowing it to be easily seen on a chest x-ray (if a barium swallow outlines the esophagus). Although the major portion of the left atrium lies posteriorly, a small "ear" (the left atrial appendage) projects around the left border of the heart. In this position, the appendage is available to the operating surgeon, who may insert his finger through it to palpate the mitral valve.

Left Ventricle (LV)

The bulk of muscular tissue of the heart is contained in the left ventricle, which propels oxygenated blood to the body. The wall of

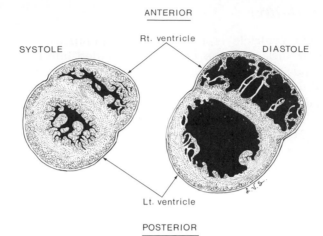

Figure 1–3. Diagram of cross section through the right and left ventricles. Note that the right ventricular cavity is crescent-shaped and that the left ventricular cavity is nearly circular.

the left ventricle is much thicker than the wall of the right ventricle, normally measuring up to 1.5 cm. It must generate enough pressure to propel blood through the relatively high-resistance systemic circuit; the LV pressure is normally 120/0–10. The inner aspect of the left ventricular wall is also crisscrossed by heavy trabeculations and the papillary muscles of the mitral valve also take their origin from these walls. Left ventricular blood has the same high oxygen saturation as the left atrial blood, 96 to 98 per cent.

There are important differences in the shapes of the right and left ventricles (Fig. 1–3). The right ventricular cavity is crescent-shaped, lying like a cap on top of the heart; its pumping action is like a bellows. In contrast, the left ventricular cavity is cone-shaped. Contraction of the left ventricle starts at the tip of the heart (the apex) and progresses toward the base, in a spiral fashion, "squeezing" blood forward into the aorta.

CARDIAC VALVES

The delicacy and flexibility of the tissues composing the cardiac valves and the amazing synchrony of their actions throughout the cardiac cycle are certainly wonders of nature. Normal valves offer very little obstruction to the flow of blood through them, yet form a blood-tight seal against the regurgitation of blood. There are two generic types of valves—the atrioventricular valves and the semilunar valves.

Atrioventricular Valves

The atrioventricular valves are situated between the atrium and the ventricle, on the left side (the mitral valve) and on the right side (the tricuspid valve) of the heart. They are composed of a fibrous supporting ring (the annulus), leaflets, supporting strands (chordae tendineae), and papillary muscles, which connect the chordae to the ventricular wall (Fig. 1–4).

Mitral valve. The mitral valve is a valve with two cusps (bicuspid) and derives its name from its resemblance to a bishop's mitre (hat). The posterior (or mural) leaflet of the mitral valve is the smaller of the two leaflets and acts as a "buttress" against which the larger anterior leaflet can abut. The anterior (or aortic) leaflet is a very flexible, delicate, and mobile structure which has a rather wide range of motion. It descends far into the left ventricle during diastole and then rapidly rises early in systole to its place of apposition against the posterior leaflet, preventing regurgitation (Fig. 1–5).

The two junctional areas where the leaflets and the annulus of the mitral valve come together are called the *commissures.* Because the mitral valve is oriented anteriorly and to the left (see Fig. 1–5), one commissure is situated anteriorly and laterally (the anterolateral commissure), while the other junctional area is placed posteriorly and medially (the posteromedial commissure). The underlying papillary muscles give off delicate chordae tendineae to the leaflets on either

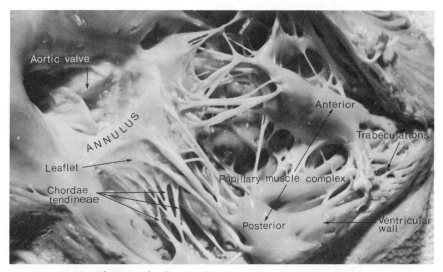

Figure 1–4. Photograph of a mitral valve and its supporting structures, as viewed from below (from the left ventricle). Note the component parts of the valve (annulus, leaflets, chordae tendineae, papillary muscles, and ventricular wall). Note also that the annulus of the mitral valve is very close to the aortic valve.

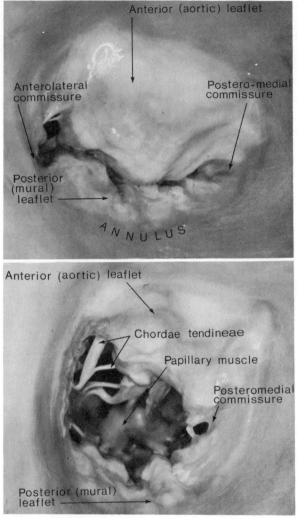

Figure 1–5. Photograph of the mitral valve in the open and closed positions, as viewed from above (from the left atrium). Note how the anterior leaflet descends into the left ventricular cavity (during diastole), revealing the anterior papillary muscle complex which provides chordae tendineae to both leaflets of the valve.

side of the commissure. The anterior papillary muscle complex thus provides chordal support to both leaflets at the anterolateral commissure and the posterior papillary muscle gives off chordae which attach to the two leaflets on either side of the posteromedial commissure.

Tricuspid valve. The tricuspid valve has three leaflets (the anterior, posterior, and septal leaflets) (Fig. 1–6). Usually, the tissues of the tricuspid leaflets are extraordinarily thin, delicate, and

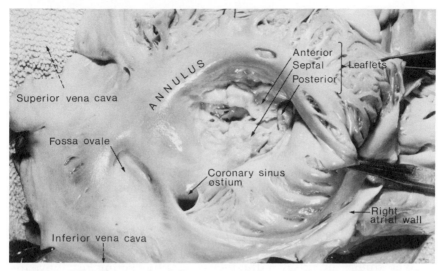

Figure 1-6. Photograph of the interior of the right atrium, showing the three leaflets of the tricuspid valve, the opening of the coronary sinus, and the fossa ovale.

flexible, as might be expected in a (relatively) low-pressure system. When the right ventricle contracts, its lateral wall (i.e., not the wall next to the interventricular septum) shortens, bringing the anterior and posterior leaflets toward the septum where they create valvular competence as they abut against the septal leaflet. The septal leaflet is anatomically important because it is in close proximity to the conducting tissue of the atrioventricular node (see discussion of cardiac nerves later) and because congenital ventricular septal defects are often found beneath this leaflet.

Semilunar Valves

Semilunar valves separate the ventricular cavities from their corresponding arterial vessels, the aorta and the pulmonary artery. These valves are composed of a fibrous supporting ring (the annulus) at the base of the aorta or pulmonary artery, three valve leaflets or "cusps," and a small recess or outpocketing above each leaflet (called the sinus of Valsalva for the aortic valve).

Aortic valve. Positionally, the aortic valve itself is an intracardiac structure, as it lies in close proximity to the right atrium, right ventricle, and left atrium; it is positioned just above the interventricular septum. A portion of its fibrous skeleton shares common tissue with the anterior part of the mitral valve annulus (see Fig. 1-4).

Each of the three valve cusps has a base which attaches to the

valve annulus and a free, or coapting, edge. During ventricular systole, the three flexible cusps float upward and toward the side walls of
the aorta, as blood is ejected from the ventricle past the cusps. Then,
during ventricular diastole, the valve cusps descend to a position
where the coapting edges come together, preventing regurgitation
through the valve.

Each coronary artery arises from a small opening in the wall of
the aorta (called an orifice or an ostium), and the cusps of the aortic
valve are named according to their association with those coronary
arteries. The left coronary artery arises from above the left coronary
cusp, the right coronary artery takes origin from above the right
cusp, and there is no coronary artery associated with the noncoronary
cusp. Each cusp normally occupies one third of the circumference of
the aortic valve. As with other cardiac valves, the junctional areas at
the valve annulus between two adjacent aortic cusps are called the
commissures (Fig. 1–7).

The sinuses of Valsalva (the recess or outpocketing just above the
aortic valve cusps) are well developed and play an important role in
coronary artery blood flow. Closure of the aortic valve prevents blood
from going from the high-pressure aorta (down to 80 mm Hg during
diastole) to the low-pressure left ventricle (down to 5 to 10 mm Hg
during diastole). During this diastolic period, however, blood flows
into and distends the sinuses of Valsalva and then flows out into the
right and left coronary arteries. Normally, at least two thirds of

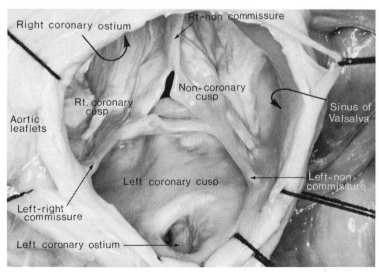

Figure 1–7.   Photograph of the aortic valve, in almost a completely closed position,
as viewed from above (from the aorta). Note the position of the valve cusps and commissures and the orifice of the left coronary artery (which is almost posterior). Only one
of the three sinuses of Valsalva has been labeled.

coronary artery blood flow occurs during diastole, while the other one third occurs during ventricular systole.

Pulmonic valve. The pulmonic valve lies just to the left and slightly anterior to the aortic valve. It separates the outflow tract of the right ventricle from the pulmonary artery (see Fig. 1–2). The anatomical features of the pulmonic valve are very similar to the aortic valve — an annulus, three commissures, and three cusps, each of which occupies one third of the circumference of the valve. Normally there are no coronary artery ostia and the sinuses of Valsalva are not well developed.

CARDIAC BLOOD VESSELS

The energy requirements of the cardiac musculature are tremendous and oxygen supply and utilization are critical. Although only about one twentieth of the cardiac output flows through the coronary arteries, there is maximal extraction of oxygen from the coronary arterial blood, even at rest. The heart extracts 70 to 80 per cent of the oxygen from the blood as compared to 20 to 25 per cent for the rest of the body's tissues. The resultant oxygen saturation of the cardiac venous blood is only about 30 per cent (a P_{O_2} of 18 to 20 mm Hg). Therefore, the amount of coronary blood flow is most important to myocardial function. Any increased demands (as during exercise) must come from an increase in blood flow rather than from an increase in oxygen extraction.

Coronary Arteries

After the coronary arteries exit from the base of the aorta, they course for a considerable distance on the epicardial surface of the heart, embedded in the fat which surrounds them. Side branches are then given off which penetrate through to the myocardium, supplying it with blood. The terminal portions of these side branches end in a collection (or plexus) of small vessels just inside the inner lining of the cardiac chambers (the subendocardial plexus). From this plexus, additional blood vessels form and pass into the trabeculations of the ventricular wall and into the papillary muscles.

Right coronary artery (RCA). The right coronary artery exits from the anterior surface of the aorta and passes diagonally toward the right side of the heart, where it descends in the groove between the right atrium and the right ventricle (the atrioventricular groove) (Fig. 1–8). In this course it provides small branches to the right atrium and a somewhat larger branch to the anterior surface of the

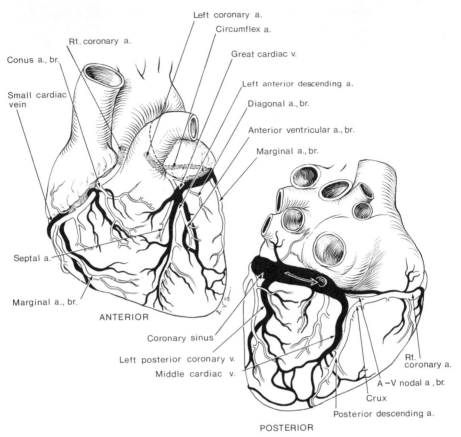

Figure 1–8. Drawing of the arteries and veins of the heart. The veins are drawn in black and the arteries are clear-colored. The major vessels are described in the text. Note how the major cardiac veins parallel the coronary arteries. The direction of the flow of blood in the coronary sinus is indicated by the arrow, whose tip is at the site of the coronary sinus ostium.

infundibulum (the outflow tract) of the right ventricle (the conus branch). Before passing around to the posterior surface of the heart it gives off its marginal branch, which descends along the lateral margin of the heart to the apex, providing branches to adjacent areas of both the anterior and posterior surfaces of the right ventricle. The major trunk of the right coronary artery then continues from right to left, high across the posterior surface of the right ventricle, where, at the site of a sharp angulation (the "crux"), it gives off a small branch to the atrioventricular node. The right coronary artery then ends in the posterior descending artery which descends in the posterior interventricular groove; it supplies adjacent areas of the right and left ventricles and the posterior part of the interventricular septum. Inferior wall myocardial infarctions may result from obstruction of the RCA.

In about 80 per cent of cases, the right coronary artery provides this posterior descending branch; the right coronary artery is then said to be "predominant." In the remaining 20 per cent, this descending branch arises from the terminal portion of the circumflex branch of the left coronary artery, which is then termed a "predominant left coronary system."

Left coronary artery (LCA). The left coronary artery exits from the posterior surface of the aorta, from the left sinus of Valsalva. Usually, there are no major branches as the main left coronary trunk passes behind the pulmonary artery, and only small twigs are given off to the upper part of the left atrium. As it emerges between the pulmonary artery and the tip of the left atrial appendage, it separates into its two major divisions—the anterior descending branch and the circumflex branch.

ANTERIOR DESCENDING BRANCH (LAD). As the name implies, this artery descends on the anterior surface of the heart, in the groove between the right and left ventricles (the anterior interventricular groove). In this course, it gives off septal branches (which supply the anterior part of the interventricular septum), anterior ventricular branches (which supply the anterior surface of the left ventricle), and a rather large diagonal branch (which supplies the lateral margin of the left ventricle). Anterior or anteroseptal myocardial infarctions are often the result of obstruction of the LAD.

CIRCUMFLEX BRANCH (CF). This vessel passes around the left atrial appendage and flows from left to right, high across the posterior surface of the heart in the atrioventricular groove, in close association with the coronary sinus (see later). Its major branch is the marginal branch which supplies much of the posterior surface of the left ventricle.

Although coronary artery branches are thought to be "end-arteries" under normal conditions, intercoronary communications are established when there is a gradual narrowing of a coronary artery (see under Pathology, this chapter). The major areas of anastomotic connections are: (1) at the posterior surface of the heart, where the terminal portions of the right coronary artery and the circumflex branch unite, giving a variable origin to the posterior descending branch; and (2) at the apex of the heart, where the terminal portions of the anterior descending artery, posterior descending artery, and the marginal branch of the right coronary all converge. Additional communications may form wherever branches from the two systems meet each other.

Cardiac Veins

As with the blood supply to most areas of the body, the venous drainage closely parallels the arterial inflow (see Fig. 1-8). Thus, there are veins that accompany each of the major coronary arteries. The great cardiac vein accompanies the anterior descending artery in the anterior interventricular groove, the small cardiac vein runs in the atrioventricular groove with the right coronary artery, the left posterior coronary vein accompanies the marginal branch of the circumflex artery, and the middle cardiac vein lies next to the posterior descending artery. All these veins flow into (and form) the coronary sinus, which is the large vein that passes from left to right, high across the posterior cardiac surface. In this course, it travels along with the circumflex artery (which is partially hidden by the coronary sinus in Figure 1–8). The coronary sinus finally ends in the right atrium (at the coronary sinus ostium) between the tricuspid valve and the opening of the inferior vena cava (see Fig. 1–6).

Cardiac nerves

Certain portions of cardiac tissue have become specialized for the rapid conduction of electrical impulses. Impulses from sympathetic and parasympathetic nervous systems "bombard" the sinoatrial node (SA Node), which is the first "way station" in this conduction system. Normally it is the site of impulse formation—the highest pacemaking center (Fig. 1–9; see also Fig. 4–2). The SA node lies at the medial aspect of the junction between the superior vena cava and the right atrium, where it is usually supplied with blood by a small atrial branch of the right coronary artery.

Transmission of the impulse from the sinoatrial node to the atrioventricular node is through the atrial musculature and three

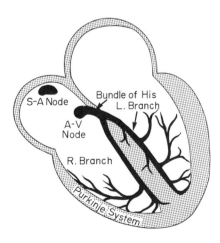

Figure 1-9. Diagrammatic illustration of the conducting tissues of the heart. Note the six major components of the system: the SA node, the AV node, the bundle of His, the right and left bundle branches, the Purkinje fibers, and finally the ventricular muscle itself.

CARDIAC CONDUCTION TISSUE

specialized "internodal" tracts. The AV node lies at the base of the atrial septum just beneath the right atrial endocardium, and rests very close to the coronary sinus ostium and to the septal leaflet of the tricuspid valve. This node receives signals from the atrium and, after a delay of about .04 seconds, sends the impulses toward the ventricle. This normal delay is important because it postpones activation of the ventricles long enough for the atria to eject their blood through the atrioventricular valves. Further, it allows only one impulse at a time to be transmitted forward toward the bundle of His.

The bundle of His is located at the junction of the atrial and ventricular septa, just beneath the noncoronary cusp of the aortic valve. In this position, it is vulnerable to inflammation and calcification in the aortic valve and to operative trauma during aortic valve operations. The bundle extends also just beneath the membranous portion of the interventricular septum. In this latter position, it poses a very real hazard to the operating surgeon during the repair of a ventricular septal defect, as the closure sutures must be placed into the lower margin of the membranous septum near to the bundle.

Shortly after the bundle of His reaches the upper portion of the muscular interventricular septum, it divides into a small right bundle branch and a much larger left bundle branch. These branches then descend in the interventricular septum where they terminate in the smaller Purkinje fibers, which carry the impulses to the ventricular musculature.

Correlation of the electrical events in this conduction system with the electrocardiographic recording of electrical activity will be made in Chapter 4.

Although the heart has the capability of spontaneous rhythmic activity, the heart rate is regulated by the autonomic nervous system through its sympathetic and parasympathetic fibers. The specialized conduction tissue and the myocardium itself will propagate the electrical impulses once they have been initiated in the highest pacemaking center (see previously).

When the sympathetic nervous system is activated (as in stressful situations), cardiac rate is increased, and conduction from the sinoatrial node through the atrioventricular node is increased. Sympathetic nerves to the heart originate in the three cervical sympathetic ganglia and pass to the "cardiac plexus," which surrounds the root and the arch of the aorta. From this plexus, nerve fibers extend to the sinoatrial node, to the atrioventricular node, and to the musculature of the coronary arteries.

Stimulation of the parasympathetic nervous system causes slowing of the heart rate and decreases conduction through the AV node. These fibers start in the medulla of the brain, pass by way of the vagus nerves to the "cardiac plexus" and from there are distributed to the SA and AV nodes.

Nervous impulses leaving the heart originate in the pain-sensitive areas in and around the heart and pass through the sympathetic plexus to ganglia in the spinal cord (at the lower two cervical and upper four thoracic levels). This distribution of nerve connections helps explain why cardiac pain is experienced in areas supplied by the lower cervical and upper thoracic nerves (neck, jaw, shoulders, arms). The impulses are finally carried to the brain, where the sensation of pain (angina pectoris) is realized.

Embryology

Every year thousands of newborn infants are born with congenital heart defects. The incidence of these defects is about 0.8 per cent of live births. Some of the defects have little effect upon the infant's cardiovascular status, while others are incompatible with life. This section will trace the embryologic development of the heart, so that specific congenital cardiac defects can be better appreciated when they are presented later in this chapter.

EARLY DEVELOPMENT

Until the embryo is two weeks old and has attained a length of 2 mm, the tissues which will later become the heart are merely indistinct bulges on the longitudinally oriented sheets of cells which comprise the three primary germ layers—the ectoderm, mesoderm, and endoderm (Fig. 1–10). The ectoderm will form the nervous system and the endoderm will differentiate into the alimentary tract and the lungs. Already the mesoderm has divided into somatic and splanchnic divisions with the body cavity (the coelomic cavity) between them. When these paired sheets of germ layers fuse in the midline, a single tubular structure is formed. The somatic mesoderm will contribute

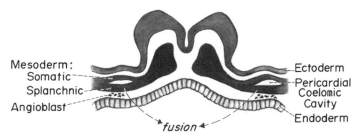

Figure 1–10. Drawing of the three primary germ layers in the two week old embryo. Note that the two sides will fuse in the midline to form tubelike structures which contribute to the different parts of the developing heart (see text).

to the future pericardial wall, the splanchnic mesoderm will form the walls of the heart itself and the coelomic cavity will become the pericardial sac. Primitive heart cells (angioblasts), which initially lie between the splanchnic mesoderm and the endoderm, will also differentiate and organize until a single longitudinal tube is formed. This tube will lie inside the tube of the fused splanchnic mesoderm and will form the endocardium, the inner lining of the heart.

During the next week, the primitive cardiac tube grows so much more rapidly than the structures surrounding it that it bends to the side and twists itself into a loop. At this stage, the cardiac loop is anchored above by the aortic arch system and below by the developing great veins which soon fuse to form the primitive collecting chamber, the sinus venosus. The external landmarks are being developed—the atria dilate rapidly and bulge out on either side of the conus arteriosus, which connects the ventricle with the truncus arteriosus (which later will divide into the aorta and the pulmonary artery). A midline groove forms at the apex of the ventricular loop, separating it into right and left sides. Thus, by the end of the first month, the major regions of the heart can already be recognized. Blood flow is still undivided, entering at the atria and sinus venosus (sinoatrial end), passing through the primitive ventricles (the atrioventricular canal), and leaving via the truncus arteriosus (Fig. 1–11).

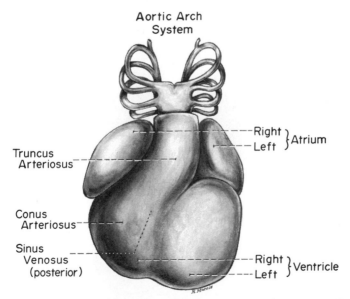

Figure 1-11. Drawing of the primitive heart at one month. Venous inflow to the heart is via the sinus venosus and the developing atria; it then passes through the primitive ventricles, and flows out through the conus arteriosus and the truncus arteriosus to the aortic arch system.

FORMATION OF CARDIAC CHAMBERS

During the second month of embryologic development, the initial phases of the partitioning of the heart into right and left sides and into atria and ventricles are begun. Sheets of tissue grow inward from the walls of the primitive heart to accomplish these divisions.

Atria

Into the common atrioventricular canal grow two masses of tissues (endocardial cushions), one from the back and one from the front. When these tissues meet together in the center of the heart, the atrioventricular canal will be separated into left and right sides. At about the same time, similar tissues grow down from the top of the common atrium and upward from the bottom of the common ventricle to begin the division of these common chambers into right and left sides (Fig. 1–12). As the developing atrial septum (septum primum) grows toward the atrioventricular canal cushions, there remains an intercommunicating hole between the two sides (ostium primum). Were the atrial division to progress to completion at this stage, the left side of the heart would become "dry," as very little blood would be returning from the undeveloped lungs and the blood returning from the placenta would remain in the right side of the heart. However, the progression of embryologic events prevents this catastrophe, as a new opening (ostium secundum) is established in the center of

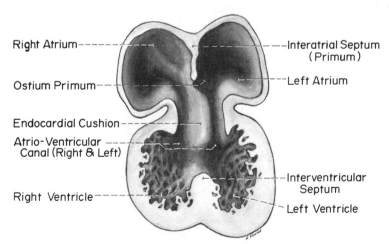

Figure 1–12. Drawing of the developing heart at two months. Note that the atrioventricular canal is being divided by the endocardial cushions, that the atrial septum is starting the division into the two atria, and that the interventricular septum is dividing the common ventricular chamber into right and left sides.

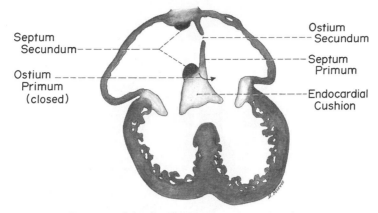

Figure 1-13. Drawing of the developing atria. Note that the septum primum has grown down to meet the endocardial cushions, thus obliterating the ostium primum. The septum primum is perforated in its upper portion by the ostium secundum. The septum secundum is just starting to develop (to the right of the septum primum).

this first atrial septum (Fig. 1–13). Subsequently, a second atrial septum (septum secundum) is formed to the right of the initial dividing wall. It is not a complete structure, as it, too, has a central hole, the foramen ovale (see Fig. 1–14). Soon the upper part of the first wall (septum primum) is resorbed, leaving the larger bottom portion to remain as a flap valve on the left side, over the opening in the second atrial wall. Blood can then flow from right to left through this foramen ovale (supplying the left side of the heart), but cannot flow in the opposite direction because of the "flap valve action" of the septum primum. It is not until after birth, when blood returns to the left side of the heart from the newly expanding lungs, that the foramen ovale is finally closed.

Ventricles

During the second month of development there is a rapid growth of the interventricular septum from the apex of the common ventricle upward toward the expanding atrioventricular canal cushions. During this growth period, the opening between the two ventricles (the interventricular foramen) becomes smaller and smaller. The final closure of this foramen awaits the downward growth of tissues from the canal cushions and from the base of the truncus arteriosus (which will go to form the aorta and the pulmonary artery). As the medial portions of the mitral and tricuspid valves become more highly differentiated, the upper portion of the interventricular septum thins out into a fibrous sheet (the membranous part of the septum). In contrast

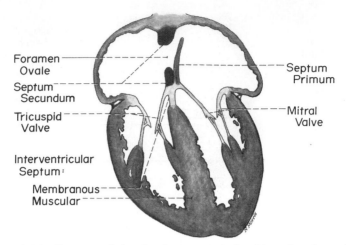

Foramen Ovale
Septum Secundum
Tricuspid Valve
Interventricular Septum:
Membranous
Muscular

Septum Primum
Mitral Valve

Figure 1–14. Drawing of the developing ventricles. Note that the endocardial cushions have fused with the developing interventricular septum to complete the division into right and left ventricles. The membranous part of the interventricular septum and the mitral and tricuspid valves have also differentiated from the endocardial cushions. The septum primum forms a "flap valve" over the opening in the septum secundum.

to the late-closing atrial septum, the interventricular septum is normally closed at this early stage of development, and the interventricular foramen is completely obliterated (Fig. 1–14).

FORMATION OF GREAT VESSELS AND CARDIAC VALVES

In the early stages of development, the outflow of blood from the ventricle passed into the truncus arteriosus, which was a single, undivided, tubular structure. As the single ventricle slowly divides into right and left portions, the truncus arteriosus also undergoes a partitioning process which will divide it into a left side (aorta) and a right side (pulmonary artery). Ridges of connective tissue, similar to the tissue of the endocardial cushions, grow in from the sides of the truncus arteriosus, until they finally meet and form a complete partition (Fig. 1–15A and B). These truncus ridges pursue a spiral course during their development so that the aorta receives the flow from the left ventricle and the pulmonary artery receives the right ventricular outflow; the aorta and pulmonary artery then assume their adult anatomic relationships.

At the base of truncus arteriosus, three small buttons of embryonic tissue grow out from each of the spiral truncal ridges. They later be-

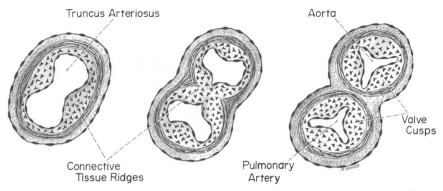

Truncus Arteriosus   Aorta

Connective
Tissue Ridges   Pulmonary
Artery   Valve
Cusps

Figure 1–15. Drawing of the formation of the great vessels and the semilunar valves. Note the connective tissue ridges growing into the truncus arteriosus, separating it into the pulmonary artery and the aorta. The truncal ridges also give origin to the cells which differentiate into the delicate cusps of the aortic and pulmonary valves.

come differentiated into the delicate tissues that form the three cusps of the aortic and pulmonic valves (Fig. 1–15C). Similarly, the atrioventricular valves (the mitral and tricuspid valves) are formed by thinning and differentiation of blunt flaps of tissue that project from the endocardial cushions and from the outer walls of the atrioventricular canal (see Fig. 1–14). The papillary muscles and chordae tendineae, the supporting structures to these atrioventricular valve leaflets, arise by modification of the muscular tissues on the inner surfaces of the ventricles.

As the ventricles and truncus arteriosus undergo partitioning, the aortic arch system also is forming its branches. Originally, there was a segmental division of the primitive blood vessel system into dorsal and ventral aortae, connected by six pairs of aortic arches. As the embryo grows and its organs and limbs develop, some of these arches increase in size while others regress and disappear. In man, the fifth pair of arches never develops and will not be considered further (Fig. 1–16).

The first two arches undergo degeneration in early stages, the third aortic arch contributes to the internal carotid arteries, and the ventral aortae become the external carotid arteries. The fourth left arch normally becomes the aorta (the right one regresses), and the sixth arch contributes to the formation of the pulmonary arteries. The right sixth arch loses its communication with the dorsal aorta, but the left-sided communicating link persists until after birth as the ductus arteriosus (see later), which shunts excess blood away from the lungs into the aorta.

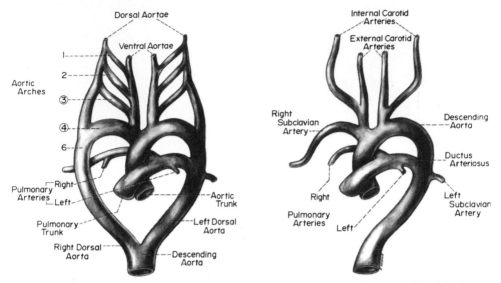

Figure 1-16. Drawings of early and late stages in the development of the blood vessel system. Note the pairs of aortic arches and the dorsal and ventral aortae. See text for discussion of the differentiation of these structures into their adult counterparts.

POSTNATAL DEVELOPMENT

There are a number of anatomic and physiologic features of the fetal circulation which must undergo rapid and radical changes when intrauterine life changes to an extrauterine existence. During fetal development, oxygenation of blood of the fetus is accomplished by the maternal placenta and the oxygenated blood enters the fetal heart via the umbilical vein, the ductus venosus in the liver, and the inferior vena cava. A prominent valve at the inferior vena caval entrance directs a considerable portion of this blood through the foramen ovale to the left side of the heart and thence to the systemic circuit (Fig. 1-17).

As the lungs are unexpanded, they have a high vascular resistance. A large proportion of the blood which is ejected from the right ventricle into the pulmonary artery is therefore shunted via the ductus arteriosus into the descending aorta, which at this time has a lower vascular resistance.

At birth, when the infant takes his first few breaths, the lungs are immediately inflated, the pulmonary vascular resistance rapidly becomes markedly reduced and pulmonary artery blood flow increases. The flow of right ventricular blood now goes to the lungs

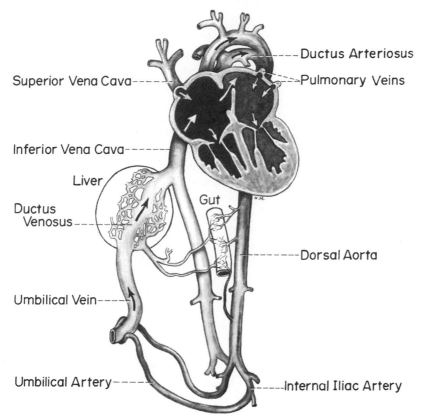

Figure 1-17. Drawing of the fetal circulation. Note that the oxygenated blood from the (maternal) placenta enters the fetus via the umbilical vein and then passes through the ductus venosus in the liver and reaches the right atrium where it is shunted to the left atrium. The small amounts of blood which enter the right ventricle and the pulmonary artery are shunted to the aorta through the ductus arteriosus, which connects the pulmonary artery to the aorta.

rather than through the decompressing ductus arteriosus. The loss of the placental blood flow decreases the right atrial pressure. Blood returning from the new pulmonary vascular bed raises the left atrial pressure above the decreased right atrial pressure and closes the atrial flap valve (septum primum), preventing left-to-right blood flow. More blood is then pumped by the left heart, the aortic pressure rises, and blood flow through the ductus arteriosus is no longer in the right-to-left direction. During the next several days, obliteration of the ductus arteriosus progresses by a combination of proliferation of its internal lining and by contraction of the smooth muscles in its wall. The permanent adult circulation is thus established.

Physiology

The first section of this chapter outlined the basic anatomy of the cardiac chambers, valves, blood vessels, and nerve tissues, and only passing reference was made at that time to the functional anatomy, valve action, or ventricular contraction patterns. In this section, the normal function of these anatomic components will be discussed in relation to three basic diagnostic modalities as seen in Figure 1–18. The electrocardiogram (ECG) reflects the electrical activity of the heart, the phonocardiogram (PCG) indicates the heart sounds, and the pressure tracings (in the left atrium, left ventricle, and aorta) depict pressure and flow events in the cardiac cycle. The ECG will be discussed in Chapter 4 and the other diagnostic modalities will be reviewed in Chapter 5.

Classically, the cardiac cycle is divided into two phases, systole and diastole. Systole is the time during which blood is ejected from the ventricles (one third of the cardiac cycle), and diastole is when the ventricles relax and fill with blood (two thirds of the cycle).

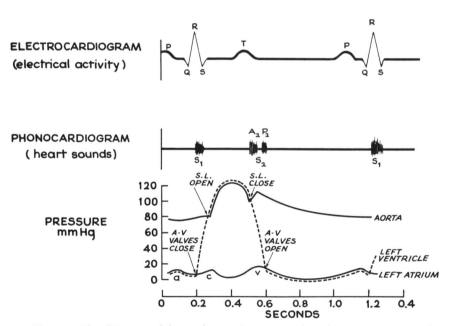

Figure 1–18. Diagram of the cardiac cycle (rate equals 60 beats per minute). The timing of the events of the electrocardiogram, the heart sounds, and the chamber pressures can be compared by relating them to time on the horizontal axis. Note that the first heart sound occurs when the atrioventricular valves close and the second heart sound occurs when the semilunar valves close. The opening and closing of the cardiac valves are related to the relative pressures on either side of the valves (see text).

Actually, the different phases of the cardiac cycle are somewhat more complicated and deserve further explanation.

Let us start the discussion of the cardiac cycle with the first phases of diastole. Only the events on the left side of the heart will be described, but the right-sided phases are very similar.

The first inscription on the electrocardiogram is the P wave, which represents depolarization of the atrial musculature (see Chapter 4). As can be seen from the horizontal time axis, this electrical activity precedes (by a brief interval) the actual mechanical contraction of the atrial muscle, which causes a rise in atrial pressure (the "a" wave on the atrial tracing). As the atrial pressure is slightly higher than the diastolic pressure in the ventricle, blood flow from the atrium to the ventricle occurs throughout ventricular diastole. This atrial contraction (sometimes called the *atrial systolic thrust*) forcefully completes the diastolic filling of the ventricle.

As with the atrial electrical activity, the depolarization of the ventricles (the QRS complex on the electrocardiogram) slightly precedes ventricular contraction. The first phase of ventricular systole is called isovolumetric contraction, which simply means that pressure is being developed in the ventricular walls without a change in the volume of blood in the ventricular lumen (no blood is entering or leaving the ventricle). Coincident with the rise in ventricular pressure is the closure of the atrioventricular valve, which is heard as the first heart sound (S_1). During this period of valve closure, the papillary muscles contract, the chordae tendineae become taut, and the valve leaflets float upward and meet each other. Closure of the mitral and tricuspid valves is so near to being simultaneous that only a single closure sound is heard (S_1).

Blood does not flow out of the ventricle until ventricular pressure exceeds the pressure in the aorta. Then, the semilunar valve opens and blood is rapidly ejected into the aorta (the rapid ejection phase). Soon, the rate of ejection slows, causing the rounding at the top of the pressure wave forms in both the ventricle and the aorta. This slow ejection phase continues until ventricular ejection finally stops, blood flow in the aorta is reversed, and the semilunar valve closes. The closure of the semilunar valve is reflected by a notch (the dicrotic notch) on the pressure wave form of the aorta and by the second heart sound (S_2) on the phonocardiogram. Normally, the aortic valve closure (A_2) occurs before pulmonic valve closure (P_2), and the two closure sounds can be heard separately. Parenthetically, repolarization of the ventricular muscle mass occurs during this time and is reflected by the T wave on the ECG.

As soon as the semilunar valve closes, there is a rapid fall in ventricular pressure, while the pressure in the aorta declines more gradually. This phase is called isovolumetric relaxation, as no blood is entering the ventricle, but the tension of the ventricular walls is "relaxing." The "v" wave of the atrial pressure tracing is caused by blood flowing into the atrium from the pulmonary circuit during this period. At the very end of isovolumetric relaxation, the upward bulging of the atrioventricular valve rapidly recedes, accounting for the initial downslope after the "v" wave.

At this point, ventricular pressure falls below atrial pressure and the atrioventricular valves will open. This event initiates the phase of rapid filling, when blood flows rapidly into the ventricle from the atrium. Shortly, the pressures in the atrium and the ventricle reach their lowest point, and ventricular filling slows considerably. During the rest of the diastole, blood flow into the ventricle is slow (slow-filling phase), until it is once again accelerated by atrial contraction. The cycle then starts all over again.

In summary, systole begins when the ventricle builds up pressure, closing the atrioventricular valves. Blood is ejected into the great vessels as the semilunar valves open and continues until those valves close, initiating diastole. The atrioventricular valves then open, allowing the ventricles to fill from the atria. The cycle then begins again.

Pathology

In the three preceding sections, the normal cardiac anatomy, embryologic development, and the physiology of normal cardiac action have been reviewed. In this section, the pathology of the different cardiac lesions will be discussed and will later be correlated with the medical aspects (Chapter 2) and the surgical therapy (Chapter 3).

INTRODUCTION

It is beyond the scope of this presentation to discuss the details of all the pathologic conditions in congenital and acquired heart disease; however, the most common lesions will be described and their clinical correlates will be briefly discussed.

CONGENITAL HEART DISEASE

Generally speaking, the different congenital cardiac anomalies impose three types of hemodynamic burdens upon the circulatory system. A *volume overload* occurs when more blood than normal enters a ventricle (usually the right ventricle, as in atrial or ventricular septal defects). To compensate for this burden, the ventricle must work harder to expel this larger load and, in so doing, undergoes hypertrophy (muscular overgrowth) and dilatation. When the hemodynamic burden is severe, ventricular failure can result. Obstruction to the outflow of blood from the heart usually causes a *pressure overload*, resulting in high ventricular pressures, severe ventricular hypertrophy, and often, cardiac failure. *Desaturation* (lower oxygen content) of circulating arterial blood results from the admixture of unoxygenated blood returning from the body with the oxygenated blood returning from the lungs. A generalized decrease in the oxygen content of the arterial blood going to the body (including the heart) often leads to poor oxygenation of the various organs which, in turn, results in acidosis. Acidosis causes decreased cardiac performance, more acidosis, and the vicious cycle starts again. Many congenital anomalies combine these different types of hemodynamic burdens and cardiac deterioration may be more rapid because of the combined burdens.

The signs and symptoms of congenital heart disease often reflect the underlying anomaly. (1) *Cyanosis* may be due to the shunting of unoxygenated blood into the left heart (e.g., tetralogy of Fallot) or may be due to poor oxygen uptake by the fluid-filled lungs in congestive heart failure. When the child cries, pulmonary pressures rise and cause increased shunting from the right side of the heart to the left; increased cyanosis results. (2) *Tachypnea* (rapid breathing) is a frequent response to low oxygen content in the blood and is detected clinically by the retraction of the intercostal spaces of the infant and by the flaring of the nares with each breath. Tachypnea is often precipitated by mild exercise. (3) *Effort intolerance* is usually manifested in the smaller child by feeding problems. The infant eats a small amount, experiences respiratory distress, coughing, sometimes vomiting; he then becomes hungry again and the cycle is repeated. The older child complains of fatigue with playing; he cannot "keep up" with his siblings or classmates. (4) *Failure to thrive* usually indicates a left-to-right shunt or congestive heart failure. The child fails to gain weight appropriately and falls well below the predicted normal values of height and weight for his age. (5) Miscellaneous findings include: (a) frequent respiratory tract infections, usually seen in atrial septal defect or patent ductus arteriosus (see later); (b) leg pains and headaches with exercise, usually indicating a coarctation of the aorta; (c) exertional chest pain and fainting, characteristic of aortic stenosis; and (d) squatting, clubbed fingers, and hypoxic "spells," most often associated with tetralogy of Fallot.

The normal flow of blood, as previously described, is represented

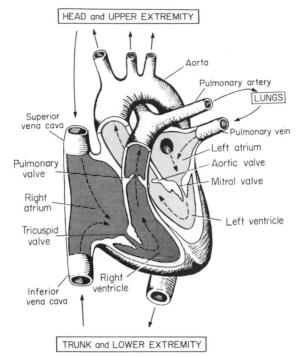

Figure 1-19. Diagram of the normal heart. Note the component structures labeled in this diagram (and abbreviated in subsequent diagrams) and the arrows indicating the direction of normal blood flow. (From Guyton, A. C.: Function of the Human Body. 3rd ed. Philadelphia, W. B. Saunders Company, 1969.)

diagrammatically in Figure 1–19, which should be compared with the diagrams of the different congenital lesions as they are presented.

For purposes of discussion, the specific congenital anomalies will be (arbitrarily) divided into left-to-right shunts, right-to-left shunts, and obstructions to the flow of blood in the pulmonary or systemic circuits. In order of frequency, the following 10 lesions are most commonly encountered: ventricular septal defect and pulmonary stenosis (either alone or combined), patent ductus arteriosus, tetralogy of Fallot, transposition of the great vessels, atrial septal defect, coarctation of the aorta, atrioventricular canal defect, aortic stenosis, and tricuspid atresia.

Left-to-Right Shunts

Left-to-right shunts are generally thought of as congenital anomalies without cyanosis (acyanotic), since oxygenated blood is shunted from the left to the right side of the heart, which then empties into the lungs.

Patent ductus arteriosus (PDA). Since the lungs remain unexpanded during fetal life, blood being pumped from the developing right ventricle is shunted into the systemic circuit through a large communication between the pulmonary artery and the descending thoracic aorta, the ductus arteriosus (see Fig. 1–17). Normally, when the lungs first expand at birth, blood is then directed into the lungs. As systemic oxygen tensions rise (because of the oxygen exchange in the lungs rather than in the placenta), the smooth muscles in the wall of the ductus cause constriction of this communication and it is usually obliterated (closed off) within a few days or weeks.

If this constrictive process does not occur, the ductus arteriosus will not be obliterated and will remain patent. Since the vascular resistance in the lungs falls sharply when the lungs first expand, the pressure in the pulmonary artery becomes much less than that in the aorta. If the ductus remains patent, blood will therefore flow from the aorta (high-pressure) to the pulmonary artery (low-pressure), causing a pressure load on the pulmonary circuit (Fig. 1–20). Right ventricular hypertrophy and constriction (narrowing) of the pulmonary arterioles result. In addition, the left-to-right shunt thus established imposes a very significant burden upon the left ventricle, causing it also to hypertrophy. If allowed to remain for many years, this patent shunt will cause marked elevations in pressure in the pulmonary circuit, sometimes to such a degree that systemic and pulmonary pressures become equal. When this point is reached, there will effectively be no shunting of blood (i.e., a balanced shunt). If the right-sided pressures exceed left heart pressures, the flow of blood may become reversed and the patient may exhibit cyanosis.

Miscellaneous extracardiac left-to-right shunts. There are a

Figure 1–20. Diagram of patent ductus arteriosus. Note the persistent connection between the pulmonary artery and the descending thoracic aorta. Abbreviations for this and subsequent diagrams are as follows: SVC, superior vena cava; IVC, inferior vena cava; RA, right atrium; RV, right ventricle; PT, pulmonary trunk; LPA, left pulmonary artery; RPA, right pulmonary artery; LPV, left pulmonary vein; RPV, right pulmonary vein; LA, left atrium; LV, left ventricle; PDA, patent ductus arteriosus; Br Art, bronchial artery. (From Kanjuh, V. I., and Edwards, J. E.: Pediat. Clin. N. Amer. *11*:55–138, 1964.)

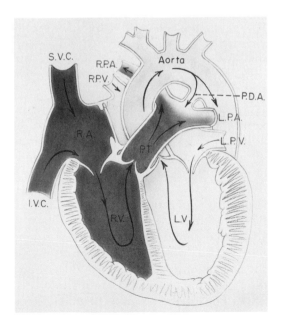

number of miscellaneous types of extracardiac left-to-right shunts which simulate the hemodynamic conditions of a patent ductus arteriosus. These include:

AORTICOPULMONARY WINDOW (A-P WINDOW).   The communication of the systemic and pulmonary circuits takes place in the proximal great vessels (just above the aortic and the pulmonary valves) rather than distally, as in a PDA.

RUPTURED AORTIC SINUS ANEURYSM.   Normally, the sinus of Valsalva of the noncoronary cusp of the aortic valve is adjacent to the right atrium and the sinus of the right coronary cusp is next to the right ventricle (see previous discussion on the right atrium); firm fibrous supporting tissue separates these adjacent structures. If the supporting tissue is deficient in its development, an outpouching, or aneurysm, may be formed in one of these sinuses and protrude toward its adjacent structure (the right atrium or the right ventricle). If the aortic sinus aneurysm were then to rupture, it would do so into the right atrium (or right ventricle), establishing a left-to-right shunt.

ANOMALOUS COMMUNICATIONS OF THE CORONARY ARTERIES. In these anomalies, the coronary arteries empty (either via a fistula or by end-to-end communication) with the coronary sinus, the right atrium, the right ventricle, or the pulmonary trunk.

Ventricular septal defects (VSD).   A defect in the interventricular septum occurs when the tissues from the base of the septum and from the endocardial cushions fail to join each other in either the muscular or membranous portions of the interventricular septum (see Fig. 1–14). Defects are more commonly found in the membranous portion of the interventricular septum, and usually lie just beneath the septal leaflet of the tricuspid valve. Ventricular septal defects may be so small that they spontaneously close in the first year of life, or they may be so large that the two ventricles form a single chamber. The different anatomic locations of ventricular septal defects are shown in Figure 1–21.

Ventricular septal defects, particularly large ones, cause the left ventricle to pump "extra" amounts of blood, as it supplies considerable blood flow to the pulmonary circuit as well as to the systemic circuit. The right ventricle is burdened with both volume and pressure loads, imposed by the left ventricle through the ventricular septal defect. Lastly, the lungs suffer from "overcirculation" (particularly in shunts in which pulmonic flow is two to three times that of systemic flow) and become congested.

Atrial septal defects (ASD).   A communicating defect between the right and left atria can occur if the complex sequence of events in the formation of the atria (as described under the section on embryology in this chapter) is interrupted. If the proliferation of cells of the endocardial cushion is insufficient to obliterate the ostium primum

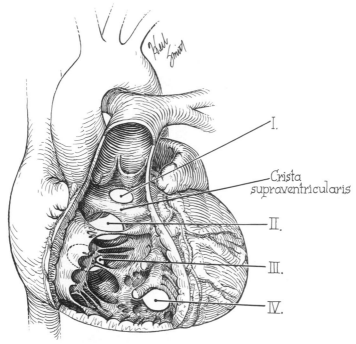

Figure 1-21. Drawing of the various types of ventricular septal defect. (From Cooley, D. A., and Hallman, G. L.: Surgical Treatment of Congenital Heart Disease. Philadelphia, Lea & Febiger, 1966.)

(see Fig. 1–12), a persistent defect will remain at the base of the interatrial septum (an ostium primum ASD). Commonly, this septal defect is accompanied by a cleft in the septal leaflet of the mitral valve (or the tricuspid valve), whose developing cells originate from the same endocardial cushion tissues as the cells which form the septum primum.

An ostium secundum ASD is encountered more frequently. The foramen ovale remains widely patent as the septum secundum is underdeveloped (see Figs. 1–13 and 1–14). The remains of the septum primum (which normally act as a flap valve over the foramen ovale) cannot cover the defect and a large interatrial communication results.

Failure of normal right and left partitioning early in atrial development can also cause the less common sinus venosus ASD. In this defect, the interatrial communication lies high on the developing interatrial septum. Abnormal drainage of one or more pulmonary veins into the right atrial side, or even into the superior vena cava, is a common accompaniment to this type of ASD (and is also known as

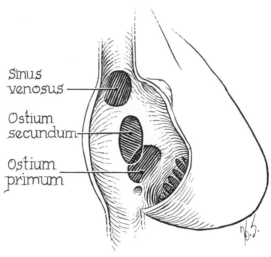

Figure 1-22. Drawing of the various types of atrial septal defect. (From Cooley, D. A., and Hallman, G. L.: Surgical Treatment of Congenital Heart Disease. Philadelphia, Lea & Febiger, 1966.)

partial anomalous pulmonary venous return) (see later). The three types of atrial septal defects are diagrammed in Figure 1-22.

The hemodynamic consequences of an atrial septal defect are not as severe as those in sizable ventricular septal defects. The shunt is at the atrial level, where the pressures are relatively low. There is no burden to the left ventricle. The right ventricle can tolerate the volume load reasonably well unless the shunt is extremely large. The lungs do have overcirculation, but the pressures in the pulmonary vessels are usually not excessive.

Atrioventricular canal defect (endocardial or AV cushion defect). In this congenital malformation, there is severe underdevelopment of the central portion of the developing heart. The faulty growth of the endocardial cushions leads to defects at the base of the interatrial septum (an ostium primum ASD) at the top of the interventricular septum, (a VSD in the membranous septum) and to loss of substance of the septal leaflets of both the mitral and tricuspid valves (Fig. 1-23). The resulting hemodynamic alterations include the shunting of blood from the left to the right atrium, from the left to the right ventricle, and sometimes from the left ventricle to the right atrium. Systolic reflux of blood through the incompetent mitral and tricuspid valves also occurs.

Most patients with complete endocardial cushion defects are severely symptomatic. The combined burdens of an atrial septal defect, a ventricular septal defect, and regurgitation through the mitral (and tricuspid) valve cause severe hemodynamic derangements,

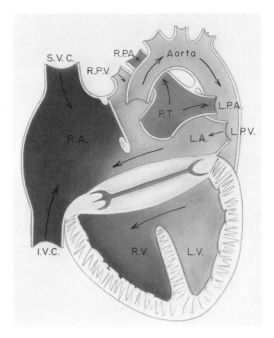

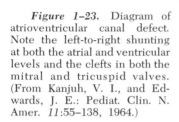

Figure 1-23. Diagram of atrioventricular canal defect. Note the left-to-right shunting at both the atrial and ventricular levels and the clefts in both the mitral and tricuspid valves. (From Kanjuh, V. I., and Edwards, J. E.: Pediat. Clin. N. Amer. *11*:55–138, 1964.)

which result in very poor forward blood flow. Repeated bouts of congestive heart failure are commonplace.

Right-to-left Shunts

Right-to-left shunts are generally considered to be cyanotic congenital anomalies, since unoxygenated (venous) blood is shunted to the left side of the heart, mixing with oxygenated blood returning from the lungs and resulting in arterial blood with a much lower oxygen content than normal. When this mixed blood is pumped to the body's peripheral tissues, they assume a deep purplish-blue color (cyanosis).

Tricuspid atresia. In this anomaly, there is no tricuspid valvular tissue, no normal exit from the right atrium, and, therefore, all the systemic venous (unoxygenated) blood shunts across an atrial septal defect to the left atrium. Usually, an accompanying ventricular septal defect allows this mixed blood to reach the underdeveloped right ventricle, which pumps the blood to the lungs. Obstruction of the pulmonary valve is common, preventing adequate blood flow to the lungs and resulting in severe cyanosis.

Tetralogy of Fallot. This complex anomaly is comprised (as the name indicates) of four anatomic defects: (1) pulmonic stenosis, the obstruction occurring at the level of the pulmonic valve or at the infundibulum; (2) ventricular septal defect, usually quite large;

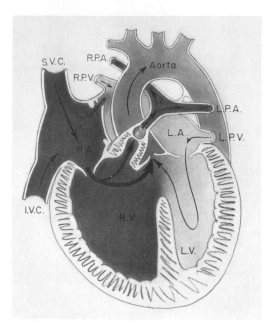

Figure 1–24. Diagram of tetralogy of Fallot. Note the aorta "overriding" the large ventricular septal defect, the pulmonic stenosis (which decreases the flow of blood to the lungs), and the right ventricular hypertrophy, both in the body of the right ventricle and in its infundibulum. (From Kanjuh, V. I., and Edwards, J. E.: Pediat. Clin. N. Amer. *11*:55–138, 1964.)

(3) the aorta taking its origin from "astride" the two ventricles, and receiving blood from each ventricle; and (4) right ventricular hypertrophy (Fig. 1–24).

The more severe the pulmonic stenosis, the more cyanotic is the child; less blood will flow to the lungs to be oxygenated and the higher resistance in the pulmonic circuit will cause more right-to-left shunting. When the child cries, the resultant rise in intrapulmonary pressures simulates an increased pulmonic stenosis; the "hypoxic fainting spell" results. When pulmonic stenosis is complete (pulmonic atresia), blood can reach the lungs only through enlarged bronchial arteries (a condition also known as a *pseudotruncus*) or through a patent ductus arteriosus. Conversely, a mild to moderate pulmonic stenosis allows more blood to enter the lungs and the right ventricular pressure is lower, resulting in less right-to-left shunting. These children are often referred to as "pink (or acyanotic) tetralogies."

Complete transposition of the great vessels (CTGV). In this anomaly, the venous connections to the heart are normal; the venae cavae empty into the right atrium and the pulmonary veins empty into the left atrium. The great vessels take origin, however, from the "wrong" ventricles; the aorta arises from the right (systemic) ventricle and the pulmonary artery from the left (pulmonary) ventricle (Fig. 1–25). In essence, there are two circulations which never meet each other. Unoxygenated blood returns from the systemic veins and is pumped out to the body by the right ventricle; oxygenated blood

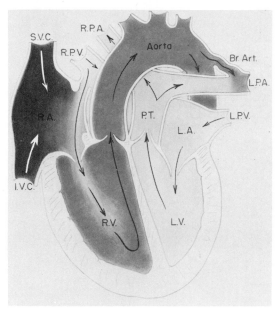

Figure 1-25. Diagram of complete transposition of the great vessels. Note the aorta arising from the right ventricle and the pulmonary artery from the left ventricle. Mixing of blood between the two circuits is achieved by the atrial septal defect and the enlarged bronchial arteries. In this diagram, the ventricular septum is intact and the ductus arteriosus is closed. (From Kanjuh, V. I., and Edwards, J. E.: Pediat. Clin. N. Amer. *11*:55–138, 1964.)

returns from the lungs and is returned there by the left ventricle. Cyanosis is intense.

Without a communication between the two circuits, the child is doomed to die, as very little oxygen would reach the peripheral tissues. Invariably, there is some communication between the two atria, even if only a patent foramen ovale. A ventricular septal defect is also present in one third to one half of the cases. A patent ductus arteriosus or enlarged bronchial arteries may add to the mixing between the two circuits.

Total anomalous pulmonary venous return (TAPVR). Partial anomalous pulmonary venous drainage was mentioned in the discussion of a sinus venosus type of ASD, in which a right pulmonary vein emptied commonly into the right atrium. In *total* anomalous pulmonary venous return, none of the pulmonary veins enter the left atrium, but an anomalous common pulmonary venous channel is formed. This common channel then enters the right atrium via a left superior vena cava, the innominate vein, and the superior vena cava (Fig. 1–26). Occasionally, the common channel empties into the coronary sinus, or makes a connection to the inferior vena cava.

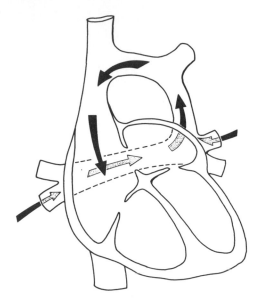

Figure 1–26. Diagram of total anomalous pulmonary venous return (right atrial entry). Note the common pulmonary venous channel behind the heart which connects to a left superior vena cava, to the innominate vein, and then to the superior vena cava. (From Norman, J. C. (ed.): Cardiac Surgery. New York, Appleton-Century-Crofts, 1967.)

Since no blood enters the left atrium directly, an atrial septal defect must be present; it shunts some of the mixture of oxygenated and unoxygenated blood to the left heart and thence to the body. Severe cyanosis results from the systemic circulation of this mixed blood.

Obstruction to Blood Flow

Obstructions to the flow of blood as it passes through the cardiac chambers and great vessels cause an elevation in pressure proximal (upstream) to the block and a resultant "pressure gradient" across the obstruction. Ventricular hypertrophy and failure of the ventricle may ensue.

Obstructions to pulmonic outflow

INFUNDIBULAR STENOSIS.   Overgrowth of the muscular portion of the right ventricular outflow tract leading to the pulmonic valve is the usual cause of infundibular stenosis; less commonly, a fibrous band or ring can lead to obstruction in this area. Infundibular muscular overgrowth may occur as an isolated congenital lesion, or it may develop as a response to stenosis at the valvular level (see Fig. 1–24).

VALVULAR PULMONIC STENOSIS.   In this anomaly, the commissures between the three cusps of the pulmonic valve become fused, thus reducing the effective orifice of the valve to a fraction of its normal size. The valve usually assumes a dome-shaped con-

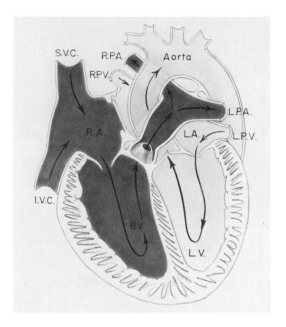

Figure 1-27. Diagram of pulmonic valvular stenosis. Note the dome-shaped stenosis of the valve, the poststenotic dilatation of the main pulmonary artery, and the right ventricular hypertrophy. In this diagram the ventricular and atrial septa are intact and there are no intracardiac shunts. (From Kanjuh, V. I., and Edwards, J. E.: Pediat. Clin. N. Amer. *11*:55–138, 1964.)

figuration with a small central orifice (Fig. 1–27). The proximal pulmonary artery usually undergoes a poststenotic dilatation as blood under high pressure is ejected into the low-pressure pulmonary artery. When the stenosis is severe, extremely high pressures (up to 250 to 300 mm Hg) are generated by the right ventricle, which hypertrophies in response to the pressure load. The infundibulum of the right ventricle often shares in this hypertrophy and contributes further to the obstruction.

Very commonly, pulmonic stenosis is combined with either a ventricular or an atrial septal defect. If the pulmonic stenosis is sufficiently severe to elevate the right ventricular pressure above the left ventricular pressure (or right atrial pressure above left atrial pressure) blood will be shunted from right-to-left, resulting in cyanosis.

Obstructions to systemic outflow

AORTIC STENOSIS. Stenosis of the left ventricular outflow can occur at the subvalvular, valvular, or supravalvular levels (Fig. 1–28). The effect is the same upon the left ventricle: hypertrophy, which in more advanced cases leads to ventricular failure.

Subvalvular Stenosis. Obstruction beneath the aortic valve generally takes two forms. In *diffuse hypertrophic subaortic stenosis,* a generalized overgrowth of the muscular tissue of the left ventricular outflow tract causes the obstruction. The hypertrophy may be part of a generalized myocardiopathy. With ventricular systole, there may be apposition of the hypertrophied musculature from both sides,

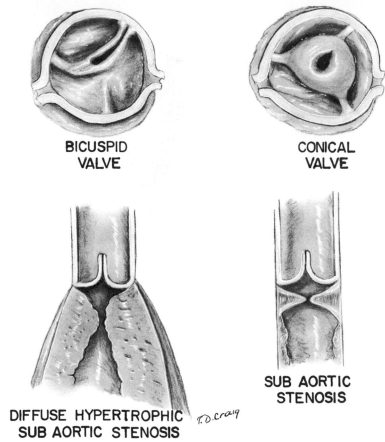

Figure 1–28. Drawing of different types of aortic stenosis. See text for description of individual lesions. (From Norman, J. C. (ed.): Cardiac Surgery. New York, Appleton-Century-Crofts, 1964.)

resulting in a high-grade obstruction to blood flow. In *subaortic stenosis,* the obstruction beneath the valve is a fibrous or membranous diaphragm which impedes blood flow.

Valvular Stenosis. Normally, the aortic valve has three delicate cusps, separated by their adjacent commissures (see Fig. 1–7). If the cusps become fused at the commissures, the orifice of the valve becomes markedly restricted, with only a small central hole remaining. In the so-called *congenital aortic stenosis,* the aortic valve is composed of only two cusps, rather than three (see Fig. 1–33). The tissues of the right and left coronary cusps are fused into a single functional cusp, with only an insignificant "shadow commissure" in the center. In addition, there usually is fusion of the commissure between the noncoronary cusp and this large combined cusp. The resultant stenotic orifice is slitlike and is eccentrically (i.e., not centrally) located. Occasionally, all three commissures are stenotic, and the three well developed cusps have thickened free margins, resulting in a "conical valve."

Supravalvular Stenosis. In this uncommon condition, there is a diaphragm-like deposition of fibrous tissue in the ascending aorta, which is usually associated with an external "hourglass deformity" in that area. This obstruction results in much the same hemodynamic abnormality as does valvular or subaortic stenosis.

COARCTATION OF THE AORTA. In this anomaly, the obstruction usually is in the aorta itself, just distal to the left subclavian artery. Two types of coarctation are differentiated by their anatomic relationship to the ductus arteriosus (or ligamentum arteriosum). In preductal (or infantile) coarctation, the obstruction occurs just proximal (upstream) to the ductus arteriosus; in postductal (or adult) coarctation, the narrowing is just distal (downstream) to the insertion of the ligamentum arteriosum. Very commonly, the lumen of the aorta is reduced to 1 to 2 mm in diameter (Fig. 1–29).

There are multiple effects upon the circulatory system in coarctation of the aorta. The left ventricle undergoes hypertrophy and may eventually fail. Intra-aortic pressure is elevated proximal (toward the heart) to the coarctation, and may cause hypertensive symptoms (headache, and so forth). Since the outflow of blood is prevented from

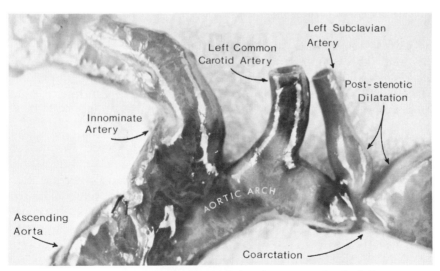

Figure 1–29. Picture of coarctation of the aorta. Note the "tight" coarctation, which in this example is just at the origin of the left subclavian artery. The lumen of the aorta is reduced to a 2 mm internal diameter. There is poststenotic dilatation of the descending aorta and the subclavian artery and marked dilatation and tortuosity of the proximal vessels (specimen from a 53 year old man who also had intercostal aneurysms, aortic valve insufficiency, and cystic medial necrosis of the aorta with an aortic "dissection").

passing directly down the descending aorta, it exits by the innominate, the left common carotid, and the left subclavian arteries and their branches, and then, after passing through collateral channels, empties back into the aorta distal (downstream) to the coarctation. These afore-mentioned vessels become large and tortuous and produce some of the characteristic findings in coarctation (notching of the ribs, pulsa-tile collateral around the shoulder girdle, and so on). The decreased peripheral blood flow yields pulses in the lower extremity which are of poor quality and are delayed in onset when timed against the upper extremity pulses. This decreased flow also leads to the classical coarctation findings of underdevelopment of the lower extremities, with exertional leg pains.

Associated with the aortic coarctation is a poststenotic dilatation of the descending thoracic aorta, which also shows a "jet lesion" in which a high-pressure stream of blood hits the opposite aortic wall. Aneurysms of the intercostal arteries at the site of reentry into the aorta are common in long-standing coarctations. A bicuspid aortic valve is associated in about four fifths of coarctations, and this valve is subject to stenosis, insufficiency, and bacterial endocarditis. Occa-sionally, aneurysms of the blood vessels in the brain may rupture, the arteries to the spinal cord may thrombose, and the aorta itself may degenerate (cystic medial necrosis) and form dissecting aneurysms.

ACQUIRED HEART DISEASE

Discussion in this section will be confined to the commonly encountered examples of valvular heart disease, arteriosclerotic heart disease (coronary artery disease) and its complications, and miscellaneous forms of acquired heart disease (including cardiac tumors, pericarditis and myocarditis, and cardiac trauma).

Valvular Heart Disease

Abnormalities of the mitral, aortic, and tricuspid valves are most commonly found in patients with rheumatic heart disease. The ini-tiating event in these lesions is one or more attacks of rheumatic fever, a disease which is still poorly understood. Acute rheumatic fever usually occurs in the aftermath of an infection with β-hemolytic streptococci; the infection usually is in the form of *strep throat*. It is seen more commonly in susceptible persons who are in the lower socioeconomic strata, who have poor nutrition, and who live crowded together. Rheumatic fever is probably not due to an actual infection of the heart with the streptococcus organism, but may rather be an antibody response to the strep infection.

Acute rheumatic carditis may involve each of the layers of the heart—the endocardium, myocardium, or pericardium. Endocardial involvement is usually limited to the endocardium of the cardiac valves—a rheumatic valvulitis. In the early stages, there is swelling of the tissues of the valve leaflets and erosion of the junctional areas (the commissures). Blood, platelets, and fibrin are deposited along the free (coapting) margins of the valve leaflets and the supporting structures of the atrioventricular valves. These deposits then undergo a process of scarring and contracture which result in the valvular lesions to be described later. Subsequent attacks of rheumatic fever cause additional valvular damage and, like the original attack, may involve one or more valves. Later, calcification may occur in the affected portions of the valves, causing them to become rigid, immobile structures.

The myocardial lesions in acute rheumatic valvulitis are called *Aschoff bodies*, which are areas of swelling, destruction of tissue, and scarring. Rarely, the coronary arteries themselves are involved. Fluid may form within the pericardial cavity and may also evoke a response from the cells which initiate the scarring process (the fibroblasts); adherence of the pericardium onto the surface of the heart may result.

The valvular lesions take the form of pure stenosis, pure insufficiency, or mixed disease of the valve. *Stenosis* means that the valve opening (orifice) is narrowed, causing an obstruction to blood flow. *Insufficiency* means that the valve is incapable of preventing retrograde blood flow; its incompetence allows blood to regurgitate through its orifice. A *mixed lesion* means that both stenosis and insufficiency are present; usually the pathologic change is advanced.

Mitral stenosis. Mitral stenosis is almost exclusively caused by rheumatic valvulitis. There is fusion of the junctional areas (the commissures), scarring of the free margins of both the anterior and posterior leaflets, and shortening, fusion, and nodularity of the chordae tendineae. These pathologic processes often cause the free margins of the leaflets to be rolled under and retracted down toward the ventricle, causing a funnel-shaped structure (Fig. 1–30).

The normal elliptical orifice of the mitral valve has a cross-sectional area of 4 to 6 sq cm (cm^2). When the mitral orifice is reduced to 1.5 cm^2, cardiac output is reduced and symptoms occur with moderate to severe exertion. At a 1 cm^2 orifice, the pressure in the left atrium is elevated, usually to between 20 and 30 mm Hg, at rest. With even mild exercise, higher pressures are required to achieve adequate flow across the valve. As the normal pressure within the pulmonary capillaries is about 30 mm Hg, acute elevations of left atrial pressure will cause this pressure to be exceeded, and fluid will flow back across the alveolar membrane into the lungs. If this fluid cannot be adequately removed by lymphatic drainage, pulmonary edema will result.

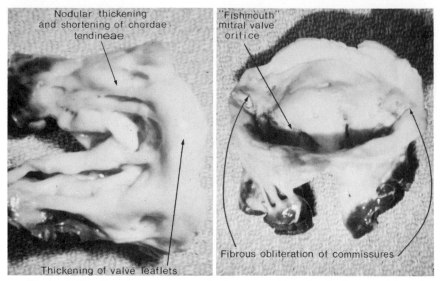

Figure 1–30. Surgical specimen, mitral stenosis. Note the thickening of the valve leaflets, the nodular thickening and shortening of the chordae tendineae, the commissural fusion, and the resultant "fish-mouthed," funnel-shaped valve orifice.

A variety of other pathologic lesions accompanies the valvular lesion of mitral stenosis. As the left atrial pressure rises, the volume of the left atrial cavity also enlarges and the atrial wall becomes thinner. When the chamber size is large enough, there is decompensation of the muscular activity of the atrial wall and the cardiac rhythm changes from a regular to an irregular rhythm (atrial fibrillation or flutter). These rhythms do not eject blood from the atrium to the ventricle, as is the case with sinus rhythm. A further decrease in cardiac output ensues. Due to the valvular obstruction and a rhythm which no longer propels blood through the valve, there is stasis of blood in the left atrium; blood clots can more easily form in the stagnant pool. When these blood clots break off into the blood stream, they form emboli which can travel to the brain, abdominal organs, or to other organs.

Elevations of left atrial pressure in mitral stenosis are transmitted back through the pulmonary veins to the pulmonary capillaries. To pump blood against these higher pulmonary pressures, the right ventricle must, in turn, generate higher perfusion pressures. In order to protect the lungs against these higher pressures, the smaller pulmonary arteries constrict, cause an increase in the resistance to blood flow (an increased pulmonary vascular resistance), and evoke even higher right ventricular pressures. Occasionally, pressures in the right ventricle exceed those in the left ventricle. As this vicious cycle progresses, the right ventricle undergoes hypertrophy and dilatation. Jugular venous distension, engorgement of the liver, peripheral edema, and ascites result when the elevated right ventricular pressure is transmitted back to the right atrium and the great veins, through a dilated, insufficient tricuspid valve (see the discussion of tricuspid insufficiency later).

Mitral insufficiency. RHEUMATIC MITRAL INSUFFICIENCY. The rheumatic process may cause such extensive scarring and calcification of the leaflets that they fail to coapt (meet each other) during ventricular systole (Fig. 1–31). Blood then refluxes through the fixed orifice in retrograde fashion back into the atrium. The left ventricle is thus subjected to a high-volume work load. Not only must it pump blood out the aorta and through the incompetent valve, but it must also receive both the normal amount of left atrial blood and the regurgitated blood as well. The usual result of this work load is ventricular hypertrophy and dilatation. Additionally, rheumatic mitral insufficiency can be caused by contracture of the involved chordae tendineae, causing the free margins of the valve to be drawn down into the ventricle where they cannot effectively prevent reflux through the valve. Occasionally chordae tendineae may rupture as a result of rheumatic involvement.

MITRAL INSUFFICIENCY SECONDARY TO BACTERIAL ENDOCARDITIS. This is a process whereby pathogenic bacteria enter the blood stream and become implanted on the valve. Dental procedures (ex-

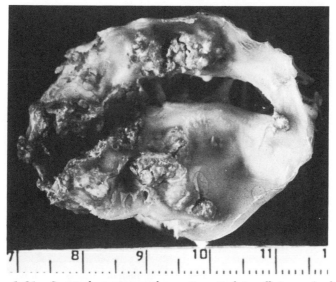

Figure 1–31. Surgical specimen, rheumatic mitral insufficiency (and stenosis). Note the calcific excrescences along the free margins of both leaflets and the scarring and calcification of the commissures which tend to keep the leaflets apart.

traction, filling, cleaning), narcotic mainlining, severe upper respiratory tract infections, and genitourinary tract manipulations (catheterizations, cystoscopy) are the usual causes of the bacteria gaining access to the blood stream. Although occasionally a normal valve becomes involved, the bacteria usually settle on a valve which has been previously damaged (congenital or rheumatic involvement).

As in other parts of the body, the bacteria cause destruction of the tissues which they infect. They may "eat away" the leaflet until a punched-out hole is formed (Fig. 1–32). Blood is then regurgitated back through this hole in the valve. The infection may also involve the papillary muscles or chordae tendineae, causing their rupture and resulting in mitral insufficiency. Further, vegetations (collections of bacteria and necrotic tissue) may form on the leaflets, preventing them from functioning normally. Very commonly, pieces of these vegetations break off into the blood stream and embolize to vital organs.

MITRAL INSUFFICIENCY FROM RUPTURED CHORDAE TENDINEAE. The support of the mitral valve leaflets which is provided by the chordae tendineae is a very important feature in maintaining competence of the valve. When this support fails because of chordal rupture,

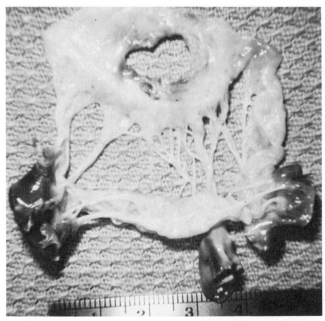

Figure 1–32. Surgical specimen, mitral insufficiency secondary to bacterial endocarditis (healed). Note the large punched-out hole in the anterior leaflet and the thickening of the leaflet tissue around the defect (the patient had a bacteremia [blood stream infection] with pneumococcus during a severe pneumococcal pneumonia).

mitral regurgitation ensues. Chordae tendineae may rupture owing to rheumatic involvement, destruction by an infectious process, or by blunt chest trauma; most commonly, however, the rupture is idiopathic (no known cause).

MITRAL INSUFFICIENCY DUE TO ANNULAR DILATATION. When the left ventricle dilates, the annulus of the mitral valve shares in this process of dilatation. A disproportion is thus established between the size of the ventricle and the mitral annulus (ventriculovalvular disproportion). The leaflets cannot come together during ventricular systole and can no longer prevent regurgitation. The most common cause of this dilatation is left ventricular failure (often from coronary artery disease), aortic valve disease (especially aortic insufficiency), and myocardiopathies (see later). This type of mitral insufficiency carries a high mortality rate because of the underlying diseases producing it.

MISCELLANEOUS CAUSES OF ACQUIRED MITRAL INSUFFICIENCY. The *floppy valve syndrome* is usually seen in patients with disorders of connective tissue (e.g., Marfan's syndrome). Degeneration of the valve leaflet tissue and lengthening of the chordae tendineae allow the leaflets to project upward far into the atrium during ventricular systole, with resultant mitral insufficiency. *Atrial myxomas*, benign tumors which arise from the atrial septum, can herniate through the mitral valve, interpose themselves between the leaflets, and produce mitral incompetence. The blood supply to the papillary muscles may become compromised during a heart attack and the muscles may undergo (ischemic) degeneration; the resultant *papillary muscle syndrome* consists of mitral insufficiency, caused by dysfunction of the papillary muscles. Finally, mitral insufficiency occasionally results *following surgical repair* of mitral stenosis, when the cleavage planes open out into the leaflet itself rather than along the commissures.

Aortic stenosis. Acquired aortic stenosis may occur at either the valvular or subvalvular level, or at both areas. Acquired *idiopathic hypertrophic subaortic stenosis* (IHSS) is similar to that seen in children (see previous discussion). It is thought to be muscular overgrowth of the left ventricular outflow as part of a generalized myocardiopathy.

VALVULAR AORTIC STENOSIS. This may be either congenital or rheumatic in origin. In the section on congenital heart disease, the typical bicuspid valve (with stenosis of the commissures on either side of the right coronary cusp) was described. As the patient grows older, calcification in these cusps progresses, making the valve inflexible and reducing the central orifice to only a small slitlike opening (Fig. 1–33). Often symptoms start to appear only between the ages of 35 and 50 years. Sometimes the calcification of the valve extends into the wall of the aorta, onto the anterior leaflet of the mitral valve, and

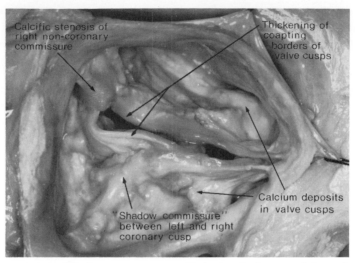

Figure 1-33. Calcific aortic stenosis. Note the thickening of the valve cusps, the "shadow commissure" between the left and right cusps, the extensive calcifications, and the small, slitlike residual orifice.

down into the ventricular septum, where it can cause heart block. As the stenosis becomes more severe, the left ventricle becomes more and more hypertrophied. Usually this ventricular hypertrophy grows inward, reducing the size of the lumen of the left ventricle while maintaining the normal external appearance of the heart. Occasionally, the valvular stenosis brings forth obstructing muscular overgrowth of the outflow tract—an acquired subvalvular stenosis. Symptoms in aortic stenosis (angina, syncope, heart failure) usually occur when the area of the valve orifice has been reduced from the normal 2.6 to 3.5 cm² to the critical range of 0.5 to 0.7 cm².

RHEUMATIC AORTIC STENOSIS. This has all the physiologic characteristics of the calcific (congenital) aortic stenosis. The valve may be heavily calcified, but usually has three cusps; the remaining orifice may be more circular and is often centrally (rather than eccentrically) placed.

Aortic insufficiency. Although there are numerous etiologies of aortic insufficiency, they all impose the same hemodynamic burden— a volume load on the left ventricle. Since the diastolic pressure in the aorta is normally about 80 mm Hg and the diastolic pressure in the ventricle is much lower (about 5 to 10 mm Hg), a very large gradient is established between these areas during diastole. Therefore, even a small area of leak would allow large volumes of blood to regurgitate back into the left ventricle. In order to accommodate this regurgitant volume, the left ventricle dilates; its volume and pressure at the end of diastole consequently increase. More blood is ejected from the left ventricle per beat (i.e., a higher stroke volume) and the systolic pressure rises, sometimes in excess of 200 mm Hg. As blood regurgitates from the aorta into the left ventricle during diastole, the diastolic arterial pressure is quite low, sometimes down to 20 to 30 mm Hg. This combination of high systolic and low diastolic arterial pressures results in an extremely wide pulse pressure, which the nurse will immediately appreciate when she takes a blood pressure reading. In addition, the wide pulse pressure results in peripheral pulses which rise and fall very quickly, a feature easily appreciated by the nurse as "full and bounding," "water-hammer" pulses.

RHEUMATIC AORTIC INSUFFICIENCY. There is thickening of the valvular tissues and shortening of both the length and breadth of the individual cusps. When the cusp tissue is so deficient that it fails to meet the other cusps (during diastole), blood will reflux through this central regurgitant orifice. Aortic insufficiency also occurs in the later stages of calcific aortic stenosis, either rheumatic or congenital. The valve becomes so heavily calcified that the valve cusps are completely immobile and cannot coapt (come together) to prevent regurgitation.

AORTIC INSUFFICIENCY FROM BACTERIAL ENDOCARDITIS. Bacterial endocarditis is a common cause of aortic insufficiency. The development and presentation of the pathologic lesions are similar to those described for mitral insufficiency from bacterial endocarditis. Vegetations on the aortic valve commonly embolize in the rapidly moving, high-pressure arterial stream. Punched-out lesions of the cusps, with thickening and retraction of free margins, may result in massive insufficiency (Fig. 1–34).

Miscellaneous causes of aortic insufficiency include involvement of the ascending aorta with *syphilis*, with resultant dilatation of the annulus of the aortic valve; *cystic medial necrosis* of the aorta, as seen in Marfan's syndrome, again with annular dilatation; and involvement of the valve in the development of a *dissecting aneurysm of the ascending aorta* or of a *sinus of Valsalva aneurysm*.

Tricuspid valve disease. The tricuspid valve is only occasionally involved by true rheumatic involvement (about 5 per cent of patients with rheumatic heart disease); mitral or aortic valve disease always accompanies the tricuspid disease. Rheumatic tricuspid stenosis and insufficiency cause high right atrial pressures. Hepatic congestion, ascites, and peripheral edema are constant findings when the pathologic change is advanced.

Functional (i.e., not organic) tricuspid insufficiency is quite common, however. When the right ventricular chamber is dilated, the papillary muscles and chordae tendineae are unable to securely anchor the leaflets of the tricuspid valve. Further, the valve ring (annulus) may also become dilated, causing a ventriculovalvular disproportion similar to that mentioned under mitral insufficiency. The

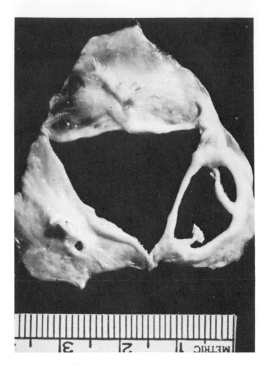

Figure 1–34. Surgical specimen, aortic insufficiency, secondary to bacterial endocarditis (healed). Note the discrete "punched-out" holes in the valve cusps, and the thickening and retraction of the tissues around these holes.

initiating event in both these mechanisms is right ventricular dilatation, which occurs when the outflow from the right ventricle is obstructed—pulmonic stenosis, pulmonary emboli, pulmonary hypertension from chronic lung disease, or elevated left atrial pressures.

Arteriosclerotic Heart Disease

Introduction. At least a half million people die every year in the United States from coronary artery disease, and tremendous effort has been applied in an attempt to determine the cause of this disease and to provide an effective treatment for it. The anatomic-pathologic problem, stated simply, is a narrowing of the coronary arteries, which prevents adequate amounts of blood from reaching the heart muscle.

There are a number of important factors which relate to the development of narrowing in the coronary arteries. Generally, this process is found in males over age 35 and females over age 50; the clinical symptoms relating to the narrowing process may not appear for 10 to 20 years after the obstructing lesion has started. The tendency of coronary disease to appear in a familial relationship may be on a true genetic basis or may be related to similarities in environment.

The effect of diet has been shown to be very important to the development of coronary artery disease. The Oriental races, living on a diet which is low in milk products, eggs, and meats, have a much lower incidence of coronary disease than does the prosperous Western man, whose diet is composed of relatively large amounts of animal fats. Diets high in saturated fats lead to high cholesterol levels in the blood while diets of unsaturated fats do not. The presence of cholesterol crystals in the pathologic lesions which block the coronary arteries (see later) emphasizes the importance of the cholesterol levels in the genesis of these lesions. Patients with diabetes mellitus generally have high serum cholesterol levels, and coronary artery disease is common in this group.

Physical exertion seems to have a somewhat protective effect against coronary disease; serum cholesterol levels are lower and heart attacks less frequent in physically active people. For example, one interesting British study showed a higher incidence of coronary disease in bus drivers (sedentary activities) as opposed to the bus conductors, who were considerably more active in their jobs. The same held true for postal clerks versus the mail carriers in an American study.

Other factors which may cause physiologic narrowing of the coronary arteries are thought to be important in producing arteriosclerotic heart disease. Cigarette smoking constricts peripheral arteries, and may constrict coronary arteries as well; and the incidence of coronary heart disease is very significantly higher in smokers as opposed to nonsmokers. Patients with hypertension are much more prone to develop coronary disease than are patients without hypertension. It has been thought that the great number of heart attacks seen in executives and other persons who are continually under stressful circumstances is related to the artery-constricting effects of the sympathetic nervous system activity in these people.

Pathogenesis (atherogenesis). The wall of the normal large coronary artery has three major divisions. The *intima* is composed of a very thin sheet of cells (the endothelium), which lines the lumen of the vessel, and also a thin fibrous lining. The *media* is a layer of smooth muscle cells separated on either side by sheets of elastic tissue (the internal and external elastic membranes). Finally, the *adventitia* is the outer supporting wall of the artery (Fig. 1–35).

Probably the earliest lesion in coronary artery narrowing is the development of an *atheroma*. Fatty material collects in the intima, causing that layer to be raised up and to project into the blood stream (into the lumen of the vessel). When observed under the microscope, this fatty material is seen to be crystals of cholesterol (the so-called cholesterol clefts). Often there is a fibrous tissue response to this lipid accumulation, and scarring of the vessel wall occurs, which may later become calcified. The atheroma (or atheromatous plaque) so developed may occupy only a small segment of the vessel or may involve its total circumference (Fig. 1–36).

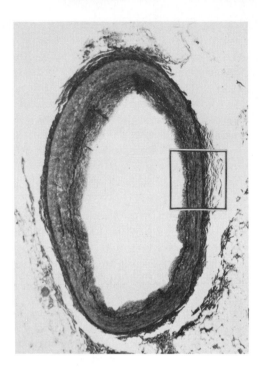

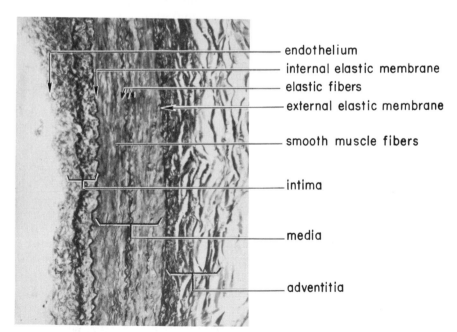

endothelium
internal elastic membrane
elastic fibers
external elastic membrane

smooth muscle fibers

intima

media

adventitia

Figure 1-35.   Microscopic section of a normal coronary artery. The insert depicts the three divisions of the vessel: the intima, the media with its two elastic membranes and smooth muscle, and the adventitia.

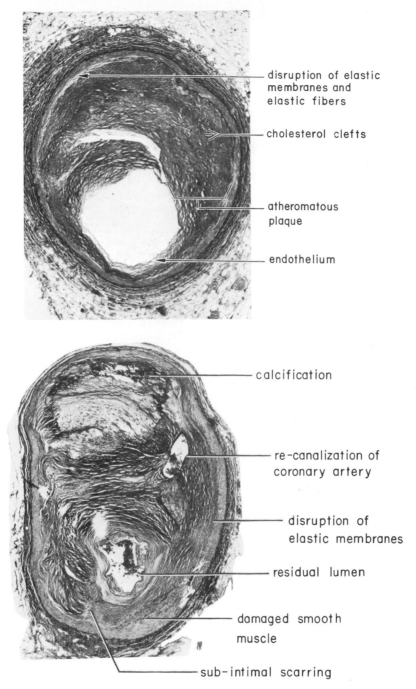

disruption of elastic
membranes and
elastic fibers

cholesterol clefts

atheromatous
plaque

endothelium

calcification

re-canalization of
coronary artery

disruption of
elastic membranes

residual lumen

damaged smooth
muscle

sub-intimal scarring

Figure 1–36. Microscopic sections of different stages of coronary artery narrowing. In the section at the top, note the encroachment on the lumen by the early atheroma; cholesterol clefts and disruption of the elastic fibers are seen. In the bottom section, the atheromatous process has almost completely obstructed the vessel. Severe scarring and even calcification of the damaged vessel wall are clearly visible. There has been "recanalization" of the artery with a new vessel.

53

As the atheroma projects into the lumen of the vessel, it causes roughening of the intima. This roughening, in turn, can cause the accumulation of fibrin and platelets—a small blood clot. Further, hemorrhage into the atheroma (either through the central blood stream or via the tiny blood vessels which supply the wall of the coronary artery itself) causes it to increase in size. Often the elastic membranes are damaged by this hemorrhage. Again, there is a fibrous tissue response.

As these processes of lipid accumulation and subintimal hemorrhage are repeated, the vessel becomes more and more narrow, limiting the amount of blood which can pass through it. Finally, the lumen becomes so narrow that a blood clot (thrombus) forms and the obstruction is then complete. The vessel is thrombosed. Sometimes, as the thrombus becomes organized with fibrous tissue, new blood vessels grow into it, allowing very small amounts of blood to flow once again (recanalization).

The narrowing process as described before may occur in the major coronary vessels or may occur even in the smallest branches. The heart muscle must have an adequate amount of blood brought to it by the coronary vessels. When that blood supply fails to meet the demands, complications ensue.

Complications of inadequate blood supply (coronary insufficiency). ANGINA PECTORIS. When the heart muscle receives an inadequate amount of blood (i.e., oxygen) to supply its needs, it is said to be *ischemic.* Of course, when there is more heart muscle to be supplied (as in the hypertrophy associated with hypertension or valvular heart disease), the needs for oxygen are greater and ischemia occurs more readily.

Just as the muscles in one's legs will cramp when running for extended periods (i.e., when the oxygen supply is inadequate), so, too, the heart muscle will produce pain when its blood supply is inadequate. Many factors increase the heart's demand for more blood, but classically they are the four E's of angina: eating, exercise, emotion, and exposure to cold. Lack of oxygen in the heart muscle will stimulate pain fibers which travel in the nerves leading from the heart. The pain impulses are perceived by the patient as *angina pectoris,* which simply means pain in the chest (see Chapter 2). As soon as the patient rests (or takes nitroglycerine), an adequate amount of blood can be supplied and the pain will stop. The reversible nature of angina pectoris means that the coronary vessels involved at that time have not been completely obstructed but merely are so narrowed that they cannot carry an adequate amount of blood during times of increased need.

MYOCARDIAL INFARCTION (MI). When a coronary artery of significant size becomes completely obstructed, it no longer can carry blood to the heart muscle supplied by it. In some cases, that particular area of heart muscle involved may also have blood coming from other nearby vessels which can take over in the time of need. These vessels, which may bring in the additional blood supply, are called *collateral vessels.*

In other cases, however, there are no collateral vessels available to bring blood to the heart muscle which has lost its supply. The muscle then becomes ischemic, now for an extended period (rather than for just the reversibly short period as in angina pectoris). This ischemia need not occur during exercise or emotion but can, and many times does, occur at rest. The prolonged ischemia leads to death of the cells in the affected area, a process called *infarction*—a myocardial infarction (MI). The infarction can involve almost any area of the heart, but usually affects the different parts of the left ventricle. It may involve the inferior wall (an inferior MI), the anterior and lateral walls (an anterolateral MI), or the septum along with an adjoining wall (anteroseptal or posteroseptal MI).

When the heart muscle dies, it acts as an irritant and the body's defenses rise to meet this new challenge. Polymorphonuclear blood cells and lymphocytes appear in the infarcted area. As the destroyed cells are slowly resorbed, fibrous tissue grows into the area, forming a scar.

Further, different areas of the ventricular wall itself may be involved in the infarction. The most vulnerable area is just inside the heart's inner lining, the endocardium (a subendocardial infarction). This subendocardial area is particularly vulnerable, because the coronary arteries must traverse the full thickness of the ventricular wall to reach it and are then furthest from their point of origin, the aorta.

Of even more serious nature is the infarction which involves the full thickness of the ventricular wall, the transmural infarction. Not only does this type of infarction involve a great deal of dead heart muscle, but it also can lead to other complications: mural thrombus, ventricular aneurysm, myocardial rupture, ischemic degeneration of papillary muscles, and myocardial fibrosis.

If the infarction is transmural (i.e., involves the whole thickness of the ventricular wall), there will be roughening of the heart's inner lining. This area does not contract briskly (if at all) and blood moves more slowly over it. This relative stasis of blood and the endocardial roughening sometimes lead to the formation of a blood clot on the inner wall of the heart—a *mural thrombus.* Occasionally these thrombi are loosened from their attachments, escape into the blood stream, and embolize to other organs (brain, spleen, kidney, and so forth).

Another complication, *ventricular aneurysm,* is usually the result of a massive full-thickness infarction of a large section of the left ventricle and involves the occlusion of at least one of the major coronary vessels (the anterior descending branch of the left coronary artery for an aneurysm on the anterolateral surface, or the main right coronary artery for a posterior ventricular aneurysm). There must be near-total replacement of the infarcted muscle by fibrous tissue. As the necrotic, dead muscle is slowly reduced to a thin sheath of fibrous tissue, it is subjected to the high pressures within the ventricular chamber. This fibrous shell then dilates and forms a non-contractile fibrotic sac which balloons out as a separate chamber, projecting from the remaining ventricle (Fig. 1–37).

Stasis of blood in the aneurysm invariably leads to mural thrombi, which often are firm and well organized next to the wall of the aneurysm, but soft and friable near the lumen of the ventricle. Embolization of this soft clot is not uncommon. Further, the aneurysm causes significant dilatation of the left ventricle; congestive heart failure is common, severe, and often leads to the patient's death. If the papillary muscles of the mitral valve happen to arise from the section of the ventricular wall that is involved in the aneurysm, mitral insufficiency can further complicate the situation.

In *myocardial rupture*, sometimes the myocardial infarction is so severe and the muscle becomes necrotic so quickly that the involved area ruptures. If the free wall of the heart ruptures out into the peri-

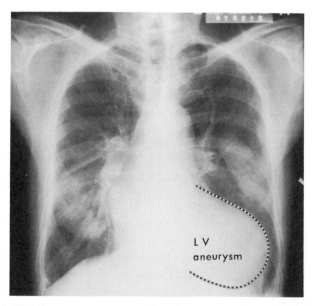

Figure 1–37. Posteroanterior x-ray film of a patient with a ventricular aneurysm. Note the huge ventricular aneurysm which projects outward from the anterior and lateral surfaces of the left ventricle (*outlined by the dotted lines*). The heart is massively enlarged and congestion of the lungs is evident.

cardium, death is usually instantaneous. Occasionally, the interventricular septum is the site of rupture. In this case, a communication develops between the high-pressure left ventricle and the low-pressure right ventricle (a ventricular septal defect). Severe heart failure is the usual sequela. If it is the papillary muscle that ruptures as the result of the infarction, congestive heart failure usually appears rapidly and is fulminant, leading to death in a short interval.

In *ischemic degeneration of papillary muscles,* very commonly the obstruction of the coronary artery which leads to infarction of the ventricular wall will prevent blood from reaching the papillary muscles of the mitral valve. A similar process of death of the cells in the papillary muscles, necrosis, and scarring will then ensue. The end result of this process is a fibrous papillary muscle which cannot contract or function effectively. Loss of papillary muscle function in turn leads to mitral insufficiency, which further complicates the myocardial infarction (Fig. 1–38).

Another complication is *myocardial fibrosis.* Just as occlusion of major coronary arteries can lead to the infarction of large segments of muscle, occlusion of smaller coronary vessels can produce death

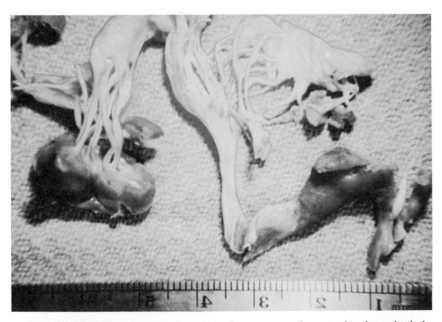

Figure 1–38. Photograph of a surgical specimen of a mitral valve which has undergone ischemic degeneration. The papillary muscle on the right has been reduced to a thin strand of fibrous tissue, while the papillary muscle complex on the left is relatively normal (the patient had an inferior myocardial infarction which involved the posterior papillary muscle and resulted in marked mitral insufficiency).

of small islands of cells. Each of these small islands of dying cells will undergo the same processes of resorption and fibrosis as described under the section on myocardial infarction, resulting in patchy islands of scarring throughout the ventricle. This diffuse type of scarring does not often lead to aneurysm formation, but it significantly impairs the ability of the ventricle to beat synchronously as an organized unit. The end result of this diffuse type of myocardial fibrosis is a dilated, flabby, poorly contracting heart; congestive heart failure is almost always the cause of death of patients with this disease.

Myocardial Disease

There are a number of important pathologic lesions of the myocardium itself, unrelated to rheumatic or arteriosclerotic heart disease. The most common of these primary myocardial diseases are myocarditis, cardiomyopathy (myocardiopathy), and idiopathic hypertrophic subaortic stenosis.

Myocarditis. Inflammation of the heart muscle itself (myocarditis) can be due to a variety of agents—bacteria, viruses, or parasites. However, the pathologic lesions in the heart are similar, no matter what the infectious agent is—cardiac dilatation and hypertrophy, mural thrombi on both the right and left sides, infiltration of circulating blood cells (mostly lymphocytes and mononuclear leukocytes) around the small coronary vessels and between the muscle fibers, and degeneration of the muscle fibers themselves.

Cardiomyopathy (myocardiopathy). The word cardiomyopathy (which simply means disease of heart muscle) is somewhat vague and nonspecific, but justly suits this pathologic entity which is similarly vague and nonspecific. Despite its lack of specificity, cardiomyopathy still forms an important and sizable percentage of patients with heart disease. The causes of cardiomyopathies are not well understood, but the disease can be loosely thought of as a nonspecific end result of an acute injury. The injury may be a vitamin deficiency (e.g., thiamine deficiency or beriberi), a bout of myocarditis, an antigen-antibody reaction, chronic alcoholic intake, or the postpartum situation.

Pathologic examination of cardiomyopathy hearts show them to be greatly dilated with varying amounts of ventricular hypertrophy. Mural thrombi, of one or both ventricles, are very common, as is thickening of the endocardium. Microscopically, there is often diffuse infiltration of fibrous tissue into the myocardium, whose fibers may have undergone degeneration.

Idiopathic hypertrophic subaortic stenosis (IHSS). This disease, which is most commonly found in young adults from ages 30 to 50, may also be thought of as a type of myocardiopathy. There is tremendous hypertrophy of the ventricular muscle, especially of the interventricular septum and the outflow tract from the left ventricle. The papillary muscles become huge pillars of tissue projecting into the left ventricular lumen. The end result of this "muscle-bound heart" is an obstruction to the outflow of blood from the left ventricle, as the hypertrophied walls meet one another during systole. The left ventricular cavity is divided at that time into two parts — the area just beneath the aortic valve (which has normal pressures) and the small high-pressure chamber at the apex of the heart, which is formed when the hypertrophied muscle masses obstruct the outflow.

Diseases of the Pericardium

Although the pericardium is not essential to life, it does function to protect the heart from trauma and infection. Normally, there is only a small amount of fluid (a few cubic centimeters) within the pericardial sac to help "lubricate" the action of the contained heart. When the amount of fluid within the pericardium increases, it is called a *pericardial effusion.* Such increases in fluid may be due to congestive heart failure, uremia, or myxedema, or may accumulate as a response to the irritation by a metastatic tumor, intrapericardial infection, or myocardial infarction.

Probably the most common type of pericarditis (inflammation of the pericardium) is the *acute idiopathic pericarditis,* so called because it comes on acutely without any apparent predisposing or causative factors. Pericarditis may also be caused by tuberculosis, pyogenic organisms (staphylococci or streptococci), or viruses (influenza or Coxsackie). The infection often produces an exudate which forms between the heart and the pericardium. Mild bleeding into the pericardial space is not unusual. When the exudate and blood become organized, fibrous tissue infiltrates the space, causing the pericardium and the heart to become adherent. As further scarring and contraction ensue, the adhesions may constrict the outflow of blood from the ventricles or impede the venous return to the atria — a *constrictive pericarditis.* There is a back-up of blood in the venae cavae, often leading to congestion of the liver and ascites, similar to that seen in severe right-heart failure. Later, calcification of the fibrotic adhesions can lead to further impairment of blood flow.

Cardiac Tumors

Tumors within the heart are not rare; they may be either primary or metastatic. The metastatic growths implanting on the heart most commonly come from primary cancers of the breast, bronchus, or lymph nodes, or from a malignant melanoma. These metastatic tumors can cause pericardial effusion and constriction or, less commonly, may grow into the heart muscle itself, impairing contractility or even obstructing blood flow.

Primary tumors of the heart are almost entirely limited to sarcomas and myxomas. A sarcoma is a malignant tumor which originates from connective tissue cells or muscle cells. When sarcomas invade the walls of the heart, they may obstruct blood flow or interrupt the normal contractions of the heart. Patients with sarcomas usually die in congestive heart failure, often with cardiac arrhythmias.

A cardiac myxoma is a benign tumor which always arises from the interatrial septum, more commonly on the left side. Myxomas, which usually form on a narrow stalk, are soft, gelatinous, friable growths which may grow to a considerable size. Because they are so friable, portions of the myxoma often break off and enter the blood stream, embolizing to a peripheral artery. The diagnosis of an intracardiac myxoma is often made fortuitously by finding the typical microscopic appearance in the specimen which is removed from an obstructed artery.

As myxomas are usually attached by a long stalk to the atrial septum, they may fall through the mitral (or tricuspid) valve. When the tumor mass thus obstructs the valve, it simulates all the clinical findings of mitral stenosis (with which it is very commonly confused). Often, with changes in body position, the tumor will "flip out" back into the atrium, relieving the obstruction and causing the stenotic murmur to disappear.

Traumatic Heart Disease

As the rate of personal injury crimes rises and the use of high-speed transportation increases, trauma to the heart is being seen with increasing frequency. Cardiac trauma may be generally divided into penetrating and blunt (nonpenetrating) categories.

About 50 per cent of persons receiving stab wounds of the heart survive to reach medical treatment, while only 10 to 15 per cent of gunshot or missile injuries are potentially salvageable. The severity of the traumatic lesion depends, in large measure, upon which part of the heart is injured and the size of the hole produced. A small, simple stab wound of the low-pressure right ventricle may cause only moderate blood loss and may seal itself off, while a laceration of the aorta usually results in a fatality. A stab wound traversing more than one chamber may cause a fistula (an abnormal communication) between the chambers, resulting in an intracardiac shunt. Laceration of a valve leaflet may cause massive valvular insufficiency.

As blood leaks out of a heart wound into the pericardial space, the patient will gradually become hypotensive due to simple blood loss. Further, the blood in the pericardial sac will cause an increased venous pressure and will limit venous return, a condition known as cardiac tamponade. If tamponade is not relieved (by needle aspirations or by operation), death may ensue. On the other hand, the high pressures within the pericardium in cardiac tamponade may stop the bleeding from the puncture site.

Blunt or nonpenetrating injury to the heart is most commonly caused by auto accidents in which the patient's sternum is crushed against the steering wheel. A variety of injuries are possible: contusions of the heart muscle, simulating the damage of a myocardial infarction; rupture of the heart with exsanguinating hemorrhage into the pericardium; rupture of chordae tendineae, papillary muscles, or valve cusps, resulting in immediate and severe valvular insufficiency. In all these circumstances, the prognosis is grave.

Bibliography

CONGENITAL HEART DISEASE

Cooley, D. A., and Hallman, G. L.: Surgical Treatment of Congenital Heart Disease. Philadelphia, Lea & Febiger, 1966.

Edwards, J. E., Carey, L. S., Henfeld, H. N., and Lester, R. G.: Congenital Heart Diseases, Correlation of Pathologic Anatomy and Angiocardiography. Philadelphia, W. B. Saunders Company, 1965.

Kanjuh, V. I., and Edwards, J. E.: A review of congenital anomalies of the heart and great vessels according to functional categories. Pediat. Clin. N. Amer. *11*:55–138, 1964.

ACQUIRED HEART DISEASE

Edwards, J. E.: An Atlas of Acquired Diseases of the Heart and Great Vessels. Philadelphia, W. B. Saunders Company, 1961.

Harrison, T. R., and Reeves, T. J.: Principles and Problems of Ischemic Heart Disease. Chicago, Year Book Medical Publishers, Inc., 1968.

Hurst, J. W., and Logue, R. B.: The Heart. 2nd ed. Part V, Diseases of the Heart and Pericardium. New York, McGraw-Hill Book Company, 1970.

Netter, F. H.: The CIBA Collection of Medical Illustrations. Vol. 5, Heart. Summit, New Jersey, CIBA Pharmaceutical Company, 1969.

CHAPTER 2

Medical Aspects

By MERVIN J. GOLDMAN, M.D.

Introduction

In this chapter on clinical heart disease, an emphasis has been placed upon the common forms of acquired heart disease as seen in a general hospital. The etiology, pathophysiology, clinical manifestations, diagnosis, therapy, and prognosis are discussed in sufficient depth to give the reader a basic understanding of the disease processes.

Congestive heart failure and cardiogenic shock are discussed separately, since these manifestations are common to many forms of heart disease and are seen in patients on medical and surgical services.

Congestive Heart Failure

The term congestive heart failure describes that syndrome which results when the cardiac output is insufficient to meet the metabolic demands of the body. The pathophysiologic causes are (1) ventricular muscle disease, as commonly results from coronary artery disease or myocarditis; (2) systolic overloading of a ventricle, resulting from increased resistance to ejection, as seen in systemic or pulmonary hypertension and aortic or pulmonic stenosis; (3) diastolic overloading of a ventricle, resulting from a volume overload, as seen in aortic, mitral, pulmonic, and tricuspid insufficiency and left-to-right shunts; and (4) those disease states which increase the body needs for oxygen, such as thyrotoxicosis, severe anemia, and arteriovenous fistulae.

The symptoms and signs of congestive heart failure are produced by two mechanisms: (1) involvement of the left ventricle by one of the previously mentioned pathologic states eventually leads to an increase in diastolic volume and diastolic filling pressure. Diastolic filling pressure further causes an increase in left atrial, pulmonary venous, and pulmonary capillary pressures. When pulmonary capillary pressure exceeds the intravascular osmotic pressure (approximately 30 mm Hg), left heart failure develops. In turn, pulmonary artery pressures are elevated, producing an increased work load on the right heart, with resulting right heart failure. (2) Reduction in cardiac output sets humoral mechanisms into play with resultant renal retention of sodium and water which increases plasma volume and, in turn, imposes an increased work load on the myocardium.

Left ventricular failure is manifested by the following symptoms: exertional dyspnea, orthopnea (shortness of breath on recumbency), paroxysmal nocturnal dyspnea (acute shortness of breath awakening patient from sleep), cough and wheezing (which may be misinterpreted as bronchial asthma), and weakness or fatigue resulting from the reduced cardiac output. Symptoms of right heart failure include right upper quadrant pain, anorexia, and nausea due to congestion of the liver and gut, oliguria during the day and polyuria at night. The signs of congestive heart failure are cardiomegaly, which is often evident on physical examination, gallop sounds (third or fourth heart sounds, or both), rales at the lung bases or throughout the entire lung fields in gross pulmonary edema, elevation of venous pressure as determined by observation of neck veins, a positive hepatojugular reflux (increase in neck vein distension elicited by abdominal compression making certain the patient is not straining), an enlarged, tender liver, and edema which may involve the ankle regions or both legs, genitalia, sacrum, and flanks. In medical and surgical intensive care units it is essential that the nurse become experienced in recognizing the early signs of failure, such as gallop sounds and pulmonary rales. Central venous pressure will usually be determined by direct measurement. The ability of the nurse to perform such examinations (a province formerly reserved for the physician alone) and to recognize heart failure in the earlier stages will result in an earlier institution of proper therapy with a resulting decrease in patient morbidity and mortality.

The chest x-ray commonly shows cardiac enlargement and pulmonary vascular congestion. The electrocardiogram is of no value in evaluation of heart failure per se, but is of obvious aid in yielding information regarding cardiac rhythm and the basic cardiac abnormality. Evaluation of serum electrolytes (especially sodium and potassium) and urine electrolytes, in conjunction with the clinical evaluation of the degree of hydration (and checked with blood volume determination when indicated), will permit an intelligent approach to fluid and electrolyte management of the patient.

Medical treatment includes the use of digitalis, sodium restriction, water restriction (especially when the serum sodium concentration is low in the presence of edema), and diuretic therapy. This will be discussed in detail in the chapter on drug therapy. In addition, therapy must be directed to specific causes and precipitating factors, e.g., hypertension, thyrotoxicosis, myxedema, anemia, infection, pulmonary infarction, and arrhythmias.

Cardiogenic Shock

In medical cardiology, shock is most commonly seen in acute myocardial infarction; however, other causes, especially blood loss and sepsis, must always be considered. The precipitating cause of cardiac shock is an acute reduction in cardiac output. Peripheral vasoconstriction and tachycardia result from an attempt to increase peripheral resistance to compensate for the falling cardiac output and to maintain blood pressure.

The symptoms and signs of shock reflect the inadequate cardiac output and insufficient perfusion. These are skin (cold and clammy), blood pressure (low and sometimes not obtainable by external arm cuff), pulse (rapid), cerebral manifestations (restlessness, disturbed sensorium, progressing to coma), renal manifestations (reduction in urinary output [below 25 ml per hour] progressing to anuria), central venous pressure (may be low or normal; if right heart failure is present it will be elevated), and arterial oxygen tension (commonly below 60 mm Hg).

The essentials for monitoring patients with cardiogenic shock are the following: An *ECG* should be taken as in any patient with acute myocardial infarction. The shock state with aggravation of myocardial ischemia or the resulting metabolic acidosis increases the risk of serious ventricular arrhythmias. *Blood pressure measurement* should be done by direct intra-arterial catheter, which will give continuous measurements and will be superior to external cuff measurements. This will also facilitate withdrawal of blood samples for determination of blood gases. Pulmonary artery diastolic pressure measurement gives a more accurate evaluation of left heart function than does blood pressure measurement or a CVP. The patient can be in left heart failure or gross pulmonary edema with an elevated pulmonary artery pressure and a normal CVP. *Intake and output* must be recorded accurately. Urine flow per hour is an essential determination. *Arterial* P_{O_2}, P_{CO_2} *and pH* are used to determine the degree of hypoxia and acidosis. As a result of tissue hypoxia, there is lactic acid accumulation resulting in metabolic acidosis. The acidosis results in further deterioration of myocardial function and increases the potential for serious cardiac arrhythmias. *Serum and urine electrolyte determinations* are essential for proper management of fluids and electrolytes. *Cardiac output* determinations are ideal, but unfortunately are not available in most units.

TREATMENT

Pain and restlessness must be controlled with morphine or meperidine. These drugs must be given in the smallest effective doses to prevent suppression of respiration and depression of myocardial function. Oxygen by reservoir mask, nasal catheter, or positive pressure apparatus (with endotracheal intubation when necessary) to maintain an arterial P_{O_2} over 70 mm Hg is essential to maintain oxygenation of all tissues.

Heart failure, if present, must be treated with adequate doses of digitalis and rapidly acting diuretics. Even in the absence of obvious signs of heart failure, digitalis may be of benefit due to its action in improving myocardial contractility.

Treatment of arrhythmias will be as indicated in any case of myocardial infarction.

In the absence of heart failure, the correction of metabolic acidosis may be attempted with IV sodium bicarbonate; however, the high sodium load may precipitate further heart failure. Tromethamine (THAM) may be preferable.

In the correction of electrolyte abnormalities, the cautious use of IV potassium is indicated if hypokalemia is present. The use of Kayexalate enemas, intravenous calcium, hypertonic glucose and insulin is required for the treatment of hyperkalemia.

The use of plasma expanders in the absence of heart failure should be considered. The use of isotonic saline, plasma, or whole blood in patients with a low or normal CVP has been disappointing in most patients with acute myocardial infarction. The major problem is in the use of the CVP as an index of blood volume. It is unreliable in cardiogenic shock as evidenced by the occurrence of pulmonary edema in the presence of a normal CVP. If there is evidence of a diminished effective blood volume (by a low pulmonary artery pressure or blood volume), cautious use of plasma expanders is indicated.

The rationale of vasopressor drugs (levarterenol, metaraminol, mephenteramine, methoxamine, and phenylephrine) is to further increase peripheral vascular resistance and hopefully increase cardiac output. Although these drugs are commonly used and result in an increase in blood pressure, the cardiac output is often unchanged or falls. The patient in shock who is cold and clammy is already maximally vasoconstricted, and these drugs have little effect improving myocardial contractility. This explains the overall disappointing clinical results from such therapy.

Isoproterenol (a beta-adrenergic stimulant), by its inotropic action on the myocardium, can increase cardiac output. This action, coupled with its peripheral vasodilating action, can improve perfusion in vital organs. The dose must be carefully adjusted to avoid undesirable sinus tachycardia or serious arrhythmias.

Large doses of corticosteroids have been advised in this shock state. There is insufficient evidence of clinical value to justify their routine use at present.

In spite of the previously mentioned measures, the mortality from shock in association with myocardial infarction remains over 60 per cent. Promising techniques to improve this dismal state include the use of extracorporeal support systems which can maintain adequate circulation for a period of hours and hopefully permit improvement in the circulatory dynamics, so that a stable state will be maintained after removing the support system.

Rheumatic and Acquired Valvular Heart Disease

ACUTE RHEUMATIC CARDITIS

Acute rheumatic carditis occurs in association with acute rheumatic fever. Although acute rheumatic fever is initiated by a hemolytic streptococcal infection, the cardiac involvement is due to a hypersensitivity reaction and not to the infection per se. The carditis is manifested by any of the following features: the development of a significant apical systolic murmur, aortic or mitral diastolic murmurs due to acute valvulitis or dilatation of the valve rings, pericardial friction rub, cardiac enlargement, and congestive heart failure. Chest x-rays will demonstrate cardiomegaly or pericardial effusion when present. The electrocardiogram commonly shows a first degree heart block and nonspecific ST and T wave changes. There is no laboratory test which is pathognomonic for acute rheumatic fever or acute rheumatic carditis. A positive throat culture for hemolytic streptococci or a positive antistreptolysin titer merely proves streptococcal infection and not necessarily rheumatic disease.

Treatment includes adequate bed rest and supportive therapy. Penicillin is indicated to eradicate the hemolytic streptococcus but will not alter the already established rheumatic process. Salicylates should be given for systemic control of fever. Corticosteroids are indicated in patients with severe carditis, manifested by cardiomegaly, heart failure, or pericarditis to reduce the acute inflammatory reaction and thereby improve cardiac function. There is no evidence that such treatment will reduce the incidence of subsequent chronic rheumatic valvular disease. Congestive heart failure is treated in the conventional manner. The prognosis is excellent for immediate recovery from acute rheumatic carditis, the mortality being only 1 to 2 per cent. However, two thirds of children with acute rheumatic carditis will have detectable valvular heart disease within 10 years. The incidence is much lower in adults.

Since recurrences of acute rheumatic fever occur most commonly within five years of the original attack, these patients should receive prophylactic penicillin therapy for a minimum of five years. If the patient is sensitive to penicillin, erythromycin is the second drug of choice. Sulfonamides now are not recommended for prophylaxis.

CHRONIC RHEUMATIC AND OTHER TYPES OF VALVULAR HEART DISEASE

Chronic rheumatic valvular disease results from one or more episodes of acute rheumatic valvulitis. This produces fusion of the commissures, fibrosis, and later calcification of the valve cusps, with shortening and fusion of the chordae tendineae. Either stenosis or insufficiency or a combination of both may result. The mitral valve is affected most commonly (60 per cent); combined mitral and aortic valve disease is seen in 20 per cent, and isolated aortic valve disease in 10 per cent. Organic tricuspid involvement occurs in less than 10 per cent and always occurs in association with mitral and aortic valve disease. Pulmonary valve disease is rare.

Mitral Stenosis

This is most commonly due to rheumatic disease. However, it may occur as a congenital anomaly (in association with an intra-atrial septal defect) (Lutembacher's syndrome). A left atrial myxoma, by obstruction of mitral valve flow, may simulate the clinical picture of mitral stenosis. Rheumatic mitral stenosis occurs most commonly in women under 45 years of age. The patient is often asymptomatic, even though physical signs of the disease are present, i.e., loud first heart sound, mitral diastolic murmur, and an opening snap (see Chapter 5). Symptoms do not occur until the mitral valve area is reduced to below 1.5 square cm and tachycardia or atrial fibrillation intervene. Reduction of the valve area below the previously mentioned critical level decreases left ventricular filling and thereby lowers cardiac output. The stenosis causes increasing pressure in the left atrium, elevating pulmonary venous, capillary, and arterial pressures (passive pulmonary hypertension). Left heart failure and later right-heart failure ensue. With tachycardia, the period of diastolic ventricular filling is reduced, resulting in a further lowering of the cardiac output. Atrial fibrillation reduces the cardiac output by the same mechanism, since the ventricular rate is usually rapid in untreated cases. The loss of atrial contraction, which significantly contributes to ventricular filling, further reduces cardiac output. In addition, some patients develop constriction of the pulmonary arterioles (active pulmonary hypertension), producing more serious overloading of the right heart and right heart failure. The early signs of mitral stenosis are an accentuated first heart sound and an opening snap, both of which indicate a reasonably pliable valve. The diastolic murmur follows the opening snap and in the presence of sinus rhythm there is presystolic accentuation. The previously mentioned findings alone are not an indication of the severity of the disease. With increasing pulmonary artery pressure, an accentuated pulmonic closure sound is evident, and with increasing right ventricular pressure, a right ventricular lift is palpable. With marked fibrosis and calcification of the valve and fusion of the chordae tendineae, mitral valve motion is seriously impeded with resulting disappearance of the accentuated first sound and opening snap. With very small valve areas, the flow is so reduced that the diastolic murmur is no longer heard. Therefore, in the advanced severe case of mitral stenosis, the typical ausculatory signs are lost and thereby the diagnosis may be overlooked. This is known as the *dumb* or *silent mitral syndrome*.

As a result of pulmonary venous hypertension, collateral veins develop between the pulmonary and bronchial veins. Large bronchial varices may develop and later rupture, producing hemoptysis.

Systemic embolization is a common complication of mitral stenosis. In 90 per cent of patients with emboli, atrial fibrillation is present. Although thrombi most commonly occur in the left atrial appendage (auricle), thrombi may occur in the main left atrial chamber near the mitral valve, or near the pulmonary veins.

The electrocardiogram may be normal in asymptomatic patients. With increasing left atrial and right heart pressures, the ECG will show left atrial abnormality (P mitrale) and signs of right ventricular hypertrophy. Atrial fibrillation, initially paroxysmal and later chronic, is common.

The chest x-rays can demonstrate enlargement of the left atrium and right ventricle and the pulmonary artery segment. The aortic shadow is usually diminutive and the left ventricular size is normal. Mitral valve calcification is best seen with fluoroscopy.

Although cardiac catheterization is not always essential to evaluate the severity of the disease and the need for surgery, it should be done whenever possible to quantitatively evaluate the degree of left atrial and pulmonary artery hypertension, the mitral valve area, and the presence or absence of associated mitral insufficiency or aortic valve disease. Left atrial or left ventricular angiography is especially valuable in evaluating the appearance and motion of the mitral cusps. This is important in the decision to perform mitral valvulotomy by a closed or an open procedure.

Medical therapy includes (1) digitalis for the treatment of heart failure or the control of the ventricular rate in the presence of atrial fibrillation, (2) diuretics as indicated for heart failure, (3) use of quinidine or electrical cardioversion to revert atrial fibrillation to sinus rhythm, (4) long-term anticoagulant therapy for treatment and prevention of systemic emboli in patients with atrial fibrillation, and (5) general supportive measures.

Surgical therapy is to be advised in any patient whose symptoms are not controlled by the previously mentioned medical therapy and in whom there is evidence of significant hemodynamic abnormalities. These abnormalities will be evidenced by significantly increased left atrial and pulmonary artery pressures and reduction in mitral valve area below 1.5 cm^2.

Closed mitral valvulotomy should be reserved for those patients with little or no calcification in the valve, evidence of a mobile valve (presence of an opening snap), sinus rhythm, and no previous arterial emboli. Patients with chronic atrial fibrillation, significant calcification of the valve, or previous mitral operations should have an open procedure. Under direct vision the surgeon can then decide whether a valvulotomy or valve replacement is indicated.

Mitral Insufficiency

Rheumatic disease is only one cause of mitral insufficiency. Others include congenital disease, bacterial endocarditis, ruptured chordae tendineae, rupture or dysfunction of papillary muscles due to myocardial infarction, and relative mitral insufficiency secondary to dilatation of the left ventricle. Rheumatic mitral insufficiency is the result of scarring and retraction of the valve leaflets and chordae tendineae (or occasionally rupture of the chordae). Blood regurgitates into the left atrium during ventricular systole, reducing forward blood flow and causing a gradual increase in left atrial volume and pressure, leading to pulmonary hypertension. Symptoms of left heart and then right heart failure ensue. Systemic emboli and hemoptysis are uncommon in mitral insufficiency. Physical findings include signs of left ventricular hypertrophy, a diminution in intensity of the first heart sound, a significant pansystolic mitral murmur, and an early diastolic gallop (S_3). Atrial fibrillation is common. The electrocardiogram may reveal left atrial abnormality or atrial fibrillation and signs of left ventricular hypertrophy. The chest x-ray film will show left atrial and left ventricular enlargement. Mitral valve calcification may be evident on fluoroscopy.

Cardiac catheterization and left ventricular angiography are necessary to quantitate the severity of the regurgitation and to evaluate the degree of hemodynamic abnormality.

Medical treatment is the same as given for mitral stenosis. Surgical treatment is indicated in patients in whom symptoms are not controlled by medical therapy and in whom hemodynamic evidence of significant regurgitation is present. This always requires open heart surgery and often requires prosthetic mitral valve replacement.

Aortic Stenosis

Although rheumatic disease is a common etiology, it is also seen secondary to congenital disease (commonly with bicuspid aortic valves) and as an "aging" process of unknown etiology. The end result of all the before mentioned etiologies is progressive narrowing of the aortic valve orifice from fibrosis and calcification.

Aortic stenosis is most commonly seen in older males. In mild to moderate cases, the patient may be asymptomatic, and, at this time, a rough aortic systolic murmur will be heard, with transmission into the carotid arteries. Signs of left ventricular hypertrophy by x-ray film and ECG may or may not be present. In more severe cases, signs and symptoms of left heart and then right heart failure develop. Dizziness and syncope may occur due to insufficient blood flow to the brain and therefore are indications for surgical therapy. Chest pain, typical of angina, is common and can result from insufficient blood supply to the myocardium and need not result from coronary artery disease per se, although both diseases may coexist. Patients with severe aortic stenosis are subject to sudden unexpected death—the exact cause of which is unknown. Physical examination in a patient with aortic stenosis reveals a left ventricular lift, a systolic aortic murmur, diminution or absence of the aortic second sound, and commonly gallop rhythms. The intensity of the murmur is not a good index of the severity of the stenosis. Patients with marked heart failure with resulting low cardiac output and low flow across the aortic valve may have a faint or absent murmur. The most important bedside sign of the severity of the stenosis is the character of the upstroke of the carotid artery, which will be delayed. X-ray films will show cardiac enlargement (principally left ventricular), and calcification of the aortic valve is commonly seen. The electrocardiogram will indicate left ventricular hypertrophy. Heart block, from involvement of the upper portion of the interventricular septum in the calcific process, is not uncommon.

Cardiac catheterization is indicated to determine the pressure gradient between the left ventricle and aorta and the cardiac output. In the absence of associated aortic insufficiency, the aortic valve area can be calculated. Areas below 1 cm^2 are hemodynamically significant and an area of 0.6 cm^2 or less is critical.

Medical therapy is the treatment of heart failure. Once heart failure ensues, the prognosis for longevity is poor, generally from one to two years. Therefore, any patient with heart failure or an aortic valve area of 0.6 cm^2 or less is a candidate for surgery. The presence of marked or progressive cardiomegaly or history of syncope indicates the need for surgery with greater valve areas up to 1 cm^2. The surgical treatment is replacement of the aortic valve with a prosthetic, homograft or heterograft valve.

Aortic Insufficiency

Aortic insufficiency is the result of disease of the aortic valves or aortic root which permits regurgitation of blood from the aorta into the left ventricle during diastole. Causes include rheumatic valvulitis, congenital lesion of the aortic valve (bicuspid valve), bacterial endocarditis, syphilitic aortitis, rheumatoid aortitis, congenital or acquired medial necrosis of the aorta, arteriosclerotic and hypertensive dilatation of the aortic root, and dissecting aneurysm of the aorta. Aortic insufficiency is often asymptomatic for years with the only finding being an aortic diastolic murmur. As the regurgitation becomes more significant, there will be progressive hypertrophy and dilatation of the left ventricle with resulting left heart failure and then right heart failure. In addition to the presence of the aortic diastolic murmur and the signs of ventricular hypertrophy, there will be changes in peripheral vascular hemodynamics. The diastolic pressure will progressively fall, at times to zero, with maintenance of a normal or rising systolic arterial pressure. This produces the typical pounding or Corrigan-type arterial pulse. The chest x-ray film will show left ventricular enlargement and widening of the aortic root in those cases of aortic root etiology. The electrocardiogram will indicate left ventricular hypertrophy. Medical treatment includes treatment of heart failure, treatment of the etiologic factor when possible (bacterial endocarditis, syphilis), and general supportive therapy.

The prognosis with medical therapy alone is poor. After signs of heart failure ensue and left ventricular enlargement is present, the average life expectancy is only two to three years. Hence, in these situations, aortic valve surgery is indicated. Cardiac catheterization and left ventricular and aortic cineangiography are indicated to (1) evaluate left ventricular size and function, (2) determine the appearance of the aorta, (3) quantitate the degree of aortic regurgitation, and (4) provide hemodynamic data regarding pulmonary and right heart pressures and cardiac output. Although aortic valve replacement will be the usual surgical therapy, in selected cases a plastic procedure on the valve or aorta may be possible.

Tricuspid Stenosis

This lesion is most commonly the result of rheumatic fever and as such is always seen in association with rheumatic mitral valve disease. It may occur as a congenital lesion or as a complication of bacterial endocarditis or the carcinoid syndrome. A myxoma of the right atrium, by obstructing the tricuspid valve, can mimic tricuspid stenosis. Since tricuspid stenosis prevents the flow of blood from the right atrium into the right ventricle, there will be a marked engorgement of the systemic venous system with hepatomegaly, ascites, and peripheral edema. Due to reduction in cardiac output, fatigue is a common symptom. In the presence of sinus rhythm, a prominent "a" wave with slow collapse will be visible in the neck veins. A tricuspid diastolic murmur and a right-sided opening snap, which are similar to those heard in mitral stenosis, may be appreciated along the left sternal border. A large right atrium will be seen on chest x-ray. Since mitral valve disease is so commonly associated with tricuspid stenosis, the physical, x-ray film, and ECG findings will be those of the combined lesions.

Cardiac catheterization will determine the presence and severity of this lesion and associated lesions. When significant, as best determined by catheterization studies, surgery is indicated and can either be valvotomy or valve replacement. In cases of rheumatic origin, associated mitral surgery will almost always be necessary.

Tricuspid Insufficiency

This lesion permits regurgitation of blood from the right ventricle into the right atrium during ventricular systole. It most commonly is a functional rather than an organic lesion of the tricuspid valve. The functional lesion is due to dilatation of the tricuspid annulus from any disease which produces heart dilatation and failure. Organic etiologies are the same as those listed for tricuspid stenosis. Physical findings include a pansystolic murmur and a third heart sound, heard best along the left lower sternal border. Both these findings will be accentuated during inspiration. Prominent regurgitant waves will be visible in the neck veins and a similar phenomenon may be seen and felt over the enlarged liver.

Cardiac catheterization will identify the lesion but may not differentiate between functional and organic disease. In patients with associated mitral valve disease who are being operated upon for the latter lesion, this determination will be made at the time of surgery. If significant organic tricuspid disease is found, annuloplasty or prosthetic valve replacement is indicated. If the lesion is found to be functional, tricuspid valve surgery is usually unnecessary, since proper treatment of the associated mitral valve (and aortic valve, if present) lesion will usually result in sufficient hemodynamic improvement in relieving the tricuspid insufficiency.

Pulmonic Stenosis

This lesion most commonly occurs on a congenital basis and is either valvular, subvalvular, or peripheral. The subvalvular type may occur in association with the carcinoid syndrome. Thromboembolic disease of the pulmonary artery may simulate pulmonic stenosis.

Pulmonary Insufficiency

This lesion may be organic or functional. Organic disease may occur on a congenital basis, secondary to bacterial endocarditis (as in addicts), diseases of the pulmonary artery, or rheumatic disease. Functional pulmonic insufficiency occurs secondary to severe pulmonary hypertension with dilatation of the pulmonic ring, as seen in mitral stenosis with high pulmonary vascular resistance and severe pulmonary or pulmonary vascular disease. Pulmonary insufficiency is sometimes seen after the repair of tetralogy of Fallot, in which an outflow patch is placed across the annulus of the valve.

Bacterial Endocarditis

Bacterial endocarditis is a bacterial infection occurring on a previously diseased (rheumatic or congenital) heart valve or on a previously normal heart valve. There are two classifications of the disease — subacute and acute. (1) Subacute bacterial endocarditis is a slowly progressive disease, resulting usually from *Streptococcus viridans* or *Streptococcus fecalis* (Enterococcus) engrafted upon a pre-existing rheumatic or congenital lesion. (2) Acute bacterial endocarditis is a more fulminating disease commonly due to *Staphylococcus aureus*, Pneumococcus, hemolytic Streptococcus, or gram-negative coliform organisms engrafted upon a normal or diseased valve.

The above classification is not absolute. Patients with subacute disease may have a rapid acute clinical illness and patients with acute disease may have a slow, smoldering clinical course.

Its clinical features are (1) fever, present in over 95 per cent of cases; (2) known pre-existing valve disease or surgery for valvular or congenital heart disease, including insertion of prosthetic devices; (3) a history of recent infection, dental work, or cystoscopy or self-administered IV drugs (addicts); (4) splenomegaly, petechiae on skin or mucous membranes, tender red nodules on fingers, palms, or toes, and changing heart murmurs; (5) systemic emboli to brain, extremities, kidneys, spleen, or bowel. This is often the initial symptom of the disease. Pulmonary or tricuspid valve disease may result in pulmonary embolization, but is relatively uncommon, except in drug addicts.

Laboratory findings consist of (1) a positive blood culture. This is essential for an absolute diagnosis. A minimum of five blood cultures should be taken within 24 to 48 hours. Unfortunately, 10 to 15 per cent of patients with bacterial endocarditis will have negative blood cultures. (2) Hematuria, anemia, and leukocytosis are often present, but do not prove or exclude the diagnosis.

Therapy is either specific or general. In specific therapy, if the blood culture is positive, the organism must be tested for its antibiotic sensitivity. Appropriate doses of single or combinations of two or more antibiotics are given parenterally. While on such therapy, the patient's blood serum is tested for its bactericidal effects on the recovered organism. If the patient's serum in a 1:10 or greater dilution prevents growth of the organism, this is good evidence of adequate therapy. The choice of agents and duration of therapy must be individualized. A patient with *Streptococcus viridans* endocarditis may be successfully treated with one to two million units of penicillin per day for two to four weeks. A patient with Staphylococcal endocarditis may require massive doses of methicillin, cephalothin, vancomycin, and so forth, singly or in combination, for six or more weeks to ensure a cure. Chloramphenicol, erythromycin, and the tetracycline drugs are not bacteriocidal, and hence should never be used as the only drugs. Patients with surgically inserted prosthetic devices (patches or valves) often require surgical replacement of these in conjunction with antibiotic therapy. In general therapy, treatment should be the same as indicated for associated heart failure, arrhythmias, and embolization. Anticoagulant therapy is contraindicated because of the danger of cerebral hemorrhage.

There may be several complications. (1) Perforation, tear, or disruption of valve-supporting structures may require emergency surgery (i.e., valve replacement) or elective surgery following bacteriologic control, depending on the clinical severity of the process. This is especially true of aortic insufficiency. (2) Emboli may continue for two weeks after adequate antibiotic treatment. When appropriate, surgical embolectomy may be indicated. Anticoagulant treatment is contraindicated (see before). (3) Local thrombophlebitis at the site of IV administration is common in all long-term IV therapy. Its incidence can be reduced by scrupulous aseptic technique, use of "scalp-vein" needles, frequent inspection of IV sites, and application of antibiotic ointment (e.g., bacitracin or neomycin) at the IV site. If plastic intracatheters are used, the site should be changed every three days, if possible. (4) Mycotic aneurysms can develop in any peripheral artery, secondary to bacterial infection in the arterial wall. When this complication can be diagnosed, as in an extremity (e.g., popliteal artery), surgical resection may be indicated.

All patients with known rheumatic or congenital valve disease or other congenital lesions which are commonly associated with endocarditis (IV septal defect, patent ductus) must receive antibiotic therapy in conjunction with dental treatments, cystoscopy, and any surgical procedures in a potentially infected area.

Coronary Artery Disease

ETIOLOGY

Coronary artery disease is most commonly due to atherosclerosis of the coronary arteries. Relatively uncommon causes are syphilitic aortitis with involvement of the coronary ostia, emboli into the coronary circulation, polyarteritis, Buerger's disease, dissection of the coronary artery, and trauma.

PREDISPOSING CAUSES

Males are predominantly affected. Before the age of 40 the incidence favors males 10:1, but by age 70 the incidence is equal. In the absence of other factors discussed below, coronary artery disease in women during the child-bearing years is a rarity. The conditions which predispose to coronary artery disease are hypertension, diabetes mellitus, the hyperlipidemic states and possibly hypothyroidism. Heredity is an important, but poorly understood, factor. Some investigators believe that certain personality patterns are correlated with this disease, namely, the compulsive, hard-working, driving individual. Obesity, per se, is not considered an etiologic factor, but the overweight state puts an added load on an already diseased heart.

CLINICAL MANIFESTATIONS

Angina Pectoris (Pain in the Heart)

This term describes the clinical symptoms which result from transient insufficiency of myocardial blood supply and hence oxygen supply to the myocardium. It most commonly occurs under those situations which increase the metabolic requirements for oxygen, such as physical exercise, emotional upsets, exposure to cold, and overeating. Associated disease states, such as anemia, polycythemia, aortic stenosis, tachycardia, hypertension, hypotension, thyrotoxicosis, and hypoglycemia all can aggravate the anginal state.

The patient's history is still the best practical means of making the diagnosis. Typically, the patient describes a squeezing or compressing sensation substernally. On occasion, the pain is described as burning in character. Radiation, if it occurs, is most commonly into the left shoulder and inner aspect of the left arm. Less commonly, radiation of pain into the right arm, both arms, neck and lower jaw, or the intrascapular region is described. Since the evaluation of the pain is so important, the questioner must spend considerable time with the patient and never use leading questions. At times, the patient will be seen to clench and unclench his fists in an attempt to describe the pain sensation, and this is a valuable clue to the constricting nature of the pain. The examiner should never be content with the term "indigestion," which the patient commonly uses to describe the symptoms, especially when the substernal pain extends into the epigastrium. The pain typically is brought on by exertion or the other factors mentioned previously and subsides within one to 10 minutes with rest or medication. The need for patience and time in evaluating these symptoms cannot be overemphasized. Musculoskeletal disease of the spine or chest wall or upper gastrointestinal tract disease may simulate the symptoms of angina. The incorrect diagnosis of coronary artery disease with its physical, emotional, and socioeconomic consequences is disastrous to the patient and his family.

Physical examination is of little value in establishing the diagnosis of coronary artery disease. If the patient is seen during an episode of pain, cautious massage of one carotid sinus may cause the pain to disappear if it is angina. The patient must not be told what to expect from this maneuver.

The electrocardiogram is most commonly normal in a patient with angina who has not had a history of known myocardial infarction, when it is taken at rest and when the patient is free of pain. Therefore, a normal electrocardiogram never excludes the diagnosis. If the ECG can be recorded during a spontaneous episode of pain, the characteristic ST and T wave changes will commonly be seen. These disappear after the subsidence of the pain. Various exercise tests have been developed to purposely put an added stress on the myocardium and evoke the previously mentioned ECG abnormalities. Such tests are not necessary for making the diagnosis if the history is considered typical. The patient must be off drug therapy (including digitalis) at the time of the test and should be under constant professional supervision during the test. Interpretation of exercise ECG can be exceedingly difficult and tragedies result from overreading. Unless the ECG changes are absolutely typical, it is unwise to make a diagnosis of coronary artery disease by this method alone.

Selective coronary cinearteriography is the best method for evaluating the pathologic status of the coronary arteries. It is essential in all cases being considered for surgery aimed at improving the coronary artery circulation, and in those cases in which the diagnosis of coronary artery disease is in doubt on the basis of history and electrocardiograms; such diagnosis is essential for the proper management of the patient. It must be emphasized that this test visualizes the coronary arterial tree and indicates the presence and severity of the vascular disease, but does not prove that the chest pain is due to coronary disease.

The anginal syndrome must never be considered as a sign of mild coronary disease. Autopsy studies and coronary arteriography indicate that such patients commonly have extensive disease involving multiple vessels.

Coronary Occlusion

Complete occlusion of a coronary artery can only be diagnosed during life by arteriography. Depending on the location and the extent of collateral circulation, occlusions can be found in asymptomatic patients, those with angina, and those with myocardial infarction.

Myocardial Infarction

This disease is the death of a portion of the myocardium resulting from insufficient blood supply. The cause may be coronary occlusion or sufficient narrowing of the coronary vessels without complete occlusion which results in sufficient restriction of oxygenation to cause death of the tissue.

Pain is the most common symptom of myocardial infarction. Its location, radiation, and character is similar to that of anginal pain but is usually more intense and persists for 30 minutes to hours, unrelieved by rest and nitroglycerine. Dyspnea, profuse perspiration, and nausea are frequently associated symptoms. At times, the latter symptoms are present without pain and should arouse suspicion of infarction. Recent prospective studies (Framingham) indicate that as many as 20 per cent of infarctions are entirely silent, i.e., not associated with any symptoms. Patients who are mentally obtunded or unconscious, as in acute cerebrovascular accidents and during anesthesia or surgery, may sustain myocardial infarction without obvious subjective complaints.

The electrocardiogram is the best laboratory test for the diagnosis of infarction. However, one single ECG must never be used to either include or exclude the diagnosis. The electrocardiogram may be normal within the first one to two days or nonspecific abnormalities may be seen which relate to the recent clinical event or to prior disease. Serial records must be taken, and a changing pattern will usually be seen.

Serum enzyme determinations (SGOT, LDH, and CPK) are of considerable value in diagnosis. Serum SGOT and LDH begin to rise after six to 12 hours. The SGOT peaks in one to two days and returns to normal in three to five days. The LDH elevation usually persists for five to seven days. The serum CPK rises earlier and returns to normal in two to three days. However, none of these enzymes are specific for heart muscle necrosis. SGOT is present in skeletal muscle and liver. Therefore, a patient with traumatized skeletal muscle, either due to intramuscular injections, accidental injury, or surgery, will have an elevated SGOT. A patient with abnormal liver function, as commonly occurs with congestive heart failure, will have elevated values. LDH is also present in skeletal muscle, liver, lung, and red blood cells, and hence abnormal function in these organs will elevate the LDH. CPK is present in the nervous system and skeletal muscle and questionably in lung. It is not present in the liver, and therefore, when elevated, aids in exclusion of liver abnormality as a cause of an elevated SGOT or LDH. The best available enzyme test is the isoenzyme analysis of LDH, which more specifically determines the cardiac, skeletal muscle, and liver components.

As a result of the necrosis of heart muscle, fever, leukocytosis, and an elevation of the sedimentation rate are commonly evident 24 to 48 hours after the onset.

COMPLICATIONS OF MYOCARDIAL INFARCTION

Arrhythmias

Ventricular arrhythmias occur in over 80 per cent of patients with acute myocardial infarction. These range from occasional unifocal ventricular ectopic beats to frequent and multifocal beats, to ventricular tachycardia, and to fibrillation. Atrial arrhythmias (atrial ectopic beats) and atrial tachycardia (flutter — fibrillation) are less common. Sinus bradycardia and varying degrees of heart block (first, second, and third degree) occur especially in patients with inferior-posterior infarctions, which are due to right coronary artery disease, the right coronary artery being the major blood supply to the AV nodal region.

Congestive Heart Failure

Signs and symptoms of left heart and then right heart failure may appear. Left heart failure (pulmonary edema) may appear acutely, but more commonly there are premonitory signs which herald its onset. It is, therefore, important for the nurse, as well as the physician, to frequently examine the patient. These signs include sinus tachycardia (in addition to the previously mentioned arrhythmias), gallop rhythm, rales at the lung bases, and elevation of central venous pressure as determined by actual measurement or by observation of the neck veins. However, elevation of CVP is a late finding and a severe degree of left heart failure can occur before it is elevated. Prompt treatment of failure in the earlier stages may prevent further deterioration of heart function.

Shock

This is the most serious complication of infarction and is still poorly understood and treated. It is clinically manifested by a fall in blood pressure, associated with cold, clammy skin due to compensatory vasoconstriction. The basic cause is deficient cardiac output with secondary changes in the peripheral arterial and venous systems. Poor perfusion to other vital organs is clinically evidenced by cerebral manifestations of mental changes progressing to coma, and renal impairment manifested by reduction in urine output. Tissue hypoxia results in metabolic acidosis which, in turn, further compromises all body functions, including the heart.

Pericarditis

The visceral pericardium is commonly involved in transmural infarction. A pericardial friction rub is heard in 20 per cent of patients. It is often transitory and therefore requires frequent examination for detection. It is a sign which a nurse should be able to recognize. In itself, this finding does not have an unfavorable prognosis. In 1 to 2 per cent of cases, sufficient pericardial bleeding (especially if the patient is receiving anticoagulants) will occur to lead to cardiac tamponade, which may require decompression.

Emboli

Systemic emboli may occur secondary to mural thrombus in the left ventricle which develops on the endocardial surface of the infarcted portion of the left ventricle several days after the onset of the disease. Pulmonary emboli are not uncommon and usually are secondary to thrombosis in leg or pelvic veins in a bedridden patient. Mural thrombi on the right side of the septum, secondary to extensive septal infarction, can also result in pulmonary embolization.

Mitral Insufficiency

The sudden appearance of a loud mitral systolic murmur with associated onset or aggravation of heart failure can result from infarction of the papillary muscle, with resulting interference of mitral valve function or actual rupture of the papillary muscle or chordae tendineae. Depending on the effect on cardiac function, immediate or late surgical intervention may be indicated.

Myocardial Rupture

Rupture of the heart has usually been considered to be invariably fatal. However, a small leak can occur which is sealed over by the overlying pericardium and escapes clinical detection. Major perforation, if such can be diagnosed immediately (by pericardial tap), could be amenable to surgical treatment. Perforation of the interventricular septum is an uncommon occurrence. It is manifested by the sudden appearance of a loud systolic murmur along the left sternal border and by signs of increasing right heart pressure and failure (distended and pulsating neck veins, hepatomegaly, and edema). It can be confirmed quickly by right heart catheterization.

Depending on the severity of the resulting heart failure, emergency or late surgical intervention may be indicated.

Ventricular Aneurysm

Although aneurysms may be evident within the first week of myocardial infarction, it usually is considered a late complication, at least as it relates to surgical treatment. However, with increasing definitive studies of patients with acute infarction, this concept is changing and surgical resection is now being considered in patients with evidence of ventricular aneurysm (including patients with a large area of infarcted and noncontractile heart muscle) associated with uncontrolled failure or shock in the acute phase of myocardial infarction.

Preinfarction Syndrome

This is a poorly defined syndrome characterized by prolonged or frequently recurring episodes of anginal-type pain, not promptly relieved by rest or nitroglycerine, but without diagnostic electrocardiographic or enzyme changes to indicate infarction. Such a diagnosis can only be made in retrospect, i.e., if infarction develops within days of the onset of symptoms. Since the symptoms indicate a worsening of the coronary circulation with the possibility of infarction in the near future, such patients should be treated exactly as one would for actual infarction, until a sufficient period of observation either excludes or establishes the diagnosis of infarction.

TREATMENT

Angina

General measures. The following are indicated: weight reduction if patient is overweight; adjustment of living habits to allow sufficient periods of sleep and avoidance of known physical and emotional stresses; continuation of sufficient physical activity, short of that which produces symptoms, to maintain a good general physical status; avoidance of smoking and excessive use of caffeine-containing beverages; treatment of associated diseases, especially hypertension and diabetes.

Specific drugs. Nitroglycerine remains the best drug for the symptomatic relief of the anginal pain. Although it is commonly thought of as a coronary vasodilator, its effect is mainly by lowering peripheral vascular resistance and thereby reducing the workload of the myocardium. The drug should be taken immediately after the onset of pain. In those situations in which a certain stimulus is known to precipitate pain and cannot be avoided, nitroglycerine can be taken prophylactically. The drug may cause a disturbing headache and hypotension. If these occur, the drug should be tried in smaller doses. So-called long-acting vasodilators (Peritrate, Cardilate and Isordil) are advocated to prevent episodes of angina. There is no convincing proof of their efficacy. Propranolol is currently being investigated for the chronic treatment of angina, and, although preliminary reports are favorable, such therapy is still investigational.

Hyperlipidemia and hypercholesterolemia. These factors are determined by analysis of the blood cholesterol, total lipids, and triglycerides and by lipoprotein electrophoresis. The most essential treatment is weight reduction in the overweight patient. Dietary adjustments to reduce the total fat content of the diet and substitution of unsaturated for saturated fats and use of lipid-lowering agents, such as clofibrate (Atromid-S), may be of value in lowering the serum level of cholesterol or lipoproteins; however, their overall value in improving the status of the coronary circulation remains to be proven. Use of thyroid analogues and estrogens in the male are entirely investigational.

Surgery. This is to be seriously considered in the patients whose symptoms are due to coronary artery disease and which cannot be controlled by the previously mentioned measures to permit the patient to live a reasonably normal and productive life. In evaluation for surgery, selective coronary cinearteriography is essential to establish the location and severity of the disease. The most popular current operation is the aortocoronary by-pass graft, in which a segment of reversed saphenous vein is interposed between the aorta and the coronary artery, downstream from its obstruction. The Vineberg procedure, which implants internal mammary arteries into myocardial tunnels, is much less effective in increasing myocardial blood flow. Other investigational surgical procedures include coronary endarterectomy and direct internal mammary-coronary artery anastomosis.

Myocardial Infarction

General measures. Hospitalization in a coronary care unit is indicated whenever possible. Sufficient meperidine or morphine should be given to relieve pain and apprehension. It must be remembered that these drugs may produce nausea and vomiting, and therefore the smallest doses to obtain relief should be used. The physician and the nurse must spend considerable time and effort to explain what is being done to alleviate the tremendous fear and apprehension which most patients experience. Sedatives and tranquilizers must be used cautiously, since they depress the myocardium and may induce hypotension.

Oxygen. Dyspnea, cyanosis, restlessness, and apprehension are all indicative of hypoxia. The best measurement to determine the degree of hypoxia is an arterial P_{O_2}. If the value is below 70 mm Hg, the patient should receive oxygen therapy, most comfortably by face mask or nasal oxygen catheter.

Bed rest versus chair rest. Once the patient is asymptomatic and all vital signs are stable, the patient may be assisted from bed into a comfortable chair with legs elevated. All clinical and electronic monitoring continues. When in bed, the patient is encouraged to perform leg movements several times a day to try and reduce venous thromboses. It is important for the nurse to enforce and supervise this activity. Leg wrapping is of no proven value, unless obvious superficial varicosities exist. When it is used, the nurse must constantly be certain that the wrappings do not act as tourniquets and constrict venous return. Attention must be paid to bowel movements, since this event requires considerable expenditure of work by the patient. Stool softeners, such as Colace or Trocinate, should be used. Whenever possible (i.e., when patient's vital signs are stable), it is preferable to assist patient onto a bedside commode rather than to use a bedpan. The latter often requires more expenditure of energy than the former.

Anticoagulation therapy. This is indicated, initially with heparin and subsequently with Coumadin, unless there is a specific contraindication to its use. This is advised to reduce the incidence of thromboembolism and not to treat the coronary artery disease per se. Unless bleeding complications occur, it should be continued till the patient is fully ambulatory.

Observation and treatment of arrhythmias, heart failure, shock, and other complications have been discussed in other sections.

After the patient's status has been stable for approximately five days, he may be transferred from the coronary care unit to the open ward. However, all the complications which are looked for in the coronary care unit may initially develop or recur after this time and hence close observation of the patient is essential. Ideally, it would be advisable to have such patients continually monitored by ECG for the next two weeks. Since it takes approximately three weeks for sufficient fibroblastic ingrowth into the area of myocardial necrosis to produce a firm scar, all patients should be kept at very restricted activity for this period of time. Absolute bed rest is not essential. Periods of rest in a comfortable chair are indicated and a few steps about the room are permissible, provided such activity does not precipitate symptoms, tachycardia, or arrhythmias. After a period of three weeks of such restricted activity, progressive ambulation is permitted again provided there is an absence of adverse signs or symptoms. Slowly increasing activity is continued for the next four to six weeks, by which time most patients will be fully ambulant and able to return to part-time or full time employment short of strenuous physical labor.

PROGNOSIS OF CORONARY ARTERY DISEASE

The prognosis is guarded and unpredictable in any patient. Patients with angina have an average survival of eight to 10 years with a yearly mortality rate of 5 to 8 per cent above those without clinical manifestations of the disease. Approximately one half of the patients die suddenly, one third die during a period of myocardial infarction, and the remainder die of congestive heart failure or other complications.

The mortality rate of patients with acute myocardial infarction is between 20 to 35 per cent of those who reach a hospital. Many die within the first few minutes, before medical assistance is available. Treatment in coronary care units has reduced this mortality by about one half, largely by early recognition and treatment of potentially life-threatening arrhythmias. The average long-term survival is 60 per cent for five years and 40 to 50 per cent for 10 years. Whether surgical revascularization procedures will substantially improve these statistics remains to be determined.

Hypertensive Vascular and Cardiovascular Disease

The basis for the diagnosis of hypertension is the determination of the blood pressure, most commonly by the indirect cuff method on the arm. Improper technique or equipment can result in false readings. Patients with very large and obese upper extremities require large (leg-type) cuffs. Conventional size cuffs in such persons can yield falsely elevated blood pressures. The proper determination of the diastolic blood pressure is debated, most physicians advising the disappearance of sounds rather than an abrupt change in intensity of the sound. In patients with a wide separation between diminution and disappearance of the sounds, both should be recorded. The exact separation between normal and high blood pressure is not clear. In general, persisting diastolic pressures over 90 mm Hg under age 50 and over 100 mm Hg after age 60 are considered abnormal. Systolic blood pressure increases with age owing to an increase in resistance from arteriosclerosis of the large arteries. A value of 100 mm Hg plus the age is a reasonable approximation of normal values. In many patients the blood pressure fluctuates markedly, related to physician observation and emotional stresses. Therefore, repeated measurements at rest and during activity are necessary to properly evaluate the range and average pressures. Blood pressures recorded by the nurse are commonly lower than those obtained by the physician, because the nurse produces less anxiety on the part of the patient. The best method of obtaining a true indication of the blood pressure is the use of a portable apparatus which can be worn by the patient day and night, by which frequent recordings are made without the values known to the patient.

The term *hypertensive vascular disease* is used to define the individual with elevated blood pressure without any evidence of cardiac involvement. Once left ventricular hypertrophy is evidenced (clinically, by an x-ray film or ECG), with or without heart failure, the proper term is *hypertensive cardiovascular disease*.

ETIOLOGY

Essential is the most common type of hypertension. The term *essential* implies that the cause is not known. It most commonly begins between the ages of 25 to 50 and is more common in females. Initially, the blood pressure is quite labile, being normal during periods of rest and raised during physical or emotional stress. Over the course of years, the tendency is toward a fixed hypertension.

In *secondary* situations a known cause is present

Renal

Parenchymal renal disease: glomerulonephritis, pyelonephritis, collagen diseases, and polycystic disease

Renovascular disease: occlusive narrowing of one or both renal arteries due to atherosclerosis, embolism, or fibromuscular hyperplasia (renin-angiotensin mechanism)

Endocrine

Primary aldosteronism

Pheochromocytoma

Cushing's syndrome

Coarctation of the aorta

Miscellaneous

Toxemia of pregnancy, increased intracranial pressure, and distention of the urinary bladder in patients with spinal cord lesions.

CLASSIFICATION

Malignant.   Malignant hypertensive patients are those in whom papilledema is present.

Benign.   This term is misleading, since it includes all patients who do not have papilledema. The severity of the disease can range from entirely asymptomatic cases to those with life-threatening complications.

EVALUATION OF THE PATIENT

The following parameters are to be investigated:

1. Determination of the range and average levels of blood pressure.

2. Diagnostic evaluation for the cause of the hypertension. It is beyond the scope of this text to discuss the investigative procedures indicated in searching for the secondary and curable types.

3. Evaluation of the effects of hypertension on target organs. This is obviously important, since they are what produces the morbidity and mortality from the disease. The major organs to be studied are the eyes, brain, cardiovascular system, and the kidneys.

SYMPTOMS AND SIGNS

Early in the course of the disease, the patient is asymptomatic. Headaches and dizziness are common early symptoms. Other symptoms and signs will result from specific target organ involvement, i.e., eyes (vascular disease of the eyes producing visible changes in funduscopic examination and varying degrees of visual impairment), brain (mental and neurologic abnormalities), cardiovascular (left ventricular hypertrophy, heart failure, and aggravation of coronary and peripheral atherosclerosis), and kidneys (progressive deterioration of renal function).

Hypertensive Cardiovascular Disease

The patient with resulting left ventricular hypertrophy, as evidenced by an x-ray film or ECG, is commonly asymptomatic for months to years. The symptoms and signs are initially those of left heart failure, which may occur abruptly with paroxysmal nocturnal dyspnea or acute pulmonary edema. In time, right heart failure ensues.

COMPLICATIONS

These are accelerated atherosclerosis, both of coronary and peripheral vascular beds and the combined effects of atherosclerosis and hypertension in the target organs mentioned before.

PROGNOSIS

Although many patients with *benign* hypertension may live 20 or more years, life expectancy is reduced and death results from heart failure, coronary heart disease, cerebral thrombosis, cerebral hemorrhage, or uremia.

Malignant hypertension, untreated, carries a mortality of over 90 per cent in one to two years.

TREATMENT

Potentially curable secondary types. Surgical repair of coarctation of the aorta or renal artery stenosis or removal of hormonally active adrenal tumors or hyperplastic adrenal glands can eliminate the inciting cause in these particular types of hypertension.

Essential type. General therapy should include overall measures to relieve those factors in the patient's environment which produce stress and anxiety. This is easier said than done, since commonly these factors relate to the patient's immediate family, his social and economic environment, and occupation. Obesity should be corrected by weight reduction. Dietary sodium restriction is indicated, the degree of restriction dependent upon the severity of the hypertension, the presence of heart failure, and the associated drugs used. The drugs include reserpine, thiazides, hydralazine, methyldopa, guanethidine, and autonomic blocking drugs. Often, combinations of these drugs are superior to single drugs. These will be discussed in detail in Chapter 7.

Malignant hypertension, because of its high mortality when not treated, requires immediate and active therapy with the previously named agents. The results are very gratifying, with most patients now living five to 10 or more years.

Hypertensive crises. These are usually manifested by cerebral symptoms, i.e., convulsions, coma, and papilledema. These symptoms constitute an acute medical emergency and require immediate measures in order to reduce the blood pressure (see Chapter 7).

Primary and Secondary Myocardial Diseases

The category of primary and secondary myocardial diseases (myocardiopathies) includes those diseases manifested by abnormality of myocardial function not owing to coronary artery disease, hypertension, acquired valvular heart disease, or congenital valvular or shunt lesions. Such diseases which have a known etiology, or at least a known associated disease entity, are classified as secondary. Those of unknown etiology are primary or idiopathic.

CLASSIFICATION

Primary

At times familial.

Secondary

Myocarditis: viral, bacterial, rickettsial, parasitic, toxic
Hypersensitivity: rheumatic fever and other collagen-type diseases
Neuromuscular: muscular dystrophy, Friedreich's ataxia and so forth
Metabolic: hyperthyroidism, myxedema, hemochromatosis, glycogen storage disease, alcoholic, thiamine deficiency
Tumor: usually metastatic
Sarcoidosis
Amyloidosis
Peripartum heart disease

CLINICAL FEATURES

Primary myocardial disease occurs most commonly in males between 20 and 50 years of age. In this country, the disease is more common in the Negro race. Alcoholism is a common factor in this group of patients, but the mechanism by which alcohol may produce myocardial disease is not known. The disease is characterized by progressive symptoms and signs of heart failure and cardiomegaly, arrhythmias, and a high incidence of pulmonary and systemic embolization. The embolization results from intracardiac thrombi in the ventricles, atria, or both. The electrocardiogram is abnormal but not diagnostic, commonly indicating left ventricular hypertrophy or intraventricular conduction defects. The arrhythmias most commonly seen are atrial fibrillation and ventricular ectopic beats. The chest x-ray film reveals generalized cardiomegaly.

The secondary myocardial diseases have a similar clinical picture. In addition, the etiology or associated basic disease will be evident.

PROGNOSIS

In the primary form, once cardiomegaly and heart failure have developed, the prognosis is exceedingly poor. The average life expectancy is three years, with death resulting from intractable heart failure, embolization, or both. The prognosis in the secondary forms will depend on the etiology and the ability to treat the underlying cause.

TREATMENT

Since the prognosis is so poor, prolonged bed rest (up to one year) has been advised, but the value of such treatment is not proven. Basic treatment should be for heart failure, control of arrhythmias, and chronic anticoagulation therapy in order to attempt to reduce the incidence of embolization. In the secondary types, additional therapy is directed at the underlying cause, if possible.

Pericarditis

The term *pericarditis* defines the disease state associated with involvement of the visceral pericardium (and usually the underlying epicardium). Thus, the term pericarditis is not an accurate description, since epicarditis and sometimes myocarditis are commonly present. Varying amounts of pericardial effusion occur.

CLASSIFICATION

1. Idiopathic: Etiology unknown; is thought to be of viral origin in most cases.

2. Infectious: Viral, tuberculous, bacterial, parasitic.

3. Hypersensitivity: Rheumatic fever, rheumatoid arthritis, systemic lupus.

4. Autoimmune: Relapsing (idiopathic), postpericardiotomy, postmyocardial infarction (Dressler's Syndrome).

5. Metabolic: Uremia, myxedema.
6. Trauma: Penetrating or blunt.
7. Malignancy.
8. Miscellaneous: In association with acute myocardial infarction, anticoagulation therapy, dissecting aneurysm of aorta, and contiguous pulmonary or mediastinal disease.

CLINICAL FEATURES

In the idiopathic or infectious groups, the common symptoms are fever and chest pain. The pain is commonly stabbing and knifelike, aggravated by deep inspiration, swallowing, or hiccoughs, and worse in the supine than in the sitting position. The pain is usually substernal but may extend laterally, especially if there is associated pleural involvement. The diagnostic physical sign is the presence of a pericardial friction rub. Additional physical signs will depend on the degree of pericardial effusion, which prevents adequate diastolic filling of the ventricles and thereby reduces cardiac output. As little as 300 ml of fluid occurring acutely within minutes to hours (as in hemorrhage) can be fatal, whereas the gradual accumulation of fluid over the course of days to weeks can distend the pericardial sac to a volume of 2000 ml or more. The syndrome resulting from restriction of adequate cardiac output is known as *cardiac tamponade.* It is clinically manifested by pulmonary rales, distended neck veins (which are further distended during inspiration [Kussmaul sign], resulting from the inability of the right heart to accommodate the increased venous return), hepatomegaly, peripheral edema, ascites, cardiomegaly, and distant heart sounds. A paradoxical arterial pulse (a fall in blood pressure with inspiration) may be present. The arterial pulse is not truly paradoxical, but an exaggeration of the normal phenomenon with a fall in blood pressure of over 10 mm Hg during inspiration.

The chest x-ray film will show enlargement of the cardiac silhouette, typically in a "water bag" configuration, but it may be impossible to differentiate between pericardial effusion and myocardial dilatation. The electrocardiogram in the early stages will usually show concave ST segment elevation, followed by T wave inversion. Atrial arrhythmias (ectopic beats, tachycardia, and fibrillation) occur in over 25 per cent of cases. As pericardial fluid increases, the voltage of the QRS and T will decrease.

DIAGNOSTIC TESTS

As stated before, the only diagnostic physical finding of pericarditis is the pericardial friction rub. If this is absent (or not detected, since it may be transitory and disappear with accumulation of pericardial fluid), a major differential can exist between pericardial effusion and myocardial dilatation. Since proper diagnosis is essential for therapy, additional studies are necessary. The simplest is a chest x-ray film taken after the intravenous injection of carbon dioxide gas with the patient lying on his left side. The gas will outline the upper border of the right atrium. If there is 1 cm or more of density between the gas shadow and the outer border of the cardiac silhouette, the test is positive. Other techniques to demonstrate pericardial effusion include radioisotope scans and echocardiography. Pericardiocentesis, when clinically indicated, will obviously prove the presence or absence of significant effusion. Cardiac catheterization will define the degree of hemodynamic impairment and is best performed in conjunction with pericardial tapping. If the right atrial pressure falls to normal with removal of the pericardial fluid, it will indicate that the effusion is the major hemodynamic abnormality. However, if the right atrial pressure remains elevated after pericardial decompression, this finding will indicate additional myocardial disease or pericardial constriction (see later).

DIFFERENTIAL DIAGNOSIS

The most common differential is between idiopathic (or viral) and tuberculous pericarditis. Since the initial clinical course (including an examination of the pericardial fluid) can be identical, tuberculosis must be considered in every case. A positive tuberculin skin test is practically always present in the latter disease, but a positive test does not prove that the pericardial disease is of tuberculous origin. Therefore, in the patient who persists with fever and other signs of pericardial disease and in whom tuberculosis cannot be excluded, an open pericardial biopsy is indicated. Prompt diagnosis and treatment of tuberculosis is essential not only to save life but to prevent the major complication, namely, constriction.

TREATMENT

Every effort must be made to establish an etiologic diagnosis with resulting specific therapy, if such is possible. In the idiopathic (or viral) group, the treatment is largely symptomatic—bed rest and salicylates. Corticoids have been advised, but are best avoided except in severely ill patients. Although corticoid therapy will often abolish the fever and the pain and render the patient asymptomatic, the symptoms and signs commonly recur with reduction or discontinuation of such therapy. Immediate closed pericardial aspiration is indicated whenever signs of cardiac tamponade are evident. If fluid continues to recur after repeated taps or if tapping does not relieve the tamponade because of loculation of the fluid or beginning constriction, open pericardial drainage or pericardiectomy is indicated.

PROGNOSIS AND COMPLICATIONS

In the idiopathic (or viral) group, death should never result from the pericardial disease per se. Death can result from cardiac tamponade, but with recognition and proper treatment, this should not occur. However, fatality may result from associated diffuse myocarditis.

The initial episode may last from days to weeks and proceed to clinical recovery. However, the disease notoriously relapses, and recurrences from every few weeks to months for one to three years are not uncommon. An autoimmune reaction is thought to be the mechanism for such relapses. Although corticoid therapy will minimize or eliminate such relapses, one will be committed to such therapy for years with all the serious complications of the corticoids. There is some evidence to suggest that pericardiectomy will eliminate the relapsing cycle.

The major complication of idiopathic (or viral and tuberculous) pericarditis is constriction. This will be discussed later.

Constrictive Pericardial Disease

Constrictive pericarditis is the sequel of one or more episodes of acute pericarditis; however, these episodes may have escaped clinical recognition, and the patient presents with constriction and without a history of prior acute attacks of pericarditis. Most commonly, constriction follows idiopathic (or viral), tuberculous, or pyogenic pericarditis. Less commonly, it is a sequel of traumatic hemopericardium, tumor, or rheumatoid disease. The thickened, fibrotic, and, at times, calcified pericardium encases the heart and prevents adequate diastolic filling of the ventricles with a resultant decrease in cardiac output. The symptoms and signs of this disease are similar to that of pericardial effusion with tamponade. Significant ascites, which precedes the appearance of leg edema, is a common finding. An early diastolic lift along the left sternal border, associated with an early sound in diastole (pericardial knock), are important findings and are due to the thrust of the heart against the chest wall during early diastolic filling of the noncompliant ventricles. The chest x-ray film is often not diagnostic unless pericardial calcification is evident. The cardiac silhouette may be small, normal, or enlarged. The electrocardiogram is also not diagnostic, usually revealing low voltages and nonspecific ST and T wave changes. Cardiac catheterization is of value, but will not be completely diagnostic since similar hemodynamic data will be obtained in some patients with primary or secondary myocardial disease.

Medical therapy includes the use of diuretic agents to reduce the edema and ascites. Digitalis is of value in control of associated atrial arrhythmias, but is probably of little value in improving cardiac output since the major abnormality is mechanical constriction of the myocardium rather than diffusely diseased myocardium.

The only definitive treatment is surgical decortication of the pericardium in order to permit adequate ventricular filling. The surgical mortality is around 10 per cent. Approximately 85 per cent of patients will be cured or greatly improved. Failures result from associated myocardial disease or inadequate pericardial resection.

Bibliography

CONGESTIVE HEART FAILURE

Gorlin, R.: Recent conceptual advances in congestive heart failure. J.A.M.A. *179*:441, 1962.
Sellor, R. H.: Refractory versus intractable congestive heart failure. Amer. J. Cardiol. *17*:631, 1966.
Seminar on congestive heart failure. Circulation *21*:95–128, 218–255, and 424–447, 1960.

CARDIOGENIC SHOCK

Agress, C. M.: Pathogeneses and management of coronary shock. Geriatrics *21*:194, 1966.
Gunnar, R. M.: Myocardial infarction with shock. Hemodynamic studies and therapy. Circulation *33*:753, 1966.
Gunnar, R. M.: Myocardial infarction with shock. Physiologic basis for treatment. Med. Clin. N. Amer. *51*:69, 1967.
Weil, M. H., and Shubin, H.: Shock following acute myocardial infarction. Progr. Cardiovasc. Dis. *11*:1, 1968.

RHEUMATIC FEVER AND RHEUMATIC HEART DISEASE

Arnoh, W. M.: The lungs in mitral stenosis. Brit. Med. J. *2*:765–770, and 823–830, 1963.
Feinstein, A. R.: The prognosis of acute rheumatic fever. Amer. Heart J. *68*:817, 1964.
Ferlic, R. M.: Aortic valvular insufficiency associated with cystic medical necrosis. Ann. Surg. *165*:1, 1967.
Gerbode, F., Keith, W. V., and Puryear, H.: Non-rheumatic acquired insufficiency of the mitral valve. Progr. Cardiovasc. Dis. *11*:173, 1968.
Hohn, A. R.: Aortic stenosis. Circulation *32*:4–12(Suppl. 3), 1965.

Jones criteria (revised) for guidance in diagnosis of rheumatic fever. Circulation *32*:664, 1965.

Kitchen, A., and Turner, R.: Diagnosis and treatment of tricuspid stenosis. Brit. Heart J. *26*:354, 1964.

Quinn, R. W., and Federspiel, C. F.: Rheumatic fever and rheumatic heart disease. A five-year study of rheumatic and non-rheumatic families. Amer. J. Epidem. *85*: 120–136, 1967.

Rees, J. R.: Hemodynamic effects of severe aortic regurgitation. Brit. Heart J. *26*:412, 1964.

Rheumatic fever in children and adolescents: A symposium. Ann. Intern. Med. *60*:1–129(Suppl. 5), 1964.

Roseman, D. M.: National history of asymptomatic and symptomatic mitral stenosis. J. Chronic Dis. *18*:379, 1965.

Shillingford, J. P.: The estimation of severity of mitral incompetence. Progr. Cardiovasc. Dis. *5*:248, 1962.

Wood, P.: An appreciation of mitral stenosis. Brit. Med. J. *1*:1051–1063 and 1113–1124, 1954.

Wood, P.: Aortic stenosis. Amer. J. Cardiol. *1*:553, 1958.

BACTERIAL ENDOCARDITIS

Lerner, P. I., and Weinstein, L.: Infective endocarditis in the antibiotic era. New Eng. J. Med. *274*:199–206, 259–266, 323–331, and 388–393, 1966.

Vogler, W. R., and Dorney, E. R.: Bacterial endocarditis in congenital heart disease. Amer. Heart J. *64*:198, 1962.

CORONARY ARTERY DISEASE

Burch, G. E., DePasquale, N. P., and Phillips, J. H.: The syndrome of papillary muscle dysfunction. Amer. Heart J. *75*:399, 1968.

Dubnow, M. H., Burchell, H. B., and Titus, J. L.: Postinfarction ventricular aneurysm. Amer. Heart J. *70*:753, 1965.

Friedberg, C. K., Cohen, H., and Donoso, E.: Advanced heart block as a complication of acute myocardial infarction. Progr. Cardiovasc. Dis. *10*:466, 1968.

Gazes, P. C.: The diagnosis of angina pectoris. Amer. Heart J. *67*:830, 1964.

James, T. N.: Anatomy of the coronary arteries in health and disease. Circulation *32*: 1020, 1965.

Katz, L. N.: Pitfalls in diagnosing coronary artery disease. Circulation *28*:274, 1963.

Killip, T., and Kimball, J. T.: Treatment of myocardial infarction in a coronary care unit. Amer. J. Cardiol. *20*:457, 1967; Progr. Cardiovascular Dis. *10*:483, 1968; and Progr. Cardiovascular Dis. *11*:45, 1968.

Levine, S. A.: Carotid sinus massage. J.A.M.A. *182*:1332, 1962.

Lown, B.: The coronary care unit. J.A.M.A. *199*:188, 1967.

Lown, B.: Unresolved problems in coronary care. Amer. J. Cardiol. *20*:494, 1967.

Mason, J. K.: Asymptomatic disease of coronary arteries in young men. Brit. Med. J. *2*:1234, 1964.

Neaverson, M. A.: Metabolic acidosis in acute myocardial infarction. Brit. Med. J.: *2*:283, 1966.

Nissen, N. J.: Evaluation of serum enzymes in the diagnosis of acute myocardial infarction. Brit. Heart J. *27*:520, 1965.

Riseman, J. E. F.: The clinical course of angina pectoris. Amer. J. Med. Sci. *252*:146, 1966.

Sampson, J. J., and Hutchinson, J. C.: Heart failure in myocardial infarction. Progr. Cardiovasc. Dis. *10*:1, 1967.

Stamlen, J.: Coronary risk factors. Med. Clin. N. Amer. *50*:229, 1966.

Walker, W. J., and Gregoratus, G.: Myocardial infarction in young men. Amer. J. Cardiol. *19*:339, 1967.

Weisse, A. B., and Regan, T. J.: The current status of nitrites in the treatment of coronary artery disease. Progr. Cardiovasc. Dis. *12*:72, 1969.

Zukel, W. J.: Survival following first diagnosis of coronary heart disease. Amer. Heart J. *78*:159, 1969.

HYPERTENSIVE CARDIOVASCULAR DISEASE (See also Chapter 7)

Breslin, D. J.: Essential hypertension: A 20 year follow-up study. Circulation *33*:87, 1966.
Finnerty, F. A., Jr.: Hypertensive emergencies. Amer. J. Cardiol. *17*:652, 1966.
Hockin, A. G.: Renovascular hypertension: Diagnosis and treatment. Arch. Intern. Med. *117*:364, 1966.
Page, I. H. (ed.): Symposium on hypertension and its treatment. Med. Clin. N. Amer. *45*:233, 1961.
Smirk, H., and Hodge, J. V.: Causes of death in treated hypertensive patients. Brit. Med. J. *2*:1221, 1963.
Symposium on cardiorenal consequences of hypertension. Amer. J. Cardiol. *17*:603, 1966.

PRIMARY MYOCARDIAL DISEASE

Burch, G. E., and DePasquale, N. P.: Alcoholic cardiomyopathy. Amer. J. Cardiol. *23*:723, 1969.
Criley, J. M.: Pressure gradients without obstruction. A new concept of hypertrophic subaortic stenosis. Circulation *32*:881, 1965.
Frank, S., and Brounwald, E.: Idiopathic hypertrophic subaortic stenoses. Circulation *37*:759, 1968.
Storstein, O.: Primary myocardial disease. Acta Med. Scand. *176*:731, 1965.

PERICARDITIS

Kesteloot, K.: Heart disease of chronic beer drinkers. Circulation *37*:854, 1968.
Schnabel, T. G.: Constrictive pericarditis. Med. Clin. N. Amer. *50*:1231, 1966.
Symposium on pericarditis. Amer. J. Cardiol. *7*:1–129, 1961.
Wolff, L., and Wolff, R.: Diseases of the pericardium. Ann. Rev. Med. *16*:21, 1965.

CHAPTER 3

Surgical Aspects

By RICHARD G. SANDERSON, M.D.

Although elective cardiac operations have been performed since the 1920s and open heart techniques have been used since 1954, the most rapid advances in cardiac surgery have been made in the past decade. Cardiac surgery is now well established as a distinct specialty, and specialized techniques, training, and equipment are necessary for its conduct.

More than any other specialty, the *team approach* in the care of the cardiac patient is tremendously important. Each member of the team is expert in his own field of endeavor and does his part toward the common goal, the successful rehabilitation of a disabled patient. Preoperative preparation, the complex operative procedure, and demanding postoperative care all require a meticulous attention to detail for a successful outcome. The cardiac nurse plays an important role in the first and third phases.

Preoperative Preparation

The goal of the preoperative preparation is to bring the patient to the operating room in the best possible condition for operation.

Many cardiac surgical patients are living on very "narrow margins" and have little reserve. When cardiac disability reduces the output of blood from the heart, other organ systems (e.g., liver, kidney, lungs, and so forth) may be affected adversely. Therefore, every effort must be made to improve the function of each of these organ systems before the operation, since this can spell the difference between success and failure in the postoperative period.

MEDICAL MANAGEMENT

Continuation and often intensification of medical management are important in achieving the optimal preoperative condition. Since control of physical activity may be decisive in attaining this goal, restricted ward activity is important in preoperative preparation. For the patients who are most seriously disabled, complete bed rest is often necessary. Because of the tendency of patients in chronic congestive heart failure to retain salt and fluids, a program of sodium and fluid restriction is usually rigorously enforced until the operative day.

There are a number of important aspects of drug therapy in the preoperative preparation of the cardiac surgical patient. Postoperative cardiac arrhythmias are commonplace, and many cardiac surgery centers have adopted the practice of discontinuing digitalis derivatives one to two days before the operation, since digitalis may cause arrhythmias at any time as a toxic side effect. The practice is not as rigidly adhered to for children with congenital heart disease, but even in these patients digitalis is often withheld the morning of operation. It is a simple matter to give additional digitalis as indications develop in the postoperative period, whereas inadvertent digitalis overdosage complicates management considerably.

Intimately related to the problem of digitalis toxicity is the patient's body stores and serum levels of potassium, since low levels facilitate and reinforce toxicity. Patients on long-term diuretic therapy (particularly mercurial compounds, thiazides, ethacrynic acid, furosemide and so on) may be potassium-depleted if adequate replacement of this ion is not maintained. Moreover, hypokalemia of itself may cause ventricular arrhythmias in the postoperative period, particularly when respiratory assist devices produce a mild respiratory alkalosis. To counteract these tendencies toward hypokalemia and ventricular arrhythmias, the administration of potassium-losing diuretics is usually discontinued many days before operation; however, potassium supplementation is continued. If renal function is adequate, superfluous and unneeded potassium will be excreted in the urine and there is little danger of potassium overload.

Careful assessment of the patient's preoperative pulmonary function may be useful in anticipating the need for prolonged respiratory support in the postoperative period. A timed vital capacity, expiratory flow rates, residual volumes, and a wasted ventilation determination will usually be adequate to predict these needs. Arterial blood should be drawn for pH, P_{CO_2}, and P_{O_2}, with the patient breathing room air and after breathing 100 per cent O_2 for five to 10 minutes. These baseline preoperative values concerning oxygen and carbon dioxide diffusion can be compared with the values obtained in the postoperative period and will help serve as a guide to the effectiveness of respiratory support.

Serum electrolyte determinations will dictate needs for fluid restriction and potassium administration. Renal and hepatic function studies may determine marginal function in these organs and warn of possible postoperative complications. The measurement of coagulation parameters can delineate clotting abnormalities so that appropriate steps can be taken to avoid postoperative bleeding problems. Some cardiac patients, particularly those who have had systemic emboli (usually from mitral stenosis and atrial fibrillation), are receiving anticoagulants. These medicines are usually stopped soon enough so that clotting mechanisms will be near normal by the time the operation is performed.

PULMONARY PREPARATION

Clinical experience has shown that the irritative effects of smoking upon the tracheobronchial tree, if continued to the day of operation, predispose to postoperative pulmonary complications. Most smokers have a chronic bronchitis of varying degree, which makes them more sensitive to the irritative effects of inhalation anesthetics. They tend to have thick and somewhat tenacious secretions. They are easily stimulated to cough and consequently present an increased hazard at the time of anesthetic intubation. For these reasons, the discontinuance of smoking is a mandatory feature in the patient's preoperative preparation. Ideally, cigarette smoking should be stopped at least three weeks before operation; many cardiac centers require this interval as a prerequisite to operation.

Preoperative pulmonary physiotherapy is a valuable adjunct in the patient's preparation for surgery. The cardiac surgical patient is taught how to deep breathe and how to cough effectively. Postural drainage is employed in those patients whose secretions are thick and difficult to raise. The patient is also taught the use of the intermittent positive pressure breathing (IPPB) apparatus, not only to help clear his lungs of any preoperative atelectasis, but also to allow him to become accustomed to this respiratory assist device. The patient will use the respirator much more effectively (and without fear) in the postoperative period if he already has practiced successfully with the device before his operation. Bronchospasm may be treated by instilling bronchodilators into the nebulizer of the IPPB device. If bronchodilators are needed for extended periods, preparations that cause tachycardia are avoided.

ELIMINATION OF INFECTION

Many cardiac surgical procedures involve the placement of prosthetic devices (e.g., Teflon patches for interventricular septal defects, tubular grafts replacing the aorta, prosthetic heart valves). Any infection involving these prostheses is a tragedy, as mortality rates subsequent to such infections are very high. Therefore, stringent preoperative efforts to help eliminate such infections are vital.

Separate cultures of the nose, throat, sputum (if any), and urine are taken. If any area shows active infection, appropriate antibiotic therapy is instituted, and the infection is cleared prior to operation.

The vestibule of the nose commonly harbors bacterial organisms, particularly in patients who have spent lengthy intervals in the hospital (and, incidentally, in professional and ward personnel). Positive culture for staphylococci are not uncommon among such patients. An antibiotic ointment placed in the nasal vestibules twice daily will usually eliminate this bacterial flora.

Cardiac operations are usually lengthy, often exceeding six hours. The opportunities for minor contaminations of the operative field from the skin incision are ever present, and should be eliminated insofar as possible. In the four or five days before operation, scrubbing of the operative sites — chest, abdomen, and groin — with a hexachlorophene soap or liquid will remove most of the superficial epithelial layers and their contained bacteria. The final skin preparation in the operating room will then be more likely to result in an aseptic field. Scrupulous examination of the skin of the operative site for acne, pimples, or furuncles should be carried out well in advance of the operation, and when present they should be eliminated.

PSYCHOLOGIC PREPARATION

An important feature of preoperative management is the psychologic preparation of the patient for the trying days of the postoperative period. The cooperation gained from the patient in this difficult period is directly related in most cases to his understanding of what will be expected from him and what will be going on around him in his intensive nursing care.

For many small children, the explanation of the details of this paraoperative experience is not easily understood. Time should be more profitably spent in establishing rapport with the child, learning what activities and toys he prefers, and discovering the little idiosyncrasies of his behavior that might make his recovery period easy or difficult. An interview with the parents is often the most direct means of getting this information.

The good judgment of the responsible attending personnel should be used in communicating with older children (six years and above) about their postoperative environment. Pertinent analogies of the anesthetic masks to space helmets, ECG monitors to movie pictures, oxygen tents to space capsules, and so forth are often appropriate.

To the adult cardiac surgical patients (and to the parents of the children), an honest and straightforward appraisal of the benefits and risks of the operation should be made by the cardiac surgeon. The major problems of the early postoperative period—cardiac arrhythmias, bleeding tendencies, the need for respiratory support—are freely discussed with the patient. Since return of the patient to the operating room for control of early postoperative bleeding is sometimes necessary, that eventuality is often discussed and placed in the appropriate perspective. Often an explanatory brochure is given to the patient which outlines these general problems.

The cardiac surgical nurse informs the patient about the ECG and other monitoring devices, the chest drainage tubes, the urinary bladder catheter, and the arterial and venous monitoring cannulae. The need for respiratory support is reviewed, as are the details of endotracheal suctioning and the "sighing" with a ventilator bag or by the respirator itself. The patient should realize that with either the endotracheal tube or a cuffed tracheostomy tube he will be unable to vocalize his needs. The patient is reassured that the nursing staff generally recognizes most of the things a patient is worried about— incisional pain, the pain when the chest tubes are "stripped," the patient's thirst, and so on—and that they will ask him questions that he can answer with a yes or no by nodding his head.

Different members of the team participate in this preoperative psychologic preparation. The surgeon discusses the benefits and risks of the operation, the generalities of the early postoperative period, when the patient can resume diet and physical activity, what additional medical treatment will be necessary, and when he might return to work. The cardiac nurse details her activities of the early postoperative period and explains how the patient will feel and might react to the many new (and sometimes frightening) experiences during his recovery period. The anesthesiologist concludes the preparatory phase by explaining how the premedications will affect the patient, what will happen as he goes to the operating room and is prepared for his procedure, and how he will be put to sleep.

THE NURSE'S ROLE IN PREOPERATIVE PREPARATION

The cardiac nurse functions intimately with other members of the cardiac surgical team in preparing the patient for his operative experience. She must be knowledgeable about the different facets of the preoperative preparation so she can participate more effectively. She must be understanding and supporting to a chronically ill patient who dislikes a diet without salt and with little liquid, who finds preoperative bed rest quite boring and who is understandably frightened by the upcoming operation. She must help the patient adjust to the routine of hospital life, calm his fears about his medical condition and its surgical treatment, ensure that he gets adequate amounts of uninterrupted sleep, and speak with the family who are concerned about the patient's welfare.

She must be on the alert for cardiac arrhythmias developing in the wake of diuretic-induced hypokalemia or when digitalis is withheld preoperatively. She often participates actively in the pulmonary preparation by teaching the patient how to cough and deep breathe, and by instructing him in the use of the IPPB apparatus. The patient who is withdrawing from his habit of heavy cigarette smoking will require considerable tact, understanding, and discipline from the cardiac nurse. Finally, she sets the stage for the postoperative phase by discussing with the patient the details of the care he will receive in the postoperative intensive care unit.

Operative Treatment

INTRODUCTION

Cardiac surgery differs from other surgical specialties in many respects. Cardiac operations require a very large and well coordinated team of highly trained personnel. Usually an open heart procedure employs at least 10 to 12 people: a four man operating team, two scrub nurses, two circulating nurses, an anesthesiologist, and extracorporeal perfusionist, a blood gas technician, and often an electronics technician (Fig. 3–1). The efforts of each person on the team must be

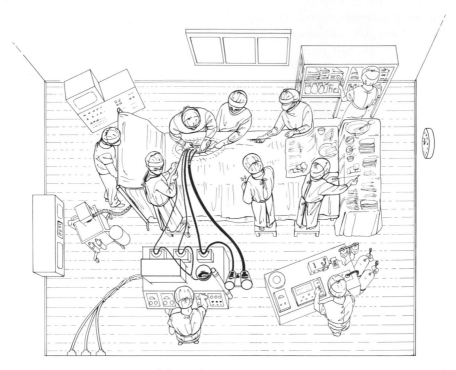

Figure 3–1.   Diagram of the cardiac operating room with the various members of the cardiac surgical team. At the operating table is the cardiac surgeon, his three assistants, and the two scrub nurses. At the patient's head is the anesthesiologist with his equipment. The extracorporeal perfusionist (the heart-lung pump technician) and the blood gas technician are shown at the bottom of the diagram. The circulating nurse is also shown at the supply cabinet. The monitoring devices and the x-ray view box are on the walls of the operating room suite.

timed and coordinated with those of every other team member if a successful result is to be achieved. Attention to myriads of small details is essential if each step in the operative process is to be done safely.

With patients who are living on "narrow margins," even minor breaks in established procedures or the neglect of a single detail can bring on serious or even fatal consequences. Few operative procedures done in other specialty fields are attended by mortality rates in excess of 2 to 5 per cent, whereas risks of 10 to 25 per cent for different cardiac procedures are commonplace. These high risks are often reflected in the tense atmosphere of the cardiac operating room.

Cardiac patients are thoroughly monitored during their operations. The electrocardiogram is continuously displayed. The patient's temperature is measured repeatedly (via esophageal and rectal thermal probes), as is the temperature of the blood in the heart-lung machine. The adequacy of extracorporeal circulation is assessed by uninterrupted monitoring of arterial and venous pressures, urine output, the electroencephalogram, and by serial blood gas determinations. The monitoring of each of these physiologic parameters involves the use of complex and expensive equipment which must always be kept in perfect running order. In addition, large numbers of specialized instruments are used during cardiac operations — perfusion and drainage catheters, tubing and connectors for the extracorporeal circuits, vascular clamps, special suction instruments, fibrillators and defibrillators, prosthetic valves, and other instruments.

HEART-LUNG MACHINE

Probably the most distinguishing piece of equipment used in open heart surgery is the heart-lung machine. In order to be able to perform delicate maneuvers inside the heart, a quiet, bloodless field is required; the function of the heart and lungs must be taken over by the heart-lung machine. As these functions are performed outside the patient's body, the machine is also called an extracorporeal support system (and the operator of the machine is an extracorporeal perfusionist).

Simply stated, the heart-lung machine drains blood from the heart, oxygenates it, and then pumps it back into the body. The drainage of blood from the body to the heart-lung machine is accomplished by inserting large cannulas through the right atrium into the superior and inferior venae cavae. Appropriate connecting tubing transports the blood returning from the heart into the *venous reservoir*. This reservoir is kept at a level lower than the heart, thus providing a siphoning effect to divert the blood. The greater the vertical distance between the heart and the reservoir, the stronger will be the siphon effect and the more complete will be the diversion of the blood. Total diversion of caval blood flow can be accomplished by encompassing the venae cavae (and their contained cannulas) with tourniquets. The right atrium can then be incised without the fear of having large amounts of undiverted blood obscuring the operative field, or of obliterating the siphon effect with an *air lock.*

The blood returning to the venous reservoir from the caval cannulas and from the coronary suction (see later) is filtered, passed on to the oxygenator and the heat exchanger, and finally is pumped back into the body (Fig. 3–2). The site of re-entry into the patient's arterial system may be either the femoral, iliac, or subclavian arteries, or the ascending aorta. The return flow of blood through the arterial routes will be retrograde, i.e., against the flow of blood as it normally comes out of the heart. When the ascending aorta is used, the flow of blood from the heart-lung machine is antegrade, or in the same direction as normal blood flow. This perfused blood then passes through

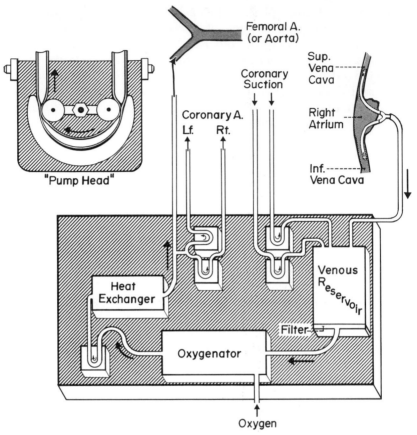

Figure 3-2. Schematic diagram of the heart-lung machine. Unoxygenated blood is drained from the heart and emptied into the venous reservoir, along with the blood retrieved by the coronary suction system. It then passes to the oxygenator, which adds oxygen to the blood until it is fully saturated. In the heat exchanger the temperature of the blood is raised or lowered. The blood is then pumped back into the body; separate circuits (like the coronary artery system) may also be perfused. The insert depicts the roller "pump head" which propels the blood forward.

the capillary beds of the various organs, muscles, and so forth, and returns to the venae cavae, where the cycle starts once again.

Despite its complexity, the heart-lung machine provides only four major functions:

Oxygenation of blood.   The conversion of dark unoxygenated venous blood to bright red arterial blood in an extracorporeal circuit occurs in the oxygenator, which provides a broad surface area for venous blood to be exposed to oxygen. This oxygen interchange may be accomplished by bubbling oxygen through a vertical column of blood (bubble oxygenator), by allowing the blood to layer out on thin permeable membranes as oxygen flows over them (membrane oxygenator), or by filming the blood onto a closely spaced series of rotating disks which dip into a reservoir of blood inside a cylindrical chamber (disk oxygenator).

Pumping. From the oxygenator, the oxygenated blood must be pumped back into the patient's body. The arterial perfusion line will provide blood flow to the entire body at rates comparable to normal resting cardiac output (about 2.4 liters per square meter body surface area per minute in high flow perfusions). However, it may be necessary to interrupt the continuity of this perfusion, in which case separate perfusion lines must be established to provide blood flow beyond the interruption in the main circuit. For example, when the proximal aorta is clamped and incised to operate on the aortic valve, separate lines may be established to perfuse the coronary arteries with blood (coronary artery perfusion circuit). Further, when the arch of the aorta is operated on, interrupting pump flow to the arteries to the brain, separate perfusion lines are established for these cerebral vessels. In order to provide these complicated perfusion circuits, the heart-lung machine must have adequate pumping capabilities.

Blood in this closed system is propelled by compression of the blood-filled polyvinyl tubing in a rotary *pump head*. Usually, each pump head has two rollers which press on the tubing nearly to occlusion, thereby forming a column of blood which is propelled forward as the next roller compresses the next segment of tubing (see insert of Fig. 3–2). The rate at which the blood is propelled forward is determined by the rate at which the rotary pump head turns, each turn of the pump delivering a certain amount of blood flow, depending on the size of the tubing.

Suction. Throughout the course of open heart procedures, considerable quantities of blood appear in the operative field (other than the blood drained via the vena caval cannulas). Residual blood in cardiac chambers which are opened during the operative procedure, blood returning from the lungs to the left side of the heart, effluent blood from coronary artery perfusion, and blood leaking from around an aortic perfusion cannula must all be removed from the operative field. The heart-lung machine must be capable of suctioning away this undrained blood and returning it to the venous reservoir; otherwise, the system would soon run dry. Just as the forward propulsion of blood is provided by the compressive action of the roller pumps on the polyvinyl tubing, a negative effect, i.e., suction, can be provided by the pump heads rotating in the reverse direction. Again, the speed of rotation of the pump heads will determine the rate at which the blood is suctioned away from the operative field.

Temperature control. It has been amply demonstrated that metabolic processes are slowed as body temperature is lowered, and relative hypoxia is better tolerated by the various organs at these reduced temperatures. For example, at 37°C the brain can tolerate anoxia for only three to four minutes without irreversible damage. At 30°C, this time interval is lengthened to eight to 12 minutes.

As a safeguard against temporary failure of the heart-lung machine and to reduce tissue oxygen requirements, the temperature of the blood in the extracorporeal circuit is lowered in the part of the machine known as the *heat exchanger*. As the cold blood is returned to the body, the tissues of the patient are slowly cooled. At the conclusion of the operative procedure, the blood is rewarmed and the body is returned to normal temperature.

In the heat exchanger, the blood is cooled (or heated) by allowing cold (or warm) water to circulate around the container in which blood is stored. The circulating water changes the temperature of the container, and, in turn, the temperature of the blood. Obviously, the blood and the water never come into direct contact. Different cardiac centers utilize different degrees of hypothermia; some prefer mild hypothermia (32°C to 36°C), others use moderate hypothermia (20° to 32°C), while only a few use severe hypothermia (18°C to 26°C).

SPECIAL CONSIDERATIONS

Certain features of the extracorporeal circuit and the conduct of the open heart operation deserve special mention, as they directly affect the patient's postoperative course.

Significant changes in the patient's clotting mechanisms are routinely encountered following open heart surgery. In order that there be no blood clotting in the extracorporeal circuit, the patient is anticoagulated with relatively high doses of heparin (usually 3 to 4 mgm heparin per kilogram of body weight). Heparinized blood is often a major constituent of the priming volume of the heart-lung machine, and is diluted with a variable amount of other nonblood solutions (Ringer's Lactate, Dextran, Albumin, Mannitol. and so forth). At the completion of the bypass, protamine sulfate is administered to reverse this heparin anticoagulation. Because of different rates of metabolism of heparin and protamine, this reversal is often imperfect. Clotting times may remain prolonged (owing to *heparin rebound*), and additional protamine may be required. Other components of the blood clotting mechanism may also be depressed after cardiopulmonary bypass. Platelets are usually rapidly depleted and do not return for a number of hours postoperatively. Labile clotting factors (prothrombin, fibrinogen, and so on) are similarly depressed, especially in patients with decreased liver function. The administration of fresh whole blood is sometimes the only way to restore these clotting factors.

Red blood cells are hemolyzed during the operation because of the mechanical trauma of the pump and suction systems and the direct exposure of the blood to oxygen (the *blood-gas interface*). The products of red blood cell breakdown impose a burden upon the liver and kidneys which metabolize and excrete them.

Embolization of calcium, air, or thrombi from the operative field into the patient's arterial system is a constant hazard in cardiac surgery, and detailed efforts are made to avoid it. Small pieces of calcium are often dislodged during resection and replacement of the aortic valve, and must be very carefully retrieved by a vacuum suction system (not the suction system of the heart-lung machine). Before completing any open heart procedure, all the air must be evacuated from the heart and replaced by blood. If the heart were to beat effectively before the air was totally removed, the residual air would be pumped out into the aorta—an air embolus. Left atrial thrombus is not an uncommon finding, particularly in patients with advanced mitral valve disease. During mitral valve surgery, great care is taken to remove all the nonadherent clot and to avoid dislodging this clot into the general circulation. Central nervous system damage may be the result of these emboli, regardless of their composition.

OPERATIVE PROCEDURES

Introduction

In the past decade, the rapid advances in patient care, diagnostic techniques, and equipment technology have been paralleled by similarly striking advances in the operative procedures for cardiac disease. Today, complex congenital anomalies may be definitively repaired, damaged valves may be repaired or replaced, coronary arteries may be repaired or bypassed, and even the heart itself can be replaced. In considering the operative procedures to repair specific cardiac defects, the reader is referred back to Chapter 1 for the illustration and discussion of the pathologic lesions.

When speaking generally of heart operations, they may be broadly classified as *closed* or *open.* Closed procedures do not involve the use of the heart-lung machine, while in open heart operations the interior of the heart can be visualized only by using the extracorporeal circuit.

Incisions

The great majority of cardiac surgery is performed through the three following incisions: median sternotomy, left lateral thoracotomy, and anterior thoracotomy.

In the median sternotomy incision, the sternum is divided down the middle with a vibrating bone saw. Retraction of the two sides of the sternum provides excellent exposure to the heart, ascending aorta, and the great vessels. This incision is well tolerated by the patient, as it is less painful and affects pulmonary function less than the thoracotomy incisions.

In the left lateral thoracotomy incision, the patient is positioned with his right side lying against the operating table and with the left side of the chest exposed. Entry into the left pleural cavity is made by making an incision between the ribs (through the intercostal muscles) or by entering through the "bed" of a rib which is removed. The lateral thoracotomy incision is particularly useful for operations on the descending thoracic aorta and is also used by some surgeons for operations on the mitral valve. With this incision, the left lung is usually compressed to gain exposure to the heart; further, the opposite lung (the *downside lung*) is often underventilated during the operation because of its dependent position. Therefore, pulmonary complications are not uncommon after thoracotomy incisions.

With the anterior thoracotomy incision, the patient is positioned supine or tilted at a shallow angle so that the anterior portion of one side of the chest is exposed. An intercostal incision is made from the sternum nearly to the axilla, but, unlike the full lateral thoracotomy incisions, the large muscles of the posterolateral chest are not divided. If additional exposure is required anteriorly, the sternum can be divided transversely and the incision extended into the opposite pleural cavity. The left anterior thoracotomy incision is particularly useful for removing the pericardium (pericardiectomy), and the right anterior thoracotomy incision is commonly used for repair of atrial septal defects.

Congenital Heart Disease

Closed procedures. Closed procedures (not using the heart-lung machine) are frequently employed in the treatment of congenital cardiac abnormalities. They are relatively simple, yet can be quite effective.

CLOSURE OF A PATENT DUCTUS ARTERIOSUS (see Fig. 1–20). The shunting of blood from the aorta to the pulmonary artery can be stopped by division of the PDA. Through a left thoracotomy incision, the ductus is dissected free. Blood flow through the ductus is prevented by placing narrow, noncrushing vascular clamps on the aortic and then the pulmonary artery ends of the PDA. The ductus is then divided and the divided ends sutured closed (Fig. 3–3). In newborn infants, emergency ligation (rather than division and oversewing) of the PDA may prove lifesaving.

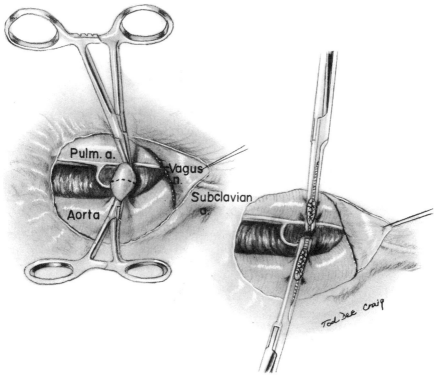

Figure 3–3. Drawings of closure of patent ductus arteriosus. In the left drawing, note the descending thoracic aorta just beyond the left subclavian artery, the vascular clamps placed on the aortic side and the pulmonary artery side of the PDA, and the proposed site of division (*dotted line*). On the right side, the ductus has been divided and the cut ends oversewn with a vascular suture. (From Norman, J. C. (ed.): Cardiac Surgery. New York, Appleton-Century-Crofts, 1964.)

REPAIR OF COARCTATION OF THE AORTA (see Fig. 1–29). In this closed procedure, the operative exposure (through a left lateral thoracotomy) is made difficult by the tremendous collateral circulation in the chest wall and in the tissues around the coarctation. One or two pairs of intercostal arteries are usually divided. As very little blood is flowing through the coarcted segment of aorta, the aorta can be safely cross-clamped above and below the coarctation. The coarcted segment is resected and the aorta reanastomosed with vascular sutures (Fig. 3–4). The lumen of the aorta should then be nearly the same size through the area of the anastomosis.

PULMONARY ARTERY BANDING. Left-to-right shunting within the heart may be great enough to cause heart failure and marked overcirculation in the lungs (almost always due to a large VSD). If this circumstance occurs within the first year of life, pulmonary artery banding is often chosen rather than a definitive repair (see later)

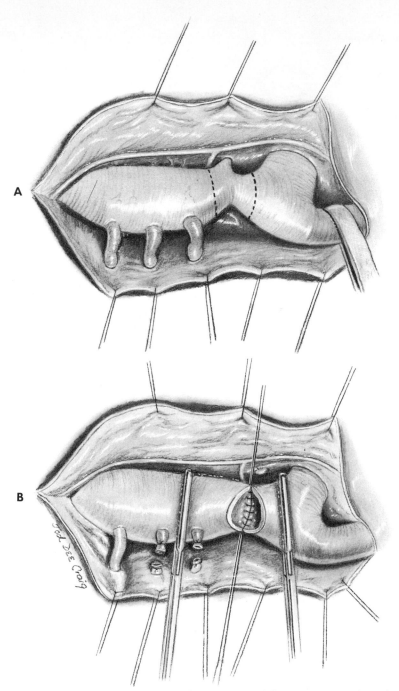

Figure 3–4. Drawings of repair of coarctation of the aorta. *A*, On the right side, note the large left subclavian artery (encircled with an umbilical tape) and the proximal aorta. In the center of the drawing, the site of the proposed resection (*dotted lines*) includes the coarcted (narrowed) segment and the ligamentum arteriosum (the obliterated PDA). On the left side, the dilated aorta and the very large intercostal arteries can be seen. *B*, Two intercostal arteries have been ligated, the noncrushing vascular clamps applied and the two sides of the aorta are being anastomosed together with vascular sutures. (From Norman, J. C. (ed.): Cardiac Surgery. New York. Appleton-Century-Crofts, 1964.)

because of the high mortality rate of open heart surgery in this age group.

Pulmonary artery banding entails dissecting free the main pulmonary artery and encircling it with a band of Teflon tape. The tape is then "tightened," causing a constriction in the pulmonary artery, until the pressure distal to the band is between one third and one half of its original value. This constricting band causes a higher pressure in the right ventricle, which reduces the left-to-right shunt from the left ventricle and thereby reduces heart failure. The lungs are also protected against the overcirculation by the pulmonary artery band.

CREATION OF LEFT-TO-RIGHT SHUNTS FOR CYANOTIC CONGENITAL HEART DISEASE. In the young infant who is too small for definitive (open heart) repair of tetralogy of Fallot or transposition of the great vessels, palliative procedures are necessary to reduce the arterial desaturation and to tide the infant over until he is old enough to undergo complete correction.

In tetralogy of Fallot (see Fig. 1–24), in which pulmonic stenosis plays such an important role in the altered hemodynamics, the purpose of the palliative procedure is to increase blood flow to the lungs. The anastomosis of a systemic artery to a pulmonary artery in order to accomplish this purpose is currently performed by either of two techniques.

The subclavian artery to pulmonary artery shunt (Blalock-Taussig procedure) involves ligating and dividing the subclavian artery at its first branching, "turning down" the vessel toward the hilum of the lung, where the end of the divided subclavian artery is anastomosed to the side of the pulmonary artery.

In the ascending aorta to right pulmonary artery shunt (the Waterston or Cooley procedure), the posterolateral wall of the ascending aorta and the pulmonary artery are isolated in a single vascular clamp and a 5 mm anastomosis is performed. Since this anastomosis is performed within the pericardium, its closure at the time of definitive open heart repair (see later) is made much easier than the aforementioned Blalock anastomosis.

In infants with transposition of the great vessels (see Fig. 1–25), the mixing of oxygenated blood from the isolated pulmonary circuit with unoxygenated blood from the isolated systemic circuit is best accomplished by creating an atrial septal defect. Recently, this atrial septal defect has been made by passing a balloon-tipped catheter through the foramen ovale to the left atrium. The balloon is inflated and the catheter is forcibly withdrawn, the inflated balloon "popping open" a defect in the atrial septum (Rashkind procedure). If this nonoperative technique fails to provide adequate mixing, a Blalock-Hanlon operation is undertaken. This procedure involves dissecting out the right pulmonary veins, placing a vascular clamp so as to isolate together the portions of the left and the right atria next to the inter-atrial septum, excising a large portion of the septum, and then re-anastomosing the lateral walls of the right and left atria.

CAVAL PULMONARY ANASTOMOSIS FOR TRICUSPID ATRESIA. There is no complete surgical correction for tricuspid atresia. In order to achieve more oxygenation of unsaturated blood, the side of the superior vena cava is anastomosed to the cut end of the right pulmonary artery (the Glenn procedure). In this way, the superior vena caval blood is diverted to the right lung, where it can be oxygenated and then returned to the left atrium.

Open heart procedures. By use of the heart-lung machine, the complex defects within the heart can be visualized and repaired. In critically ill newborn infants and children under one year of age, open heart surgery is attended by a rather high mortality and, when available, closed palliative procedures are preferred, leaving defini-tive repair until an age when the child can better tolerate the open heart procedure.

CLOSURE OF AN ATRIAL SEPTAL DEFECT (see Fig. 1–22). When the atrial septal defect is small (usually a secundum defect), it can often be closed without tension by simply suturing together the sides of the defect. However, if the secundum defect is large or if the defect is of the septum primum or sinus venous types, closure is usually accomplished by using a patch of pericardium or Dacron (Fig. 3–5).

CLOSURE OF A VENTRICULAR SEPTAL DEFECT (see Fig. 1–21). Open heart repair of a ventricular septal defect is performed through a median sternotomy incision. Usually the defect is exposed by mak-ing an incision in the right ventricle (although a right atrial approach is occasionally used). If the defect is small and has a firm fibrous rim, it may be closed by simple interrupted sutures. Usually, however, closure of the defect requires a patch of Teflon or Dacron cloth. The lower rim of a ventricular septal defect is very close to the conduction bundle and great care is exercised in the placement of sutures in this area, in order to avoid heart block. If a pulmonary artery band had been placed at a previous palliative procedure, it is removed and the pulmonary artery enlarged if necessary.

REPAIR OF ATRIOVENTRICULAR CANAL DEFECT (see Fig. 1–23). Since this complex defect involves the lower portion of the atrial septum and the upper portion of the ventricular septum, it is best approached through an incision in the right atrium. The clefts in the mitral (and tricuspid) valves are repaired first and the sutures are left long. A patch of pericardium or Dacron cloth is used to close the ventricular and atrial defects, while the septal portion of the mitral (or tricuspid) valve is buttressed against the patch using the retained

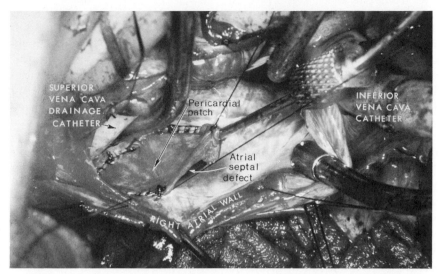

Figure 3–5. Photograph of repair of a sinus venosus atrial septal defect; view looking into the right atrium. An incision has been made through the atrial wall to expose the defect. The vena cava drainage catheters are listed. In the center of the photograph, the pericardial patch has been sutured to the atrial septum over three fourths of the circumference of the atrial septal defect, which lies beneath the patch.

sutures. Only rarely does the pathology in the mitral valve require prosthetic valve replacement.

TOTAL CORRECTION OF TETRALOGY OF FALLOT (see Fig. 1–24). The total correction of Fallot's tetralogy in many regards is similar to a VSD closure, but with some important variations and additions. If a Blalock-Taussig or Waterston anastomosis has been performed previously, that shunt is closed first so that the blood flow from the shunt will not return through the pulmonary artery and obscure the operative field. When the right ventricle is opened, the hypertrophied, obstructing muscle of the right ventricular outflow tract is resected and the pulmonic valve is opened, if necessary. If the outflow through the pulmonic valve is then still too small, a gusset of pericardium is sutured over this area to enlarge it. Since the aorta "overrides" the ventricular septal defect, great care is exercised in placing the VSD closure patch so as to avoid injury to the aortic valve.

TOTAL CORRECTION OF TRANSPOSITION OF THE GREAT VESSELS (see Fig. 1–25). The most widely used operation for total correction of TGV is the Mustard procedure. In this complex procedure, a "baffle" of pericardium is constructed in such a way that the blood returning from the venae cavae is shunted over to the left atrium (and thence to the left ventricle and out the pulmonary artery) and the blood returning from the pulmonary veins is diverted to the right atrium (and thence to the right ventricle and out the aorta).

CORRECTION OF TOTAL ANOMALOUS PULMONARY VENOUS RE-
TURN (see Fig. 1–26). The correction of TAPVR is designed to
reroute the pulmonary venous blood away from the right atrium back
to the left atrium. It involves the anastomosis of the posterior wall of
the left atrium to the common pulmonary venous channel behind the
heart. If the ascending left superior vena cava is then ligated, all the
blood from the lungs will then enter the left atrium and the patient's
cyanosis will be eliminated.

PULMONIC VALVULOTOMY FOR PULMONIC STENOSIS (see Fig.
1–27). The fact that the main pulmonary artery is usually dilated
beyond the stenotic pulmonic valve makes relief of this obstruction
relatively simple. An incision in the dilated pulmonary artery easily
exposes the dome-shaped valvular stenosis, which is then incised,
relieving the obstruction. The overgrowth of infundibular muscle
which develops in response to valvular stenosis will usually recede
with relief of the valvular obstruction. If the major obstruction is
primarily in the infundibulum, the obstructing muscle can be resected
as is done in the repair of tetralogy of Fallot.

RELIEF OF LEFT VENTRICULAR OUTFLOW OBSTRUCTION (see
Fig. 1–28). As described in Chapter 1, the obstruction to the outflow
of blood from the left ventricle may be at a level below the aortic
valve, at the valve, or above the valve.

If the obstruction below the aortic valve is a fibrous or membranous diaphragm, it can be removed through an opening in the
aorta. If the subvalvular stenosis is due to an overgrowth of muscle,
this tissue can be either resected or simply incised, preventing the
muscle from constricting the outflow tract.

In children, when the obstruction is at the level of the aortic
valve, the commissures between the aortic valve cusps are usually
fused together in fibrous union. Only with advancing age does the
valve become calcified. By incising this fibrous fusion of the commissures, the opening (orifice) of the valve can be greatly increased
and the obstruction relieved. Replacement of the valve is usually
unnecessary unless calcification makes valvulotomy and reconstruc-
tion impossible.

The obstruction which lies above the aortic valve is usually from
a waistlike constriction, and repair of this defect involves removing
some of the obstructing tissue on the inside of the aorta and enlarging
the ascending aorta with a "gusset" of Teflon or Dacron.

Acquired Heart Disease

Closed procedures.   MITRAL COMMISSUROTOMY FOR MITRAL
STENOSIS (see Fig. 1–30). When the patient's history and the

diagnostic studies indicate that the leaflets of the mitral valve are flexible and noncalcified, that the mitral stenosis is unaccompanied by mitral insufficiency, and that there are probably no clots within the left atrium, the closed procedure of mitral commissurotomy may be performed. In many centers the closed procedure has now given way to *open mitral commissurotomy* (see later).

Through a left thoracotomy, the left lateral side of the heart is exposed. A purse-string suture is placed around the left atrial appendage. When the base of the appendage is clamped, the tip of the appendage is removed and the surgeon's finger can then be introduced into the left atrium. Loss of blood from the atrial incision is prevented by pulling the purse string tightly around the finger. Often the fusion of the mitral leaflets can be split apart by forcibly pressing the exploring finger against the commissure — the so-called *finger fracture*. When the finger fracture technique fails to make an adequate opening, an expandable *dilator* is introduced into the apex of the left ventricle. By directing the position of the dilator with the palpating finger (through the atrial appendage) it can then be expanded, causing the fused commissure to "crack open" (Fig. 3–6). It is expected that the area which splits open under this pressure will be the commissure; if the cleavage plane extends instead into a mitral leaflet, immediate mitral insufficiency will result. For this reason the heart-lung machine is ready at "standby" so that valve replacement can be accomplished without delay.

REPAIR OF TRAUMATIC LESIONS OF THE HEART. Repair of puncture wounds of the heart caused by knives, ice picks, and other sharp instruments can often be accomplished without the use of the heart-lung machine. Exposure is provided through a median sternotomy or left anterior thoracotomy incision. If the patient is still alive, the puncture hole is usually small enough to be occluded by the surgeon's finger. With the bleeding site thus isolated, the hole can be sutured closed. Traumatic damage to the cardiac valves or shunts within the heart will require open heart techniques for repair.

PERICARDIECTOMY FOR CONSTRICTIVE PERICARDITIS. The removal of a thickened, adherent, constricting pericardium from the surface of the heart is a tedious, delicate operation which can almost always be accomplished without pump support. Usually the left ventricle is freed first so that when right ventricular output to the lungs is increased, the left heart can handle the new "load."

PACEMAKER INSERTION FOR HEART BLOCK. When the passage of electrical impulses through the specialized conduction tissues of the heart is interrupted (heart block) and the cardiac rate falls to 30 to 50 beats per minute, the patient may become quite symptomatic (fainting spells and so forth). Usually the patients with complete heart block are elderly (from 70 to 80 years old), and a thoracotomy

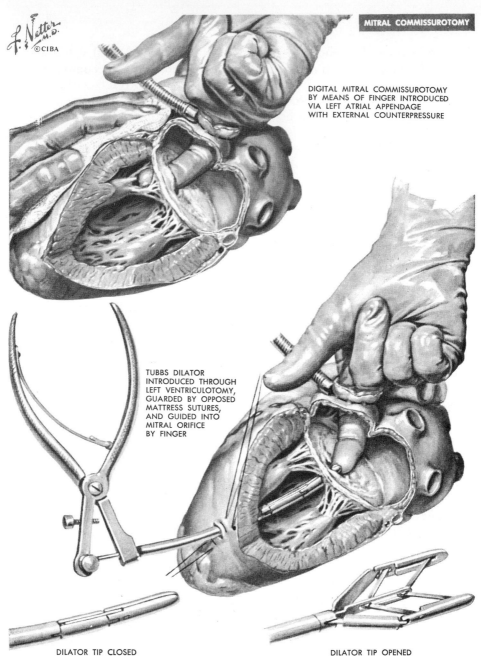

DIGITAL MITRAL COMMISSUROTOMY
BY MEANS OF FINGER INTRODUCED
VIA LEFT ATRIAL APPENDAGE
WITH EXTERNAL COUNTERPRESSURE

TUBBS DILATOR
INTRODUCED THROUGH
LEFT VENTRICULOTOMY,
GUARDED BY OPPOSED
MATTRESS SUTURES,
AND GUIDED INTO
MITRAL ORIFICE
BY FINGER

DILATOR TIP CLOSED

DILATOR TIP OPENED

Figure 3–6. Drawing of closed mitral commissurotomy. In the upper drawing, the surgeon's finger has been introduced into the left atrium through the purse-string suture. The finger is being pressed against the commissure, "fracturing" it apart. External counterpressure from a hand against the heart facilitates the commissurotomy. In the lower drawing, a small incision in the left ventricle has been made between opposing mattress sutures. The tip of the closed dilator has been guided through the mitral orifice by the finger in the atrium and is properly aligned. When the dilator tip is opened, its sides will press forcibly against both commissures, "dilating" them apart. (Copyright 1969 CIBA-GEIGY CORPORATION, reproduced, with permission, from THE CIBA COLLECTION OF MEDICAL ILLUSTRATIONS by Frank H. Netter, M.D.)

for the placement of pacemaking wires directly onto the surface of the heart is rarely warranted.

The insertion of a permanent transvenous pacemaker starts with the isolation of a central vein (usually the cephalic vein near the shoulder or the external jugular vein at the base of the neck). Through this vein the permanent electrode is passed, and under fluoroscopic control it is advanced into the right atrium, past the tricuspid valve and then out into the tip of the right ventricle, where it becomes entrapped by the trabeculations. The other end of the electrode is then connected to the pulse generator, a compact device powered by nickel-cadmium batteries, which provides a pacemaking stimulus at a certain rate. The pulse generator is then buried in a "pocket" in the subcutaneous tissues or beneath the pectoral musculature (see Fig. 8–12). The pulse generator usually will last 18 to 30 months before the batteries run down, requiring replacement of the pulse generator (but usually not of the pervenous endocardial electrode).

Open heart procedures. OPEN MITRAL COMMISSUROTOMY. It is thought in many quarters that direct visualization of a stenotic

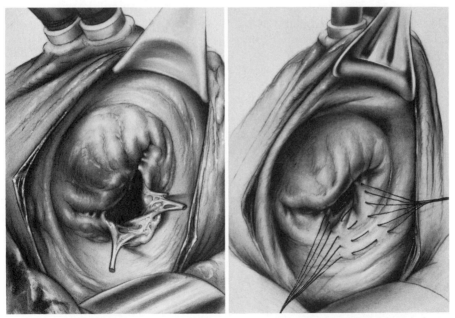

Figure 3–7. Drawings of repair of mitral valve for ruptured chordae tendineae. On the left, the "flail" portion of the posterior leaflet and the ruptured chordae can be easily visualized. Repair is affected by suturing together the sides of the flail portion of the leaflet and by decreasing the circumference of annulus with the "annuloplasty" sutures (the bottom three sutures in the right drawing). (From Gerbode, F., Kerth, W. J., Hill, J. D., Sánchez, P. A., and Puryear, G. H.: Surgical treatment of nonrheumatic mitral insufficiency. J. Cardiovasc. Surg. (Torino) *10*:103, 1969.)

mitral valve can provide a better repair than that accomplished by closed techniques. The left atrium is opened widely, any clot within the atrium is safely removed, and the commissures can be visualized, sharply incised, and then "teased apart." Often there is fusion of the chordae tendineae, which can be gently separated under direct vision.

MITRAL VALVULOPLASTY. Sometimes replacement of an insufficient mitral valve can be prevented by a careful repair. For example, rupture of chordae tendineae supporting the posterior (mural) leaflet of the valve can be effectively treated by eliminating the "flail" section of the leaflet and by reducing the circumference of the annulus of the valve (an annuloplasty) (Fig. 3–7).

MITRAL VALVE REPLACEMENT (Figs. 1–30 to 1–32). When the mitral valve is not amenable to repair, when the leaflets have no flexibility, when there is extensive calcification, when marked mitral insufficiency is present, when the chordae tendineae are so thickened and fused that the leaflets are pulled down into the ventricle, when the papillary muscles are infarcted, when there is active bacterial infection in the valve, or when repair techniques do not make a hemodynamically acceptable valve, then valve replacement is resorted to. The irreparably damaged valve is removed and a prosthesis (an "artificial heart valve") is sutured into place. The relief of the hemodynamic burden by the valve replacement may be rapid and very gratifying (Fig. 3–8).

AORTIC VALVE REPLACEMENT (see Figs. 1–33 and 1–34). In adults, reparative procedures on the aortic valve are not highly successful and replacement of the valve is most commonly chosen. Stenotic valves are often heavily calcified and no repair procedure could make them functional again. Insufficient valves in the high-pressure aorta can only rarely be successfully repaired.

Replacement of the aortic valve has been accomplished with a variety of devices—prostheses (artificial heart valves made of metal and cloth or other synthetic materials [Fig. 3–9]), homografts (cadaver aortic valves), heterografts (aortic valves from other animals like pigs or sheep), and fascia lata grafts (valves fashioned from the fascia of the patient's thigh muscles). The choice of one or another of these devices is for the most part a personal preference of the surgeon.

In the operative procedure of aortic valve replacement, after cardiopulmonary bypass is established, a vascular clamp is placed across the ascending aorta so that blood pumped in from the heart-lung machine will not reach the area of the aortic valve. The aorta is incised below the cross-clamp exposing the aortic valve whose destroyed cusps are removed. In many centers, the coronary arteries are perfused with blood during the valve replacement via separate *coronary perfusion lines.* Sutures are placed radially around the

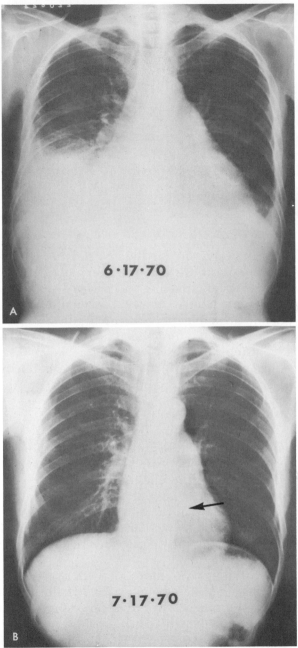

Figure 3–8. X-rays of a patient with mitral insufficiency from bacterial endo-carditis: preoperative and one month after operation. (The pathologic change of this patient's valve is shown in Figure 1–32.) On the preoperative film, note the enlarged heart and the large effusion in the right pleural cavity (from heart failure). The post-operative film one month later shows a clearing of the heart failure, a smaller cardiac size, and a prosthesis in the mitral position.

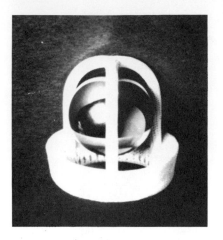

Figure 3–9. Photograph of an aortic valve prosthesis, a Starr-Edwards aortic valve, model 2320. The sewing ring of the valve is made of Dacron and Teflon, the poppet is a highly polished metal alloy (Stellite), and the cage struts are Stellite, covered with Teflon cloth.

annulus of the aortic valve and are then passed through the prosthesis (or homograft). The prosthesis is lowered into place, the sutures tied, and the aorta closed (after removing the coronary cannulas).

TRICUSPID VALVE REPLACEMENT.   As mentioned in Chapter 1, Section D, organic involvement of the tricuspid valve is unusual, but tricuspid insufficiency on a "functional" basis (i.e., due to dilatation of the right ventricle from end-stage mitral valve disease) is not uncommon. Severe tricuspid insufficiency occasionally requires valve replacement, usually accomplished with a prosthesis similar to a mitral prosthesis.

REPLACEMENT OF THE ASCENDING THORACIC AORTA.   Sometimes aortic valvular insufficiency is accompanied by diseases of the ascending aorta, such as dissecting aneurysms, Sinus of Valsalva aneurysms, or syphilitic aneurysms. In these instances, the aorta is cross-clamped well above the aneurysm, the aneurysm is removed and a Teflon or Dacron tubular graft is sutured distally to the aorta and proximally to the base of the aorta or to the aortic prosthesis itself. Occasionally, in patients with aneurysms of the ascending aorta requiring graft replacement, the aortic valve may be uninvolved and may not require any treatment.

RESECTION OF LEFT VENTRICULAR ANEURYSM (see Fig. 1–37). When a patient has repeated bouts of heart failure secondary to a ventricular aneurysm, removal of the aneurysm often eliminates the heart failure or makes it much more manageable.

With well developed ventricular aneurysms, the pericardium is usually densely adherent to the thin wall of the aneurysm, providing major support to the heart wall. Separation of the aneurysm from the pericardium involves considerable handling of the heart which would expose the patient to the danger of breaking off a clot from the inside of the aneurysm into the blood stream. Therefore, full cardiopulmonary bypass is established prior to this dissection and the heart is intentionally fibrillated (put into ventricular fibrillation) so that this clot cannot be ejected by the beating heart. An opening is then made into the aneurysm, and the walls of the aneurysmal sac are removed. By visualizing the inside of the left ventricular chamber directly, damage to the mitral valve can be avoided, all remaining blood clot can be carefully removed, and accurate placement of the sutures to bring the ventricle wall back together can be assured (Fig. 3–10). After reconstituting the wall of the ventricle with a double row of sutures, the patient is removed from cardiopulmonary bypass, usually without difficulty.

AORTOCORONARY SAPHENOUS VEIN GRAFT FOR OBSTRUCTION OF THE CORONARY ARTERY (see Fig. 1–36). Patients with angina pectoris usually have obstructions in one or more of their coronary arteries. Techniques to bypass the coronary obstruction have been highly successful in bringing new blood flow to the coronary arteries beyond the blockage.

A segment of the patient's saphenous vein is removed from its position in the subcutaneous tissues of the upper thigh. This saphenous vein graft (SVG) is reversed so that the venous valves will not

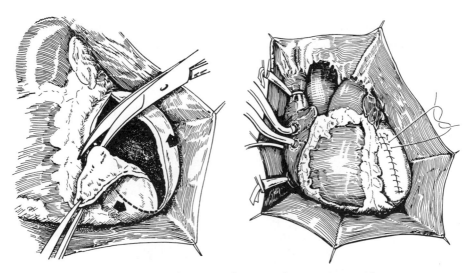

Figure 3–10. Drawings of repair of ventricular aneurysm. After instituting cardiopulmonary bypass, the aneurysm is dissected free from its overlying and adherent pericardium. On the left, the aneurysm is being excised at the line of demarcation between the thin wall of the aneurysm and the healthy heart muscle. A small rim of scar tissue is left at the base of the aneurysm to provide a firm support for the sutures which close the ventricular wall. On the right, the walls of the aneurysm have been brought together with a double layer of sutures. The vena caval drainage catheters are seen on the left; the pericardium is elevated by sutures to localize and contain the blood lost during the operation. (From Favaloro, R. G., et al.: Ventricular aneurysm— Clinical experience. Ann. Thorac. Surg. 6:227, 1968.)

obstruct blood flow. One end of the SVG is anastomosed to the side of the ascending aorta, just above the opening of the patient's own coronary arteries. Then, an opening is made into the coronary artery downstream from the obstruction and the other end of the SVG is connected to this opening. Blood can then flow from the aorta through the SVG and into the coronary artery, thus bypassing the obstruction (Fig. 3–11). Sometimes multiple arteries are blocked and two or even three SVGs are used to bring new blood flow to the ischemic heart muscle.

PULMONARY EMBOLECTOMY FOR PULMONARY EMBOLI. The formation of blood clots in the veins of the legs or the pelvis is usually associated with thrombophlebitis in those areas. Although part of the clot becomes fixed to the vessel wall, there is often a "tail" of the clot lying in the stream of moving venous blood. When this part of the clot breaks off, it travels through the venous system to the right side of the heart. It then advances into the pulmonary artery, or one of its branches, where it then becomes lodged. In this position, the clot obstructs pulmonary blood flow to that portion of the lung supplied by the blocked pulmonary artery. Life-endangering changes in the heart and lungs usually occur when more than 50 per cent of the pulmonary arterial tree is blocked, as demonstrated by a pulmonary arteriogram.

The operative procedure to remove these blood clots is relatively straightforward. Cardiopulmonary bypass is established and an inci-

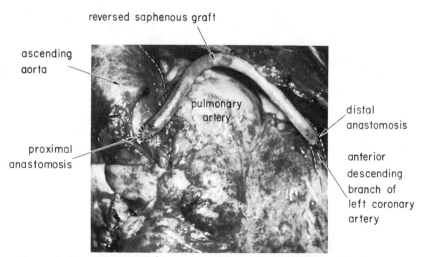

Figure 3–11. Photograph of aortocoronary saphenous vein graft (SVG) (the patient had a high-grade obstruction in the first portion of the anterior descending branch of the left coronary artery). Note the reversed SVG with one end anastomosed to the ascending aorta and the other end to the anterior descending artery downstream from the obstruction. In its course, the SVG travels over the pulmonary artery.

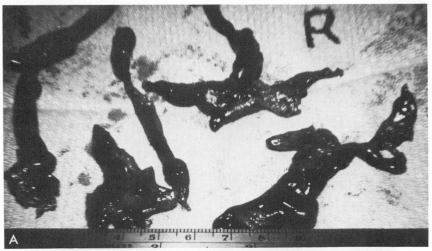

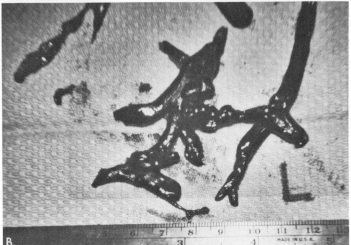

Figure 3–12. Photographs of emboli removed from the pulmonary artery. Note that the clots removed from the right (*A*) and left (*B*) pulmonary arteries conform to the branching of these vessels. (Specimen from a 75 year old man who had about 60 per cent of his pulmonary arterial tree blocked with these clots; he continues to do well three years after the operation.)

sion is made in the lower portion of the main pulmonary artery. The blood clots are extracted with forceps, with suction, or by "squeezing" them out of the lungs (Fig. 3–12). When as many clots as possible are removed, the incision in the pulmonary artery is sutured closed. This cardiac part of the procedure is then followed with a ligation of the inferior vena cava to prevent any further clots from traveling to the lungs.

Postoperative Problems

The first few days following cardiac operations are the most critical in terms of the patient's survival. The safety with which he can be conducted through this crisis period is largely dependent upon minute-to-minute observations and interventions made by the cardiac nurse. She is really the first line of defense in detecting and treating changes in the patient's condition; she must exercise good judgment in knowing when to inform the physician of a change or when to take care of the problem herself.

The patient's safety in this period is also dependent upon careful clinical and laboratory observations, effective medical management, and avoidance of predictable complications. As each organ system plays an important role in the patient's final outcome, each system will be considered separately.

Cardiac complications

The major postoperative cardiac problems are arrhythmias, low output syndrome, and tamponade. They may occur separately, but are often closely interrelated.

Arrhythmias

Prevention of cardiac arrhythmias in the postoperative period is important because of the deleterious effects the arrhythmias have upon cardiac performance. Ventricular fibrillation and prolonged ventricular tachycardia are incompatible with life, and multiple or multifocal premature ventricular contractions often precede these fatal arrhythmias. Cardiac output is decreased up to one third by atrial fibrillation or atrial flutter as compared to sinus rhythm. Synchronized atrial contractions result in more effective filling of the ventricle, and a larger stroke volume results. As maximum cardiac performance is both desirable and often necessary for recovery, the elimination of undesirable arrhythmias holds a high priority in postoperative care.

Operative trauma may engender or contribute to postoperative arrhythmias. The trauma of surgery includes the general effects of a lengthy anesthesia, multiple blood transfusions, total circulatory support with a nonpulsatile pumping system, and unphysiologic spreading apart of the ribs or the sides of the divided sternum. More specific trauma includes incisions into a ventricle, cannulation of the venae cavae or cardiac chambers, retraction of the atrial or ventricular walls to provide exposure, and placement of sutures to repair valvular or septal defects. The cardiac conduction pathways may be traumatized during the removal of calcified aortic valves, during resection of muscular tissue, or during repair of septal defects. The presence of a rigid prosthetic heart valve in a relatively small ventricle may cause direct trauma to the ventricular septum, initiating additional arrhythmias. Coronary arteries may be damaged directly by cannulation and perfusion, in the placement of sutures for a mitral valve replacement, or during myocardial revascularization procedures. The resultant myocardial anoxia may cause rhythm disturbances.

Other causes of undesirable postoperative arrhythmias include hypotension, hypoxemia, potassium imbalance, or digitalis excess. Hypotension is usually accompanied by poor perfusion and impaired function of the liver, lungs, kidneys, and heart. A decrease in coronary artery perfusion may result in arrhythmias directly, or indirectly by causing a fall in cardiac output with attendant metabolic acidosis. The use of sympathomimetic amines (e.g., Isuprel and epinephrine) to support the falling blood pressure may also predispose to ventricular arrhythmias, and ineffective blood flow to vital organs may ensue.

Hypoxemia may also cause postoperative arrhythmias. Lowered oxygen tensions in systemic arterial blood prevents normal oxygen utilization by the vital organs; diminished organ function and systemic acidosis are the expected sequelae. Atelectasis and pulmonary edema are common causes of hypoxemia and effective countermeasures are necessary to prevent the vicious cycle of hypoxia, acidosis, arrhythmias, more hypoxia, more acidosis, more arrhythmias, and so on.

Potassium imbalance has very adverse effects on cardiac conduction. Excess potassium delays AV conduction and intraventricular conduction and, if severe enough, can result in cardiac arrest, in standstill. Hypokalemia prolongs repolarization and increases cardiac automaticity and irritability (see Chapter 4).

Often inseparable from the arrhythmia problems of hypokalemia is digitalis excess, since patients with chronic heart failure are often receiving both digitalis derivatives and potent diuretics. Many of the most effective diuretics cause increased potassium losses in the urine, resulting in lowered serum levels. When hypokalemia supervenes, susceptibility to digitalis-induced cardiac arrhythmias is increased and vice versa. The use of Mannitol during the operative procedure (causing high urine flows and potassium losses) and of mechanical ventilation in the postoperative period (with its resultant respiratory alkalosis) accentuates the hypokalemia-digitalis arrhythmia problem.

Therefore, very careful attention is paid to repleting body stores of potassium and also preventing digitalis excess before the operation. Oral potassium supplements are given continuously until the day of operation (even if serum potassium values are normal), while digitalis derivatives are generally withheld one to two days before the cardiac procedure. Experience indicates that the difficult-to-treat, digitalis-induced arrhythmias have been significantly decreased by such a program.

Careful monitoring of serum potassium levels and arterial pH values in the postoperative period are mandatory. If renal function is adequate, aggressive potassium replacement is indicated. As postoperative urine commonly contains in excess of 100 milliequivalents of potassium per liter, large amounts of potassium are often necessary to maintain the serum level in a normal range (4.0 to 5.0 mEq/L). Serious arrhythmias can be avoided by this aggressive potassium supplementation program.

Hyperkalemia is less common, but also poses significant arrhythmia problems. Renal failure, systemic acidosis, and the breakdown of red blood cells may all contribute to hyperkalemia. Withholding the potassium supplementation, lowering serum potassium levels (by ion exchange resins or with glucose and insulin), and providing a mild alkalosis (by hyperventilation or the administration of sodium bicarbonate) will reduce the hazard of serious arrhythmias.

Following cardiac surgery, the most common *atrial arrhythmias* are rapid atrial fibrillation and atrial flutter. Discontinuing digitalis one to two days before operation reduces the chance of digitalis toxicity, but sometimes allows the ventricular rate to escape from digitalis control in the early postoperative period. Ventricular rates of 140 to 160 per minute are not uncommon. The degree of expediency required to bring these arrhythmias under control depends upon the patient's hemodynamic status. If the clinical signs of adequate cardiac performance are reasonably well maintained, rapid intravenous supplementation of existing digitalis levels can be used. Digoxin in 0.25 mgm or 0.50 mgm doses is given about every one and one half to two hours until appropriate rate control is achieved (90 to 110 beats per minute). Larger initial doses may be used if the patient has not been digitalized preoperatively. Interestingly, postoperative atrial flutter often requires rather high doses of digoxin, in the range of 2.0 mgm to 3.5 mgm, to achieve adequate atrioventricular block and control of the ventricular rate. Rapid deterioration of cardiac performance as a result of these arrhythmias sometimes dictates the need for cardioversion with a synchronized direct current countershock. The patient is usually momentarily anesthetized with a short-acting agent (Pentothal or Brevital). Atrial flutter may be converted with as little energy as 50 to 100 watt-seconds (joules), while atrial fibrillation usually requires 200 to 300 watt-seconds. Sometimes rapid digitalization or direct current countershock not only controls the ventricular response but provides the added benefit of changing the rhythm to a normal sinus mechanism. At other times, these measures are ineffective and a beta-adrenergic blocking agent, propranolol (Inderal), is used to supplement the digitalis. As propranalol may dramatically depress ventricular function (particularly in patients with advanced ventricular disease), it is always used with great care. Intravenous administration of 1 mgm doses is given every one to two minutes until a response is obtained; usually 3 to 7 mgm is sufficient. Obviously, the electrocardiogram and the arterial blood pressures should be continuously monitored through this critical period. When conversion from atrial fibrillation or flutter to sinus rhythm is achieved, quinidine in doses of 0.8 to 1.6 gm daily will usually prevent recurrence of the arrhythmia.

Bothersome *nodal rhythms* are also observed postoperatively. At rates below 60, nodal rhythm often causes significant depression of cardiac performance. An intravenous drip of isoproterenol (Isuprel) at a rate of one to two μgm per minute will usually speed the rate to more acceptable levels. If this technique fails to bring about the desired response, electrical pacemaking may be used. Pacemaking wires are often affixed to the epicardium of either the right atrium (near the sinus node) or the right ventricle at the time of operation, in expectation that rate control might become necessary in the postoperative period. When bradycardia occurs, an increased rate can be achieved by connecting the epicardial wires to an external battery-powered pacemaker. Rapid nodal tachycardias are usually the result of excessive digitalis and may be treated by withholding digitalis and administering potassium, diphenyl-hydantoin (Dilantin), or both.

Heart block is occasionally seen in patients undergoing repair of tetralogy of Fallot, ostium primum atrial septal defects, and ventricular septal defects, or after the replacement of a calcified aortic valve. Often the block is transient and is due to local swelling caused by sutures placed near the conduction tissue. Temporary pacemaking through the epicardial pacing wires is generally sufficient to maintain an adequate rate until the edema subsides. Rarely, the heart block is permanent and requires the placement of permanent endocardial or epicardial electrodes with an implanted battery-powered pulse generator at a second operation.

The occurrence of *premature ventricular contractions* (PVCs) in the postoperative period is a warning sign that should not be neglected. Frequent PVCs are not only detrimental to cardiac performance, but they also are commonly a prelude to more serious ventricular arrhythmias. Often, PVCs can be attributed to an easily corrected cause, such as hypokalemia, hypoxemia, excessive digitalis, or respiratory alkalosis. Correcting the underlying abnormality will often eliminate the PVCs. At other times, there is no obvious cause for them. When they occur in runs of two or more, arise from multiple ventricular foci, appear at rates of greater than five to 10 per minute, or cause bigeminy, they should be controlled by suppressive agents. Lidocaine (Xylocaine), being a short-acting antiarrhythmic agent, is usually used first. If a bolus of 50 to 100 mgm of lidocaine stops or significantly reduces the PVCs, and they recur after the agent is metabolized (five to 15 minutes), an intravenous drip of the agent (1 to 3 mgm per minute) usually will prevent their subsequent recurrence. If longer-acting agents are desired, procaineamide (Pronestyl) or quinidine may be used. If none of these agents is effective, propranolol or diphenylhydantoin may be tried.

The occurrence of *ventricular tachycardia* demands immediate and effective treatment, as the rapid reduction in cardiac output invariably leads to cardiovascular collapse if the arrhythmia is not terminated. If lidocaine does not reverse the arrhythmia in a few moments, direct current countershock (200 to 300 watt-seconds) should be applied immediately. Once the ventricular tachycardia has been stopped, suppressive agents (lidocaine, procaineamide, quinidine, and so forth) should be given to prevent its recurrence, and an underlying cause for the arrhythmia should be searched for assiduously.

Ventricular fibrillation demands immediate defibrillation with an electrical shock to the precordium, complete resuscitation, and a thorough search for underlying causes.

Low Output Syndrome

The *low cardiac output syndrome* seen after cardiac operations is simply the result of an inadequate amount of blood flowing to the body's tissues. As a result of the poor tissue perfusion, the following clinical manifestations are usually seen: a cold, clammy, mottled skin; a narrow pulse pressure (the difference between systolic and diastolic pressures); thready peripheral pulses; low urine output; cerebral disorientation; and labored respirations. Distension of jugular neck veins, rales in the lung bases, and regurgitation through the mitral and tricuspid valves are also often found.

Laboratory findings which corroborate the clinical impression of the low output state include a severe metabolic acidosis (large-base deficits), lowered arterial oxygen tensions (low $P_{a_{O_2}}$), a very dark, desaturated venous blood (indicating high extraction of oxygen by the poorly perfused tissues), and cardiac enlargement and pulmonary engorgement as seen on the chest x-ray film.

The clinical setting of the postoperative low cardiac output syndrome is usually seen in a patient with severe and long-standing cardiac disease. The ventricles have been compromised by scarring from rheumatic myocarditis, by inadequate coronary blood flow because of coronary artery disease, by ventricular overload from outflow obstruction, or by pulmonary hypertension. Operative considerations in the production of this syndrome are prolonged extracorporeal perfusion, aortic cross-clamping with less than optimal coronary artery perfusion, incomplete surgical correction of existing anatomic abnormalities, and hemodynamic deficiencies imposed by valvular prostheses which are too large for the cardiac chambers in which they are placed. Contributions to the low output state in the postoperative period include arrhythmias, cardiac tamponade, hypoxemia, metabolic acidosis, depressant drugs, and electrolyte abnormalities, such as hypokalemia, hypocalcemia, or severe hyponatremia.

The treatment of the low output state is both prophylactic and supportive. Patients likely to develop the syndrome can usually be identified by preoperative evaluation. Preparation for their cardiac operation must be optimal in every respect. Efforts must be made to provide maximum support to the heart during the operative procedure and to eliminate any significant residual anatomic abnormality. Adequate drainage of the mediastinum is provided to help eliminate the possibility of cardiac tamponade. The need for prolonged respiratory assistance is recognized and optimum mechanical ventilation is provided. Epicardial pacemaking wires (atrial, ventricular, or both) are placed in expectation that they will be used in the postoperative period. The means for careful monitoring of physiologic parameters should be provided.

Specific supportive therapy for the low output syndrome involves many and varied parameters. Blood volume replacement must be adequate, as the failing heart usually requires higher filling pressures (higher ventricular end-diastolic pressures) for optimum cardiac output. The central venous pressure is the most commonly used parameter to monitor the status of the blood volume, but it is not altogether reliable, nor does it always reflect the status of the left side of the heart. In the absence of mitral valve disease, the left atrial pressure is a better monitor of left ventricular function. Correct replacement of blood volume is critically important in these cases, as undertransfusion prevents optimum cardiac output and overtransfusion compounds the problem of cardiac failure. Hypovolemia may be treated by the infusion of packed cells, whole blood, or a noncolloid solution. The therapy of hypervolemia involves phlebotomy or the administration of a rapid-acting and potent diuretic, such as ethacrynic acid (Edecrin) or furosemide (Lasix).

Ionotropic agents are commonly used to support the failing heart, and play a very important role in treating the low output state. Digitalis preparations have usually been given for many months or years and are usually circulating in adequate amounts. Potent beta-adrenergic stimulating agents, especially isoproterenol (and epinephrine), are very useful because they increase the force of ventricular contraction and reduce peripheral resistance. The consequent improvement in cardiac output and the increased peripheral perfusion decrease the accompanying metabolic acidosis. The use of these valuable agents is not without hazard, however. Both isoproterenol and epinephrine increase cardiac rate and this is sometimes detrimental to cardiac performance, particularly in patients with valvular prostheses. Ventricular irritability is another undesirable side effect and may limit the dose that can be given safely. Both of these ionotropic agents tend to become less effective as time goes on and dosage requirements increase (tachyphylaxis). High-dose epinephrine can cause peripheral and visceral vasoconstriction, another unwanted side effect.

Other supportive measures for the low output syndrome include the following: careful maintenance of acid-base balance with respiratory support, sodium bicarbonate, or tromethamine (THAM-E); adequate ventilatory support; elimination of cardiac arrhythmias; and adequate sedation.

Cardiac Tamponade

Cardiac tamponade indicates a compression of the heart, caused by excessive amounts of blood clots (collecting between the heart and the anterior chest wall) which are inadequately removed by the chest drainage tubes. The return of venous blood to the right atrium and the output of blood from either ventricle may be very significantly impaired.

The clinical picture of cardiac tamponade includes a falling blood pressure, a narrowing pulse pressure, a rising central venous pressure (often with plethora of the upper extremities), a falling urine output, and a "paradoxical pulse pressure" of greater than 10 to 15 mm Hg (see Chapter 5). A widened mediastinal shadow is usually seen on a chest x-ray film. As bleeding into the mediastinal space is the usual cause for the postoperative cardiac tamponade, patients with coagulation defects, patients who have been taking anticoagulants, and patients with poor liver function (resulting in decreased production of coagulation factors) are prime candidates for this complication.

By comparing the clinical findings of cardiac tamponade with those of the low output syndrome, it can be appreciated that they are very similar. In fact, cardiac tamponade is one of the causative factors in the low output syndrome; the differentiation between these two complications is often extremely difficult.

At the time of operation, certain precautions can be made to help avert cardiac tamponade: meticulous hemostasis, appropriate reversal of the heparin administered for the extracorporeal circulation, thorough drainage of the mediastinal space, and a wide open pericardium (incised to allow full drainage into a pleural cavity).

If cardiac tamponade is suspected on the basis of clinical observation and the appearance of the chest x-rays and the patient's condition is deteriorating, reoperative exploration and evacuation of the compressing mediastinal hematoma can be lifesaving. Procrastination in this regard is very dangerous, as profound circulatory collapse may occur very rapidly. If adequate blood volume replacement has been maintained, the risk of this operative procedure is slight.

The cardiac nurse plays an extremely important role in the care of the patient with postoperative cardiac complications. Her observations and interventions very often spell the difference between a smooth and a stormy postoperative course. Knowledge of arrhythmia patterns, the clinical findings of the low output syndrome and cardiac tamponade, and the modes of treatment of these three complications are essential.

First, the nurse is constantly observing both the patient and his monitoring devices. She notes the appearance of an arrhythmia, tries to document it with a recording of the electrocardiogram, and attempts to relate the arrhythmia with some change in the patient's condition or his care. Perhaps the patient had a brief run of ventricular tachycardia as the nurse performed endotracheal suction; nodal tachycardia may have been precipitated by an untoward increase in the rate of isoproterenol administration; or perhaps the patient's agitation precipitated a bout of rapid atrial flutter. Any significant change in the patient's rhythm should be communicated to the physician. Should the patient develop severe bradycardia, the cardiac nurse should be able to make appropriate connections of the epicardial pacemaking wires to the battery-powered pacemaker, turn on the pacing circuit, and "capture" the patient's rhythm at a faster (and appropriate) rate. Further, the well trained cardiac nurse must be prepared to administer a direct current countershock to the chest should ventricular fibrillation or persistent ventricular tachycardia suddenly appear.

Second, the cardiac nurse must be very careful and very accurate in the way she administers medications to the patient. The intravenous drip rates of potent ionotropic drugs (like isoproterenol and epinephrine) must be meticulously monitored to avoid too fast or too slow an infusion. Prescribed digitalis derivatives must be accurately prepared and administered. Xylocaine is prepared in a labeled syringe and held "at the ready" in the event of multiple PVCs or a run of ventricular tachycardia. The concentration (in the IV bottle) and the rate of infusion of potassium chloride must be accurate, even though the dosage may be frequently altered by the physician in response to changes in the level of serum or urinary potassium.

Third, the nurse must keep an accurate account of the amounts of fluids and blood administered to the patient and the amounts of drainage from the chest tubes and the urinary catheter. She must prevent hypovolemia by infusing blood in amounts at least equal to the amount draining from the chest tubes. She must intermittently "strip" the tubes to ensure their patency and prevent the accumulation of blood in the mediastinum.

Respiratory complications

A high percentage of patients undergoing cardiac surgery have impaired pulmonary function. Pulmonary hypertension from long-standing mitral valve disease, left ventricular failure, or chronic lung disease is frequently seen. Restrictive lung disease is common in patients with pleural fibrosis or effusion, in massive cardiomegaly and prolonged heart failure, or following previous thoracotomy. Recurrent pulmonary infections as a sequel to congenital or acquired heart disease leave their toll upon overall pulmonary function. Providing optimum pulmonary management to these patients is an essential feature of their survival.

Preoperative assessment of pulmonary function and pulmonary preparation for the operative procedure has been previously discussed. The elimination of the tracheobronchitis which accompanies cigarette smoking, preoperative pulmonary physiotherapy including IPPB training, and optimum medical management are the most essential features of this preparatory program.

Certain operative considerations bear upon postoperative pulmonary complications. Unless hyperventilation is accomplished intermittently by the anesthesiologist during and at the completion of the operative procedure, atelectasis can easily occur. When a lateral thoracotomy approach is used, the *downside lung* (the dependent lung) is compromised by the mediastinal structures, and the lung on the operated side is usually compressed in gaining exposure to the operative field. Secretions tend to pool in the tracheobronchial tree during a lengthy procedure and must be removed by suctioning. Both thoracotomy and median sternotomy incisions are painful for the patient, and cause him to "splint" his respiratory efforts, adding to the incidence of atelectasis. The cuff of the endotracheal tube often remains inflated throughout the low output conditions of cardiopulmonary bypass and ischemic necrosis of the tracheal mucosa may result occasionally. Dry, irritative anesthetic gases can produce a mild inflammation of the respiratory mucosa, compounding postoperative pulmonary problems.

The value of continued postoperative respiratory assistance in the care of critically ill cardiac patients is now unchallenged. The anesthetic endotracheal tube may be left in place for two to three days or a tracheostomy can be performed, either at the time of operation or when the endotracheal tube is removed. Ventilatory support with a volume-cycled or a pressure-regulated respirator ensures appropriate ventilation and reduces fatigue, as the patient is relieved of the "work of breathing." Suctioning of the patient's secretions is facilitated by the easy access to the tracheobronchial tree provided by the endotracheal tube.

However, a program of respiratory support has its hazards. Complete ventilatory control with a respirator and cuffed endotracheal tube leaves the patient at the mercy of the oxygen supply; should the supply run out, unnoticed by the attending personnel, the patient would asphyxiate. Occasionally a soft endotracheal tube can kink in the oropharynx, causing respiratory obstruction. Unless the tube is carefully taped to the face, it could slip into a bronchus, resulting in overventilation of one lung and atelectasis of the other. The endotracheal tube, if improperly positioned, can rub on the gum margins and cause ulcerations of the oral mucosa. Unless adequate humidification of the inspired gases is provided (preferably by ultrasonic or heated-water humidifiers), the tracheobronchial mucosa will become dehydrated and inflamed (tracheitis sicca). Constant pressure by the cuff of the endotracheal or tracheostomy tube can cause ischemic necrosis of the tracheal mucosa; postintubation tracheal stenosis may result unless the cuff is deflated intermittently. Obstruction of the tip of the endotracheal tube by inspissated mucus or clotted blood can usually be prevented by frequent suctioning. Metal tracheostomy tubes sometimes are supplied with cuffs which can move up or down on the cannula; if the inflated cuff slips over the end of the tube, respiratory obstruction can result. The nursing personnel must be constantly vigilant and should assign the highest priority to averting these complications.

Monitoring of arterial blood gases and pH is essential to proper postoperative management. There are many causes for depression of the arterial oxygen tension. First, the ventilator may be delivering an inadequate minute volume. This occurs when the patient is "fighting the respirator," when pulmonary compliance is reduced by left ventricular failure and high left atrial pressures, or when the rate, volume, and pressure settings of the respirator are set too low. Concomitantly, the arterial pH is usually lowered and the carbon dioxide tension is increased (respiratory acidosis). This abnormality can be corrected by sedating the patient (with small doses of intravenous morphine), correcting left ventricular failure, or by increasing the rate, volume, or pressure settings of the respirator.

In atelectatic segments of lung, pulmonary arterial blood is shunted into the pulmonary veins without being exposed to alveoli. Such blood remains unoxygenated (AV shunting) and contributes to overall hypoxemia, i.e., a decreased arterial P_{O_2}. Causes of postoperative atelectasis include bronchial obstruction by a mucous plug, pulmonary edema, insufficient ventilatory volumes, and compression of lung by pleural effusion, mediastinal hematoma, or a dilated heart. Blood gas study typically confirms that there is a large difference between the oxygen tension in the inspired air that enters open alveoli and that found in the arterial blood (an increased alveolar-arterial P_{O_2} gradient). To return the arterial P_{O_2} to normal, the inciting cause should be removed (suction the mucous plug, improve left ventricular function, remove compressing fluid or clot, or increase ventilatory volumes). Until the etiology can be determined and effectively treated, the hypoxemia can be lessened by raising the oxygen tensions of the inspired air. Prolonged ventilation with high percentage oxygen can be hazardous, however, as *oxygen toxicity* can result and cause further respiratory embarrassment.

One type of respiratory insufficiency seen in patients after cardiopulmonary bypass is the so-called *pump lung,* also known as *hemorrhagic atelectasis syndrome* or *respirator syndrome.* There is a marked reduction in lung distensibility, and diffusion of oxygen from alveoli to blood is impaired, again resulting in alveolar-arterial P_{O_2} gradients. Pathologically, there is interstitial edema, hemorrhage, and inflammation. Whether the syndrome is due to loss of pulmonary surfactant, to microemboli settling in small pulmonary vessels, or to some other cause is still uncertain. The early use of controlled lung inflation with high oxygen mixtures in the inspired air may reverse the process.

An important decision in the course of postoperative pulmonary management is the removal of the endotracheal or tracheostomy tube. One cannot remove abruptly the continuous ventilatory support before adequate pulmonary dynamics are assured. First, the patient is allowed short intervals (five to 10 minutes) off the respirator and breathes room air. Observation of the patient's color, ease of respiration, and ECG pattern help determine if he is ready for extubation. Further, the patient should be able to cooperate in breathing deeply and in coughing effectively. When doubt remains, further trials of 15 to 20 minutes off the respirator are conducted. If the vital signs do not change and the arterial P_{O_2} is above 60 mm Hg on room air, the patient will probably tolerate removal of his endotracheal or tracheostomy tube. Professional responsibility does not stop at this point, for the patient often feels insecure without the respiratory assistance and he must be observed closely and encouraged in the postextubation period. Hoarseness and paroxysms of coughing are common at this time. Additional intermittent support with the IPPB apparatus and with a reservoir oxygen mask are extremely useful expedients during this transition period. Reintubation (or tracheostomy) should be accomplished if there is evidence of significant hypoxemia in spite of these measures.

The prevention of respiratory complications is another important task for the cardiac nurse, as she is the person most intimately involved with the care of the patient. The maintenance of a patent airway is a prime consideration — she must suction away obstructing mucous plugs, prevent kinking of the endotracheal tube, or keep a tracheostomy tube meticulously clean. The diligence with which she exercises proper sterile technique in suctioning the patient's airway may well prevent a pulmonary infection. The oxygen supply must always be adequate; many respirators utilize the oxygen as their "driving force." Deflation of the cuff of the endotracheal or tracheostomy tube and proper inflation (just enough air injected to barely occlude the trachea) are mandatory if the serious complication of tracheal stenosis is to be avoided.

Auscultation of the chest which was once the sole province of the physician is now an integral part of the cardiac nurse's responsibility in the respiratory care of her patient. She should be able to detect atelectatic areas of the lungs, bronchospasm, pulmonary edema, or pleural effusions. Her evaluation of the auscultatory findings should guide her in her respiratory care — suctioning, encouraging the patient to cough and deep breathe, "cupping" the chest wall to free up obstructing mucous plugs, and using the IPPB apparatus. She should also be able to evaluate the clinical responses to her interventions in respiratory care.

Finally, the cardiac nurse must make a careful evaluation of her patient in terms of his needs for sedation. She should adequately alleviate pain and anxiety by judicious use of morphine or other sedatives ordered for the patient, yet must not oversedate him and depress his respiratory drive or prevent his alert cooperation. Cerebral disorientation, actual hallucinations, or obstreperous behavior are often cardinal signs of hypoxemia and should not be misinterpreted as a simple need for more sedatives.

RENAL COMPLICATIONS

When cardiac output has been poor prior to surgery or postoperatively, renal function is often compromised. Elevated levels of blood urea nitrogen and creatinine and depressed creatinine clearances are then common. Moreover, additional burdens may be added to the kidneys during the operation. Trauma to red blood cells by the pumping, oxygenation, and suction systems in the heart-lung machine cause hemolysis and many of the breakdown products are excreted in the urine. If urine flow is low or if acid hematin is formed in the renal tubules in an acid urine, renal tubular damage can result. Low cardiac output both during cardiopulmonary bypass and after the operation results in poor renal perfusion, and in combination with prolonged hypotension, predisposes to renal shutdown. Further reduction in renal blood flow is occasioned by lowered body temperatures and by the use of vasopressor agents like levarterenol, metaraminol, or epinephrine. High dosages of certain nephrotoxic antibiotic agents can also precipitate renal failure.

Postoperative monitoring of urine volumes, specific gravity, and pH allows rough estimates of renal perfusion, function, and acid-base balance. Determinations of blood urea nitrogen, serum electrolytes, and creatinine, urinary electrolytes, and urinary urea nitrogen are also used to follow the course of the renal function.

In the postoperative period, if hourly urine volumes fall below 15 to 20 cc, the possibilities of hypovolemia and low cardiac output should be investigated before treatment for renal shutdown is started. Infusion of blood or fluids while monitoring the central venous or left atrial pressures both tests for and corrects low blood volume. Ionotropic agents or rapid-acting and potent diuretics may also be useful adjuncts for increasing urine output.

If oliguria (low urine output) persists in spite of these efforts to improve urine flow, if there is a high concentration of sodium and a low concentration of urea nitrogen in the urine, if red cell casts are seen in the urinary sediment, or if serum potassium values rise above 5 to 6 mEq/L, renal failure is probably present.

Renal shutdown in the postoperative cardiac patient, as in any other patient, is treated by fluid restriction, and any administered fluids must be potassium free. The dosage of drugs excreted by the kidney is reduced or eliminated when possible. Careful monitoring of serum potassium levels is essential and the use of ion-exchange resin enemas (Kayexalate) may be used to lower serum potassium. If there is continuing fluid overload or if hyperkalemia progresses, early peritoneal dialysis or hemodialysis is indicated. If the underlying cardiac abnormality is corrected and there is improvement in cardiac output, the renal failure will usually be only transitory and the patient will survive.

Infection of the lower urinary tract can result if careful prophylactic techniques are not followed. The drainage tubing should not be disconnected from the indwelling urinary catheter, since any break in the system is a potential entry site for infecting bacteria. A closed collection system is therefore most advantageous. The urethral meatus, especially in males, should be cleansed routinely with an antiseptic solution, since it is another potential site of entry for bacterial infection.

BLEEDING COMPLICATIONS

Bleeding after cardiac surgery is commonplace and relates intimately to the care of the cardiac patient. Postoperative blood loss may be due to preexisting clotting abnormalities, to problems of surgical hemostasis (e.g., vascular suture lines), or to clotting abnormalities produced by the heart-lung machine. No matter what the cause, blood lost into the mediastinum has a direct effect on the patient's hemodynamic status; the simple blood loss may lead to hypovolemic cardiovascular collapse, while cardiac tamponade (from undrained blood clots) is a life-threatening complication.

Pre-existing clotting abnormalities are often due to a damaged liver which is unable to manufacture sufficient quantities of clotting factors, such as prothrombin, proconvertin, or fibrinogen. Chronic right heart failure commonly causes this hepatic dysfunction. Preoperative anticoagulant therapy with Coumadin (for pulmonary or systemic emboli or for prophylactic treatment because of a previously inserted valve prosthesis) can also predispose to postoperative bleeding problems.

In the operating room, every effort is made to achieve exacting surgical hemostasis in the operative area. The suture lines (closing incisions in the aorta, atria, or ventricles) are carefully inspected for bleeding points. The many small bleeders along the sternum, pericardium, and in the subcutaneous tissues are carefully coagulated. Closure of the sternotomy or thoracotomy incision is attempted only after adequate hemostasis is obtained. Often, however, a diffuse *oozing* is apparent, without any detectable specific bleeding points being identified. In large measure, this oozing is due to changes in the coagulation mechanisms brought on by the heart-lung machine.

Cardiopulmonary bypass poses some special problems to the patient's coagulation mechanisms. In order to prevent blood from clotting in the extracorporeal circuit, the patient is fully anticoagulated with heparin. At the completion of the procedure, the anticoagulant action of the administered heparin is neutralized with protamine sulfate. However, there are individual variations in the metabolism of heparin and protamine, and the reversal is sometimes inadequate. A significant decrease of circulating platelets is usually evident owing to their sequestration, dilution, and destruction; platelet counts well under 100,000 per ml are common during the bypass. Fibrinolysin titers in the blood are often elevated after cardiopulmonary bypass, causing a decrease in serum fibrinogen.

Other labile protein-bound coagulation factors (e.g., prothrombin, proconvertin, and so on) are also decreased as a result of the heart-lung bypass.

When a patient demonstrates excessive postoperative bleeding, an immediate evaluation is made. A prothrombin time is obtained to check for low levels of prothrombin in the blood. The Lee and White clotting time is performed; if it is prolonged, the heparin may have been inadequately neutralized or, conversely, there may have been a *heparin rebound.* A protamine titration test (clotting times done on a control blood sample and on blood samples with protamine added) will help determine if additional protamine is needed. A platelet count may indicate thrombocytopenia (decreased platelets). When a sample of blood is allowed to clot in a test tube and if the clot disintegrates within one to four hours, fibrinolysins are suspected. A serum fibrinogen determination showing low levels also raises the suspicion of circulating fibrinolysins.

The restoration of these abnormal coagulation factors toward normal is, in large measure, dependent upon the body's ability to manufacture them. Usually a period of four to six hours is sufficient for the bone marrow and the liver to manufacture sufficient quantities of platelets and protein-bound clotting factors, if there is no additional bleeding. However, if bleeding continues, the body may be unable to keep up with the current demands (continued bleeding) added to the deficits imposed by the heart-lung bypass.

Fresh, whole blood (the fresher the better) is the mainstay of treatment in these coagulation defects. If the blood is not freshly drawn, the labile coagulation factors will be destroyed by storage. For platelet function, the blood should be less than eight hours old; rarely are platelet concentrates necessary to reverse thrombocytopenia. Blood drawn within 24 hours is adequate for prothrombin, proconvertin, and fibrinogen. If fibrinolysins are present, epsilon-aminocaproic acid (Amicar or EACA) is administered in an attempt to restore the fibrinogen level to normal. Depressed prothrombin formation may be treated by the administration of small doses of vitamin K. Special care is required in patients with valvular prostheses, however, as the vitamin K may cause an increase in the state of coagulation (hypercoagulability), resulting in thrombus formation on the prosthesis.

If, in the absence of a recognizable coagulation abnormality, blood loss from the chest tubes continues at a rate of 200 cc per hour for four to six hours, reoperation for bleeding is indicated. The unavailability of cross-matched blood in the presence of persistent bleeding or the appearance of cardiac tamponade lends urgency to the decision to re-explore the operative area. Many times re-exploration reveals large amounts of clots, diffuse oozing, but no specific bleeding points; simple evacuation of the clots almost always stops subsequent bleeding. At other times, specific bleeding points are found, usually in high-pressure vessels like the aorta, an intercostal artery, or a coronary artery; careful suture ligation of the vessel will usually satisfactorily stem the bleeding.

COMPLICATIONS OF THE GASTROINTESTINAL TRACT

Although gastrointestinal disease is sometimes seen in cardiac patients, it is seldom a consequence of the cardiac abnormalities. Hepatic dysfunction (including cardiac cirrhosis) as a result of right heart failure and tricuspid insufficiency is a notable exception.

Postoperative gastrointestinal complications are not unusual. Gastric dilatation occurs so frequently that it is checked for routinely by abdominal examination and by portable chest films. Usually a simple in-and-out nasogastric aspiration and gentle lavage with saline will suffice. If the distension recurs, the tube should be left in the stomach and connected to intermittent suction.

The hazard of ulceration of the upper gastrointestinal tract, brought on by the stress of surgery or by underlying peptic disease, is greatly increased in patients who undergo anticoagulation for their valvular prostheses. Upper gastrointestinal bleeding can assume very significant proportions, sometimes requiring operative intervention, a highly undesirable measure in critically ill patients. Prophylactic treatment with antacids, either by mouth or through the nasogastric tube, will help to reduce this hazard.

Complications of lower sections of the gastrointestinal tract are occasionally seen. Hypertension and a necrotizing arteritis after repair of coarctation of the aorta sometimes occurs. This arteritis commonly results in a postoperative ileus lasting four to six days, and occasionally progresses to gangrene of the small and large bowel. Immediate control of the hypertensive crises with sympatholytic agents is essential in preventing this complication. Intestinal ischemia is also occasionally seen in patients whose low output state is treated by potent vasopressors. The small bowel is highly vulnerable to an abrupt decrease in mesenteric blood supply, and an acute abdominal emergency may result. The prognosis of this condition is very poor, as there may be gangrene of long segments of small bowel; extensive bowel resections in critically ill patients are poorly tolerated.

Varying degrees of hepatic dysfunction, evidenced by elevations in serum bilirubin or transaminase levels, occasionally occur in the postoperative period. Jaundice is usually detected clinically at bilirubin levels in excess of 3 mgm per cent. Serum hepatitis (from previous transfusions or needle punctures), toxic hepatitis (from certain anesthetics, phenothiazines, e.g., Thorazine, or other drugs), and poor hepatic perfusion (from low output states and the use of vasopressors) are common causes of hepatic failure. Supportive therapy with a high carbohydrate, low protein, high vitamin diet and with avoidance of salt or fluid overload is the treatment used for the milder cases. When massive hepatic necrosis occurs (with trans-aminase levels in the thousands), treatment with massive steroid support (1000 mgm of prednisone per day) may be helpful.

CENTRAL NERVOUS SYSTEM COMPLICATIONS

Postoperative cerebral dysfunction unfortunately is not a rare occurrence, but only occasionally are these complications fatal. At times, there may be only a localized deficit (a hemiparesis, for exam-ple), but generalized depression may also be seen. During the operation, mild cerebral edema can result from the extracorporeal perfusion or from the cooling and rewarming of the body (and the brain). Emboli of calcific debris, blood clot, and air are always a possibility, and are prevented only by assiduous technique. Post-operatively, the release of platelet debris, fibrin, or blood clots from prosthetic heart valves constitutes additional hazards. Treatment of these embolic phenomena is directed against cerebral edema and its complications. The use of corticosteroids, mannitol, or urea has been advocated for this purpose. Total body hypothermia between 32° and 34°C has been useful in decreasing the oxygen requirements of the brain and in reducing brain swelling. Remarkable recoveries from severe CNS deficits and restoration of cerebral function have been observed on many occasions, so that ongoing supportive therapy (mouth and skin care, prevention of decubitus ulcers, physical therapy, and so on) should not be inhibited by feelings of hopeless-ness.

Psychologic aberrations, including paranoid delusions, dis-orientation, and hallucinations, are even more frequent than organic cerebral depressions. It is thought that sleep deprivation, a wide variety of confusing sensory inputs (oscilloscope tracing, respirator noises, ECG "beepers"), and the constant, aggressive nursing care are major causative factors. Thorough preoperative education of the patient to the ICU environment has been helpful in reducing the incidence of this *postpump psychosis.* Children seem to respond to the familiar stimuli of a favorite toy, pictures of their immediate family, radio programs, or even a clock. If preoperatively the patient has met and gained confidence in the nurses who will care for him after the operation, his fears will be allayed, and consequently his postoperative course will be smoother.

Specific treatment of these psychologic syndromes revolves around gentle reassurance, attention to the patient's physical needs, mild sedation with phenothiazines, and restraints, if necessary. Often, removing the patient from the confusing, unfamiliar, and harassing ICU environment will be all that is required to eliminate the psychosis.

Bibliography

Austen, W. G., Corning, H. B., Moran, J. M., Sanders, C. A., and Scannell, J. G.: Cardiac hemodynamics immediately following aortic valve surgery. J. Thorac. Cardiovasc. Surg. *51*:461–467, 1966.

Austen, W. G., Corning, H. B., Moran, J. M., Sanders, C. A., and Scannell, J. G.: Cardiac hemodynamics immediately following mitral valve surgery. J. Thorac. Cardiovasc. Surg. *51*:468–473, 1966.

Beller, B. M., Frater, R. W. M., and Wulfsohn, N.: Cardiac pacemaking in the management of postoperative arrhythmias. Ann. Thorac. Surg. *6*:68–76, 1968.

Fisch, C., Knoebel, S. B., Feigenbaum, H., and Greenspan, K.: Potassium and the monophasic action potential, electrocardiogram conduction and arrhythmias. Progr. Cardiovasc. Dis. *8*:387–418, 1966.

Fishman, N. H., Hutchinson, J. C., and Roe, B. B.: Controlled atrial hypertension. A method for supporting cardiac output following open-heart surgery. J. Thorac. Cardiovasc. Surg. *51*:307–325, 1966.

Hazan, S. J.: Psychiatric complications following cardiac surgery. Parts I and II. J. Thorac. Cardiovasc. Surg. *51*:307–325, 1966.

Hedley-Whyte, J., Corning, H. B., Laver, M. B., Austen, W. G., and Bendixen, H. H.: Pulmonary ventilation-perfusion relations after heart valve replacement or repair in man. J. Clin. Invest. *44*:406–416, 1965.

Kirklin, J. W., and Rastelli, G. C.: Low cardiac output after open intra-cardiac operations. Progr. Cardiovasc. Dis. *10*:117–122, 1967.

McIntosh, H. D., and Morris, J. J., Jr.: The hemodynamic consequences of arrhythmias. Progr. Cardiovasc. Dis. *8*:330–363, 1966.

McQueen, J. D., and Jeanes, L. D.: Influence of hypothermia on intercranial hypertension. J. Neurosurg. *19*:277, 1962.

Mundth, E. D., and Austen, W. G.: Postoperative intensive care in the cardiac surgical patient. Progr. Cardiovasc. Dis. *11*:229–261, 1968.

Phillips, L. L., Malm, J. R., and Deterlin, R. A., Jr.: Coagulation defects following extracorporeal circulation. Ann. Surg. *157*:317–326, 1963.

Rasmussen, T., and Gulati, D. R.: Cortisone in the treatment of postoperative cerebral edema. J. Neurosurg. *19*:535, 1962.

Sanderson, R. G., Ellison, J. H., Benson, J. A., Jr., and Starr, A.: Jaundice following open-heart surgery. Ann. Surg. *165*:217–224, 1967.

Spodick, D. H.: Acute cardiac tamponade, pathologic physiology, diagnosis, and management. Progr. Cardiovasc. Dis. *10*:64–96, 1967.

Suramicz, B.: Role of electrolytes in etiology and management of cardiac arrhythmias. Progr. Cardiovasc. Dis. *8*:364–386, 1968.

Yeh, T. J., Brachrey, E. L., Hall, D. P., and Ellison, R. G.: Renal complications of open-heart surgery, predisposing factors, prevention and management. J. Thorac. Cardiovasc. Surg. *47*:79, 1964.

SECTION II

The Methods

CHAPTER 4

Electrocardiography

By THOMAS P. FORDE, M.D.

Introduction

Common to all phases of the evaluation and care of the cardiac patient is the use of the electrocardiogram as a diagnostic tool and as a moment-to-moment check on the activity of the heart. The cardiac nurse will be most concerned with electrocardiography in the monitoring of the patient in the intensive or coronary care unit. In this setting, the electrocardiogram is most often used to detect disturbances in cardiac rhythm, i.e., the arrhythmias. To function most effectively, the cardiac nurse must not only be able to appreciate the appearance of an arrhythmia, but should also be able to diagnose the more common arrhythmias, be aware of the significance of these arrhythmias in terms of their effect on cardiac function, and recognize the hazards each holds for the immediate welfare of the patient. In addition, she should be aware of the usual treatment that is applied when one of the more common arrhythmias occurs. A solid understanding of basic electrocardiography is essential to the specialist in cardiac nursing.

145

Basic Electrophysiology of the Heart

In order for the heart to function as a pump, the heart muscle must contract effectively and in an orderly and rhythmic fashion. Contraction is accomplished by means of electrical impulses which are conducted through specialized pathways in the heart, and which then spread out through the heart muscle cells themselves. The electrical impulse causes the cells to change their electrical charge from negative to positive owing to a rapid influx of sodium ions into the heart muscle cell from the fluid outside the cells (Fig. 4–1). This process, termed *depolarization,* initiates the shortening of the myocardial cells. Potassium ions then leave the cell as the process of repolarization, by which the cell returns to the resting electrical state, begins. As repolarization is completed, sodium-potassium exchange occurs across the cell membrane, the potassium re-entering the cell as the sodium is pumped out.

During the process of repolarization, a second impulse reaching the cell may be unable to initiate another depolarization; the cell is

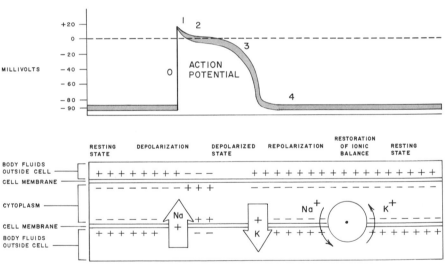

Figure 4–1. The process of depolarization and repolarization. *Above,* The action potential of a single myocardial cell. Phase 0 is the rapid depolarization of the cell from a negative charge to a slightly positive charge. Phases 1, 2, and 3 represent repolarization; during this time the cell is refractory to a second depolarization. Phases 1 and 2 are periods of absolute refractoriness; during phase 3 the cell is relatively refractory. Phase 4 is the resting phase; repolarization is complete and the cell can be depolarized by another impulse. *Below,* The ionic shifts which occur with depolarization and repolarization. Sodium ions rapidly enter the cell with depolarization; as the cell repolarizes, potassium ions leave the cell, restoring the net negative electrical charge. Ionic balance is then restored by a sodium-potassium exchange across the cell membrane. (After Netter, F. H.: The Ciba Collection of Medical Illustrations. Heart. Vol. 5. Ciba, 1969.)

then said to be refractory. Early in the repolarization cycle, the cell is completely refractory — no matter how strong the impulse, it will not cause depolarization. As repolarization progresses, the strength of the impulse required to effect depolarization decreases until the resting state is reached, at which point the susceptibility to a second depolarization is stable. It is apparent, therefore, that if a second impulse reaches an area of the conducting system through which a previous impulse has recently passed, it may not be able to depolarize the cells in this area and no further conduction of the impulse will occur, or the impulse may be conducted by a different pathway. The greater the duration of repolarization in any given cell, the longer it will be refractory to a following impulse.

Specialized conducting tissues in the heart have the capability of spontaneously depolarizing and thereby initiating an electrical impulse which then spreads to the rest of the heart muscle. The speed at which this spontaneous depolarization normally occurs is different in the various areas of the conduction system and determines the frequency with which an impulse is spontaneously generated by an area. The area of the heart which has the most rapid rate of spontaneous depolarization becomes the *dominant pacemaker,* and the impulse spreads from this area through the conducting system to the remainder of the heart.

In the normal heart, the role of dominant pacemaker belongs to the sino atrial (SA) or sinus node. This area of the heart normally has the most rapid rate of spontaneous depolarization, and the impulse generated in the sinus node normally has a rate between 60 and 100 times per minute. From the SA node, which is located high on the wall of the right atrium at its junction with the superior vena cava, the impulse travels to the atrioventricular (AV) node by means of three bundles of specialized conducting tissues (Fig. 4–2). These bundles are called the anterior, middle, and posterior internodal tracts. Another pathway, called Bachmann's bundle, carries the impulse from the SA node to the left atrium.

The AV node is situated close to the junction of the atria and ventricles on the floor of the left atrium. From the AV node, the impulse passes through the common bundle, or bundle of His, along the membranous interventricular septum. At the top of the muscular part of the interventricular septum, the common bundle divides into the right and left bundle branches, which extend beneath the endocardium of the right and left ventricular aspects of the interventricular septum, respectively. The left bundle soon divides into multiple branches which can be divided into two groups, the anterior and posterior divisions of the left bundle. As the right and left bundles extend beneath the endocardium of the ventricles peripherally, they subdivide into multiple smaller branches and form the Purkinje net-

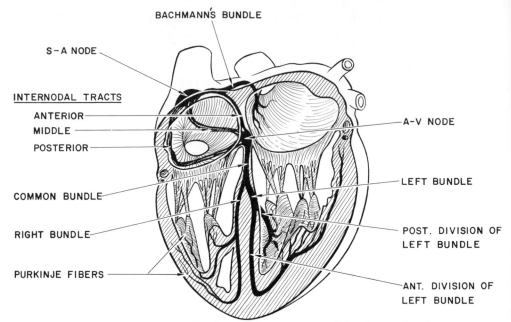

Figure 4-2. The specialized conducting tissues of the heart, showing cross sectional representation in the frontal plane. See text for explanatory details.

work of fibers, which extend a variable distance into the ventricular walls and are in continuity with the ventricular muscle fibers.

Normal conduction then consists of an impulse arising in the SA node, spreading through the atria by means of Bachmann's bundle and the internodal tracts, with depolarization of the atria as the impulse travels to the AV node. Conduction through the AV node is slow; the impulse then emerges in the common bundle and spreads via the right and left bundles to the ventricles, which are then depolarized.

The Electrocardiogram

The sum of the changes in electrical charge occurring in the many individual cells of the heart gives rise to an electrical voltage which can be recorded at the surface of the body, and this is what is recorded by the electrocardiogram. It is important to note that only the changes in voltage generated by the heart muscle cells in the atria and ventricles can be detected by the body surface electrocardiogram; the changes in voltage of the specialized conducting tissues—the SA node, the intranodal pathways, the AV node, the bundle of His, the right and left bundle branches, and the Purkinje network—are not of sufficient magnitude to be recorded at the body surface.

Thus, the normal electrocardiographic tracing of an electrical cycle or heart beat consists of a number of deflections which are representative of the electrical events as they occur within the heart, and these deflections have been assigned arbitrary designations (Fig. 4–3).

As mentioned before, the depolarization of the SA node is not recorded at the body surface and the electrocardiographic tracing is flat or *isoelectric* during this event. Then there follows depolarization of the atria, which is represented by the P wave. Following the P wave, the electrocardiographic tracing again becomes flat or isoelectric, as the impulse travels through the AV node and bundle of His out to the ventricular myocardium. Then another deflection appears, designated the *QRS complex,* which represents the depolarization of the ventricles. This complex is followed by another brief period when the electrocardiogram is isoelectric and then repolarization of the ventricles is recorded as the *T wave.* Ordinarily, atrial repolarization is not recorded as a separate deflection, as it is lost in the large QRS complex. Occasionally, following the T wave,

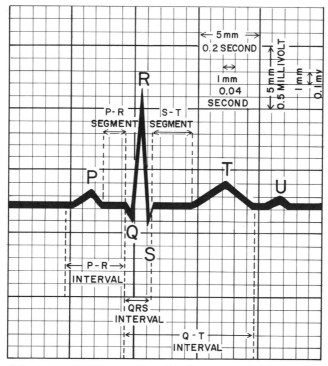

Figure 4–3. Normal ECG complex. The designations of the various deflections and intervals are indicated. The complex is superimposed on the standard electrocardiographic paper at customary amplitude (1 mm = 0.1 mv) and paper speed (25 mm per sec).

another deflection called the *U wave* is recorded. The origin of the U wave is not well understood.

The isoelectric interval from the *end* of the P wave to the *beginning* of the QRS complex is termed the *PR segment*. The interval from the *beginning* of the P wave to the *beginning* of the QRS complex, i.e., the P wave plus the PR segment, is called the *PR interval*. The QRS complex may consist of a number of positive (upward) or negative (downward) deflections in any particular electrocardiographic lead. The initial negative deflection, if present, is termed the *Q wave*; the initial positive deflection is termed the *R wave*. If a negative deflection follows the R wave, it is termed the *S wave*. If a second positive deflection occurs it is denoted as R′ (R prime). Following the QRS complex, the normally isoelectric segment before the T wave is termed the *ST segment*. The interval from the *beginning* of the QRS complex to the *end* of the T wave is called the *QT interval*.

By convention, the terms used to designate the various deflections and intervals are written in capital letters. Often, in attempting to describe in writing the form of the QRS complex, small letters are used to describe the deflections of small magnitude and capital letters are used to describe the major deflections (Fig. 4–4).

In order to standardize the recording of the electrical potential

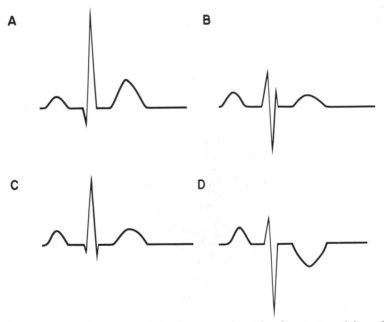

Figure 4–4. Various forms of the QRS complex. The description of these forms, indicating the amplitude of the deflections, would be as follows: A, qR; B, RSr′; C, qRs; and D, rS.

of the heart at the body surface, a number of conventions have been adopted. The paper on which the electrocardiogram is recorded is run at a standard speed, usually 25 mm per sec so that the time duration of the various deflections and intervals can be measured and compared. The paper is therefore ruled in 1 mm and darker 5 mm spaced lines, both horizontally and vertically. The vertical lines will then represent time intervals, the space between each 1 mm vertical line representing 0.04 seconds and the space between each 5 mm vertical line representing 0.2 seconds.

The heart rate can thus be determined by measuring the time between two successive QRS complexes—the *R-R interval*—provided the rhythm is regular. The duration of the various components of each cycle can also be measured and compared to normal values. In adults, the normal values for the most commonly measured variables are: PR interval, 0.12 to 0.20 seconds, and QRS complex, 0.06 to 0.10 seconds.

The QT interval varies with changes in heart rate, increasing as the heart rate decreases. Normal values for the QT interval must be related to the heart rate or R-R interval. These values can be obtained from a table of normal QT intervals for different heart rates, or calculated from the formula:

$$QTc = \frac{QT}{\sqrt{R\text{-}R}}$$

where QTc is the "corrected" QT interval, and QT is the measured interval. Upper limits of normal for the QTc have been estimated by various authors to be between 0.425 and 0.445 seconds.

Vector Concepts

Thus far, we have considered the electrocardiogram as recording electrical voltages as related to time. In addition, the electrical voltage has two other dimensions—direction and amplitude.

As the electrical waves of depolarization and repolarization spread through the heart, the sum of the electrical voltages which is recorded by the electrocardiogram at any given time will proceed in a given direction. The direction of this net voltage in space is termed the *cardiac vector*.

The direction of the waves of depolarization and repolarization (the P, QRS, and T vectors) is three-dimensional. In order to determine them by means of electrodes at the surface of the body, a number of different vantage points or leads are used in recording the

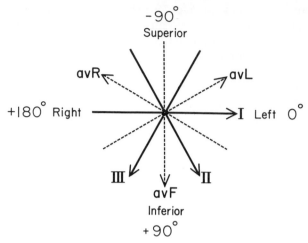

Figure 4–5. The limb leads. The six limb leads detect the direction of the electrical impulses in the frontal plane—right, left, superior, and inferior. The orientation of these leads in the frontal plane is indicated. The arrow heads indicate the positive pole of each lead. The direction of an impulse in this plane can be denoted in terms of the number of degrees of the angle which it makes with the lead I axis. Clockwise from lead I is positive, counterclockwise is negative.

standard electrocardiogram. Each lead is oriented in a different direction, and has a positive and a negative pole. As the electrical impulse approaches the positive pole of any given lead, an upright or positive deflection is recorded; as the impulse goes away from the positive pole, a negative deflection is recorded. If the impulse is traveling perpendicular to this particular lead, i.e., neither approaching it nor going away from it, no deflection is recorded and the lead is flat or isoelectric at that moment.

The routine electrocardiogram consists of 12 leads. There are six limb leads, which are the *frontal plane leads*; i.e., they detect the direction of the electrical impulse as it travels in the frontal plane — right and left, superior and inferior (Fig. 4–5). There are also six precordial leads, which detect the direction of the electrical impulse as it travels in the *horizontal plane*, i.e., right and left, anterior and posterior (Fig. 4–6).

Let us review the sequence of normal depolarization. As the impulse leaves the SA node, the atria begin to depolarize, the wave of depolarization spreading from the area of the SA node through both atria in a leftward, inferior, and anterior direction and the P wave vector will have this direction. Looking at our frontal plane leads (Fig. 4–7) the leftward and inferior direction of the P wave will result in positive P waves in leads I, II, III, and avF. It will be almost perpendicular to avL, and, therefore, may be flat, or slightly positive or negative in this lead. It will be negative in avR.

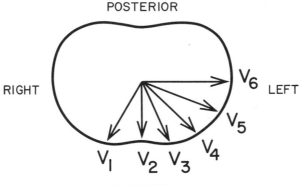

Figure 4–6. The unipolar limb leads. Leads V_1 to V_6 detect the direction of the electrical impulses in the horizontal plane—right, left, anterior, and posterior. The orientation of these leads in the horizontal plane is indicated. The arrowheads denote the positive pole of each lead.

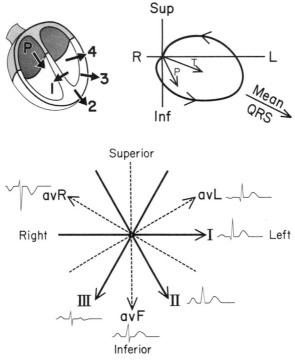

Figure 4–7. Sequence of depolarization in the frontal plane. *Upper left,* Schematic frontal plane cross section of the heart. P represents the net direction of atrial depolarization. Arrows 1, 2, 3, and 4 represent the sequence of changes in the net direction of the QRS vector. *Upper right,* Depiction of the mean P, QRS, and T vectors and the sequence of ventricular depolarization (QRS vector loop) in the frontal plane. *Below,* The P, QRS, and T vectors as recorded by the frontal plane leads. See text for details.

The precordial or horizontal plane leads view the heart from the anterior (V₁–V₃) and then from progressively more left lateral (V₄–V₆) vantage points. The P wave vector being left and anterior will be positive in all these leads (Fig. 4–8).

The impulse that has been conducted from the SA node via the internodal tracts to the AV node reaches the bundle of His after a delay in the AV node. It then spreads to the ventricular muscle by means of the right and left bundle branches and the Purkinje system. Normally, the first part of the ventricular muscle which is depolarized is the interventricular septum, and this depolarization gives rise to the initial part of the QRS complex. Depolarization of the interventricular septum commonly occurs from left to right, inferiorly and anteriorly. In the frontal plane leads (Fig. 4–7), this rightward and inferior vector will result in a small negative deflection, or Q wave, in leads I and avL, and positive deflections or R waves in the other leads. The initial QRS vector in the horizontal plane will be to the right and anterior, giving rise to an initial positive deflection or R wave in the

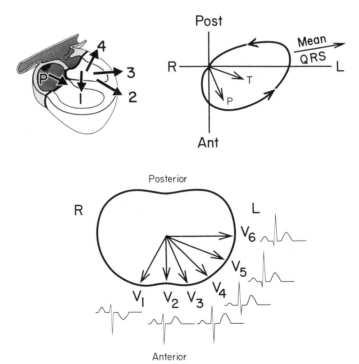

Figure 4–8. Sequence of depolarization in the horizontal plane. *Upper left,* Schematic horizontal plane cross section of the heart. P represents the net direction of atrial depolarization. Arrows 1, 2, 3, and 4 represent the sequence of changes in the net direction of the QRS vector. *Upper right,* Depiction of the mean P, QRS, and T vectors and the sequence of ventricular depolarization (QRS vector loop) in the horizontal plane. *Below,* The P, QRS, and T vectors as recorded by the horizontal plane leads. See text for details.

anterior leads (V_1–V_3) (Fig. 4–8). A small initial Q wave may be inscribed in the more lateral leads (V_4–V_6).

After depolarization of the interventricular septum has begun, both ventricles depolarize simultaneously. The left ventricle, having the greatest bulk of myocardium, contributes the greater share of the net voltage and determines the net direction of the remainder of the QRS vector. Depolarization of the left ventricle occurs first left and inferior and anterior, then continuing leftward the wave of depolarization swings posteriorly and perhaps slightly superiorly.

Looking at our frontal plane leads (Fig. 4–7) after septal depolarization and as the QRS vector swings to the left and inferiorly, an R wave will appear on leads I and avL and an S wave in avR. Continuing to the left, the QRS vector may then swing slightly superiorly with inscription of S waves in leads III and avF (and possibly lead II) before returning to the baseline.

In the horizontal plane (Fig. 4–8) as the QRS vector swings leftward and anteriorly, R waves will be present on all the precordial leads. Finally, as the vector, continuing leftward, swings posteriorly, S waves will appear in the more anterior leads (V_1–V_3), while the more lateral leads (V_4–V_6) will record progressively taller R waves before returning to the baseline.

We have just described the moment-to-moment, or instantaneous QRS vectors in the normal heart. There is some variation among normal hearts, however, in the direction of the instantaneous QRS vector, especially in the frontal plane. The wave of depolarization may spread in a clockwise fashion, rather than in the counterclockwise direction described. Nevertheless, the resultant of these instantaneous vectors, i.e., the predominant direction of the net QRS vector, will be similar. The predominant direction of the QRS vector is called the *mean QRS vector*; normally it is to the left, inferior, and somewhat posterior (Figs. 4–7 and 4–8).

The wave of ventricular repolarization, or T wave, also has a direction or vector. Normally, this vector is very similar to the mean QRS vector, i.e., leftward, inferiorly, and posteriorly. In the frontal plane (Fig. 4–7), the leftward and inferior T vector will result in a T wave which is positive (upright) in leads I, II, and avF, and negative in avR. The T wave may be positive, flat, or negative in leads III and avL. In the horizontal plane, the T wave, being leftward and posterior, is generally upright from V_2 through V_6, and may be upright or inverted in V_1 (Fig. 4–8).

Other Lead Systems

Mention should be made of the availability of other lead systems in addition to the standard electrocardiogram. Vectorcardiographic lead systems have been developed which can give a better representation of the instantaneous vectors in three dimensions, and which picture the vectors as loops rather than merely positive and negative deflections.

Special leads are often of value when the P waves are not well seen in the standard electrocardiogram. These leads include the Lewis lead (which is taken with the right and left arm electrodes on the right and left sides of the anterior chest), the esophageal lead (which the patient swallows), and the intra-atrial lead (which is a lead passed via an arm vein directly into the right atrium).

In many coronary and intensive care units, electrocardiographic monitoring is accomplished by means of a simple bipolar chest lead, which consists of positive and negative electrodes and a ground electrode. Often the positions of electrode placement are chosen quite arbitrarily; however, many units favor the *modified chest lead I* (MCLI) configuration because of its superiority in detecting diagnostically important changes in QRS configuration, and because it leaves the left precordium unobstructed for physical examination of the heart and the application of counter shock. This lead approximates the precordial lead V_1 and is obtained by placing the positive electrode in the V_1 position (fourth right interspace at the right sternal border) and the negative electrode near the left shoulder. The ground electrode is usually placed near the right shoulder.

Myocardial Infarction

When a patient suffers an acute myocardial infarction, the blood supply to a specific area of the ventricular myocardium is lost. Deprived of oxygen and nutrients, the myocardial cells in the affected area become acutely ischemic, and then undergo necrosis. Subsequently, the infarcted area is invaded by inflammatory cells and eventually fibrous tissue is laid down with the formation of a fibrous scar.

This chain of pathologic events is mirrored in a series of abnormalities in the electrocardiogram, which allows us to diagnose the occurrence of a myocardial infarction, and also to localize the area of the ventricular muscle involved. It must be remembered, however, that not all patients suffering a myocardial infarction will develop the classic electrocardiographic pattern. In some, the full sequence of events may take place rapidly and may not be observed in sequential routine electrocardiograms. In others, the infarction may not involve the entire thickness of the ventricular wall; i.e., it may not be "transmural," and the complete electrocardiographic pattern may not develop. In still others, the classic pattern may be obscured by other electrocardiographic abnormalities, such as previous infarctions and conduction disturbances.

With the development of the initial acute ischemia in an area of the myocardium, the first change that is seen is elevation of the ST segment, often accompanied by "peaking" of the T wave. This pattern is often termed the *current of injury.* The ST segment, normally isoelectric or flat in all leads, should have no net direction or vector. With the development of the current of injury, the ST segment elevation now allows us to determine an ST segment vector. The ST segment will be positive, i.e., elevated, in those leads whose positive poles point to the area of infarction; the ST vector is, therefore, *toward* the area of infarction.

Following the development of ST segment elevation, T wave abnormalities develop. The mean T wave vector changes so that it has an abnormal direction, and this direction is *away from* the area of infarction.

Subsequently, with the necrosis of the myocardial tissue, there is a change in the instantaneous QRS vector. The necrotic tissue is no longer electrically active, and depolarization of the involved area is no longer reflected in the surface electrocardiogram. The result is a loss of initial positive QRS forces in the area of infarction (the initial QRS vector will point *away from* the area of infarction, giving rise to abnormal initial negative deflections or Q waves in the leads whose positive poles point to the area of infarction). In the standard electrocardiogram, these pathologic Q waves generally have a duration of 0.04 seconds or greater.

Consider then, the sequence of electrocardiographic events which might occur in a patient with an acute infarction involving the inferior, or diaphragmatic, surface of the heart. The first change would be the development of an ST vector pointing *toward* the infarcted area or inferiorly, giving rise to ST segment elevations in the leads whose positive poles are inferior (leads II, III, and avF). There may be reciprocal ST segment depression in the other frontal plane leads. Then the T vector changes so that it points in an abnormal direction and *away from* the area of infarction; it is no longer left and inferior, but is now left and superior. This change will result in T wave inversion in the leads whose positive poles face the infarction (leads II, III, and avF). Finally, the initial QRS forces will point away from the area of infarction, i.e., the initial QRS forces will be superior rather than inferior and pathologic Q waves will be seen in leads II, III, and avF.

Other areas in which a myocardial infarction commonly takes place are the anterior and anterolateral walls of the left ventricle, and the same sequence of changes described before will be seen in the electrocardiographic leads which have their positive poles oriented toward the area of infarction. In an anterior infarction, the anterior leads in the horizontal plane, leads V_1 to V_4, will be affected (Fig. 4–9). In an anterolateral wall infarction, the leads in the frontal plane which are orientated toward the left lateral wall, leads I and avL, and the lateral leads in the horizontal plane, leads V_4 to V_6, will be affected.

With healing and scarring of the area of myocardial infarction, the abnormal ST segment vector usually returns to normal. Often, the abnormal T vector also returns to normal. The abnormal initial QRS vector, however, may persist permanently, reflecting the fact that in the area of the infarction the functioning myocardial cells have been replaced by a fibrous scar.

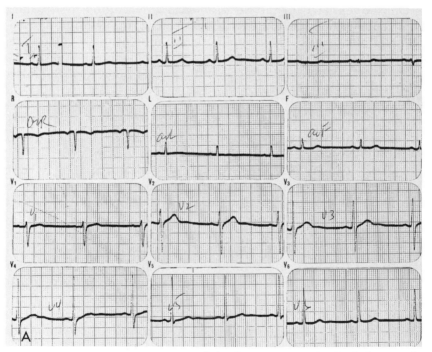

Figure 4–9. Acute anterior myocardial infarction. A, Twelve lead electrocardiogram prior to myocardial infarction. Slight ST segment and T wave abnormalities are present. B, Electrocardiogram taken shortly after the onset of chest pain. Note the ST segment elevation present in lead avL and strikingly apparent in leads V_1 to V_5. Reciprocal ST segment depression has occurred in leads I, II, and avF. C, Electrocardiogram taken later that same day. T wave inversion has now occurred in leads V_1 to V_4, and the ST segments are returning toward the baseline.

(Illustration continued on opposite page.)

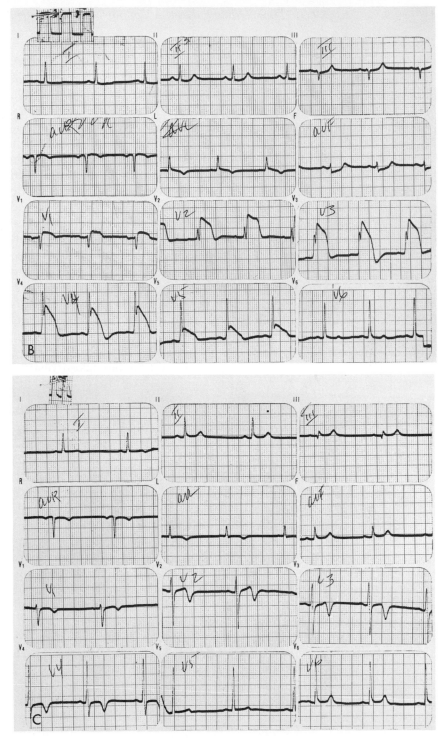

Figure 4-9. Continued.

Myocardial Ischemia

If the demand of the heart for oxygen exceeds the supply available to it through diseased coronary arteries, ischemia of the myocardial cells occurs. Often this ischemia is transient, as when a patient exerts himself and brings on the clinical syndrome of angina pectoris. Usually, such ischemia is not limited to a single geographic area of the heart, but diffusely involves the subendocardium of the left ventricle. The electrocardiographic pattern which is seen with such episodes of ischemia consists of generalized ST segment depression, which reverts toward normal if the ischemia is relieved. Rarely, in the variant type of angina pectoris (Prinzmetal angina), there is marked ST segment elevation, giving rise to an ST segment vector which points *toward* a specific area of the heart. This electrocardiographic pattern is indistinguishable from that of the ST segment elevation of an acute myocardial infarction involving the area of the heart toward which the ST segment vector points. The distinction can be made only after the ischemic pain subsides, at which time the electrocardiogram rapidly returns to the preangina tracing with variant angina, but develops the usual evolutionary pattern of myocardial infarction when an actual infarction has taken place.

Myocardial Hypertrophy

If one of the chambers of the heart is subjected to an excessive workload, one of the means by which it responds to this load is by hypertrophy — an enlargement of the heart muscle cells. For example, in a patient with hypertension or aortic stenosis, if the left ventricle is subjected to an increased pressure load, it must generate a greater than normal systolic pressure. In a patient with aortic insufficiency, the left ventricle must handle a greater than normal volume because of the regurgitant flow through the incompetent valve, and is subjected to volume overload. Similarly, in a patient with mitral insufficiency, both the left ventricle and left atrium are subjected to volume overload. In all these situations, the affected chamber hypertrophies. The increase in the mass of the chamber wall is reflected in the electrocardiogram.

The electrocardiographic changes in hypertrophy include an increase in the amplitude and duration of the electrical forces. Previously, it was mentioned that the electrocardiogram has been standardized as to the speed of recording, so that the vertical lines represent specific time intervals. Similarly, the electrocardiogram is standardized as to the amplitude of the deflections. This is accomplished by introducing a standardization signal of known electrical potential (1 mv) and adjusting the deflection obtained to 10 mm on the ECG paper. Thus, each 1 mm horizontal line on the ECG paper represents an electrical force of 0.1 mv, and any electrocardiogram can then be compared to normal standards for amplitude.

ATRIAL HYPERTROPHY

Hypertrophy of the atria leads to electrocardiographic abnormalities in the P wave. In right atrial hypertrophy or enlargement, the P wave becomes tall and peaked, exceeding 2.5 mm in height. In left atrial hypertrophy, there is a delay in conduction through the left atrium. This results in a P wave that is prolonged to 0.12 seconds or greater; often it is bifid (shows a double hump) in the frontal plane leads. In the horizontal plane, the terminal vector of the P wave is directed posteriorly, resulting in a biphasic P wave deflection in V_1, initially positive, then negative.

VENTRICULAR HYPERTROPHY

Hypertrophy of either of the ventricles results in an increase in the electrical voltage generated by that ventricle. This change in voltage is reflected in the QRS complex of the electrocardiogram by an increase in its amplitude and often by a change in the QRS vector.

In right ventricular hypertrophy (Fig. 4–10), the normal predominance of left ventricular depolarization in determining the magnitude and direction of the QRS vector is modified by an increase in the electrical potential arising from the right ventricle. Since depolarization of the right ventricle occurs to the right and anteriorly, in the frontal plane the presence of right ventricular hypertrophy causes the QRS vector to shift rightward; in the horizontal plane, there is an increase in the anterior forces.

In left ventricular hypertrophy (Fig. 4–11), there is an increase in the amplitude of the normally predominant leftward forces and the QRS vector becomes more posterior in orientation. In the frontal plane, this results in increased amplitude of the positive deflections in those leads with positive poles to the left, i.e., leads I and avL, and an increased negative deflection in those leads with positive poles to the right, i.e., leads III and avR. In the horizontal plane, there is an increase in left lateral and posterior forces, often with some loss of anterior forces. There is, therefore, an increase in the amplitude of the S wave in the anterior precordial leads V_1 through

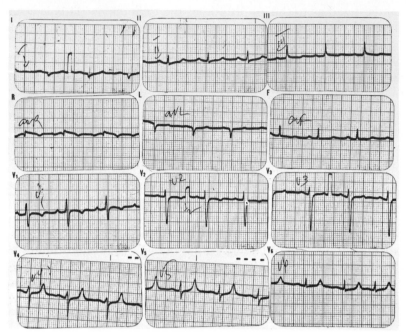

Figure 4–10. Right ventricular hypertrophy. In the frontal plane, the mean QRS vector has shifted to the right of +90 degrees, with an rS complex in lead I. In the horizontal plane there is an increase in anterior forces, with prominent R waves in leads V_1 and V_2 (lead V_2 taken at one half standardization). Prominent S waves extend to lead V_5.

V_3, often with the diminution of the R wave in these leads. The amplitude of the R wave in the lateral precordial leads, V_4 through V_6, increases.

With progression of ventricular hypertrophy, ST segment and T wave abnormalities appear and their vectors are pointed in a direction opposite to the QRS forces generated by the hypertrophied ventricle. In right ventricular hypertrophy, the abnormal ST segment and T wave vectors are directed posteriorly, resulting in ST segment depression and inverted T waves in the anterior precordial leads, V_1 through V_3. In left ventricular hypertrophy, the abnormal ST segment and T wave vectors are directed anteriorly and to the right, resulting in ST segment depression and inverted T waves in leads I, avL, and the lateral precordial leads, V_4 through V_6.

Various criteria for the electrocardiographic diagnosis of ventricular hypertrophy have been evolved, but the accuracy of these criteria is far from perfect. Some criteria are relatively sensitive in detecting early ventricular hypertrophy, but are not very specific; i.e., too many normals are included as "false positives." Other criteria are very specific (few "false positives" are included) but are insensitive, detecting only gross degrees of hypertrophy.

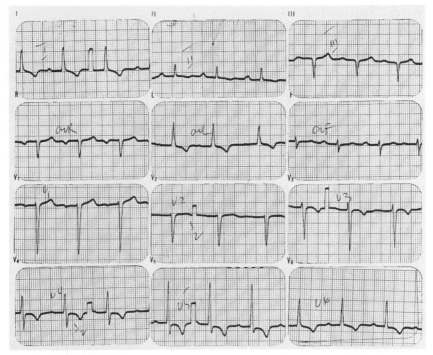

Figure 4–11. Left ventricular hypertrophy. In the frontal plane, there is increased amplitude of leftward QRS forces. R avL equals 11 mm. ST segment depression and T wave inversion are present in leads I, II, and avL, and the T wave in avR has become upright. In the horizontal plane, the increased posterior forces are evident. S V₁ plus R V₅ equals 48 mm. ST segment depression and T wave inversion are present in leads V₃ to V₆. (Leads V₂ and V₄ are one half standardization). First degree atrioventricular block is also present. (PR interval equals 0.28 seconds.)

Commonly employed criteria for right ventricular hypertrophy include the following:

1. Right axis deviation of the mean QRS vector in the absence of a ventricular conduction defect.

2. An R or R¹ in V₁ of 5 mm or more, with a ratio of R wave amplitude to S wave amplitude of V₁ of 1.0 or greater.

3. Persistence of large S waves in the left lateral precordial leads (V₅ and V₆).

For left ventricular hypertrophy, many sets of criteria and scoring systems have been employed. In common use are the following:

1. The sum of the R wave in lead I and the S wave in lead III is 25 mm or greater.

2. The R wave in lead avL is 11 mm or greater.

3. The sum of the R wave in lead V₁ and the S wave in V₅ or V₆ is 35 mm or greater.

The Arrhythmias

Detection and diagnosis of disturbances in cardiac rhythm are usually the prime purposes of electrocardiographic monitoring of the cardiac patient. It must be realized however, that although a rhythm disturbance can be rapidly detected with a monitoring system, the analysis of the exact type of arrhythmia may often require a write-out of the monitor pattern on electrocardiographic recording paper. Sometimes interpretation of the arrhythmia may require the recording of a conventional 12-lead electrocardiogram or even the use of specialized leads. Indeed, even then, some arrhythmias may be quite difficult, if not impossible, for even the most experienced of electrocardiographers to diagnose.

Nevertheless, the vast majority of arrhythmias which occur can, with some experience, be readily interpreted. A systematic approach to the arrhythmia is essential.

Differential diagnosis of the arrhythmias is facilitated if the electrocardiogram is examined for four specific points:

1. **The QRS complex.** Is it normal in configuration and duration; does it resemble the complex recorded when the patient was in normal sinus rhythm?

In general, if the pacemaker of any given heart beat arises in the ventricles, the QRS complex will be widened and deformed. If the impulse is normal in configuration and duration, it arises above the ventricle and is supraventricular in origin.

In some instances, however, supraventricular beats will have a deformed and widened QRS complex. This configuration may be due to a preceding conduction disturbance, such as bundle branch block, or may occur if the supraventricular beat is abnormally conducted through the ventricle. This *aberrant conduction* may occur if the supraventricular beat follows the previous beat at an interval which is so short that all the conduction pathways in the ventricle have not yet fully repolarized and some are therefore refractory to being depolarized again.

2. **The P waves.** Can P waves be seen? Do they appear similar to those present when the patient was in normal sinus rhythm? How many P waves are present for every QRS complex, and is their relation to the QRS complex constant or changing? Are there any P waves hidden in the QRS complex or in the T waves? What is the PR interval?

3. **Rate.** What is the rate of the P waves and of the QRS complexes: is the arrhythmia a tachycardia (rate greater than 100) or a bradycardia (rate less than 60)?

4. **Rhythm.** Is the rhythm perfectly regular, slightly irregular, or grossly irregular? Determine this for both the P waves and the QRS complexes.

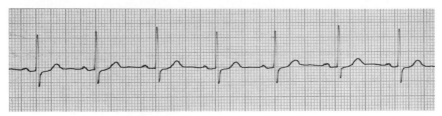

Figure 4–12. Normal sinus rhythm at a rate of 75 per minute.

NORMAL SINUS RHYTHM (Fig. 4–12)

Applying the above approach to normal sinus rhythm it will be noted that (1) the QRS complex is normal in configuration and duration; (2) the P waves are visible, have a normal appearance and a normal vector, and have a constant 1:1 relationship to the QRS complexes. The PR interval is normal (0.12 to 0.20 second) and does not vary. (3) The rate is between 60 and 100 beats per minute and (4) the rhythm is basically regular, although there might be a slight variation in the R-R and P-P intervals from beat to beat.

PREMATURE BEATS

Premature beats are beats which occur early, i.e., before the next beat of the underlying basic rhythm would be expected to occur. They may occur singly, may follow every normal beat (bigeminy) or every two normal beats (trigeminy), or may appear without a discernible pattern. A number of premature beats may occur in succession; if three or more do occur in succession, a brief run of tachycardia arising from that focus may be said to be present.

Premature beats may arise from any of the specialized conduction tissues of the heart—in the atria, around the AV node, and in the conduction pathways in the ventricles. The varieties of premature beats are therefore three: atrial, nodal or junctional, and ventricular.

Atrial Premature Beats (APB, APC, PAC) (Figs. 4–13 to 4–16)

These beats arise in the specialized conducting tissues of the atria. From here the impulse spreads through the atria and the AV node to the ventricles (antegrade conduction) and also up to depolarize the sinus node (retrograde conduction).

The QRS complex is usually normal in configuration and duration; however, an early APB may be aberrantly conducted through the ventricle, giving rise to a widened, deformed QRS complex.

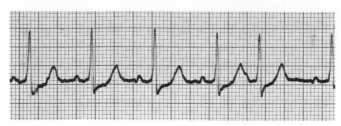

Figure 4–13. Atrial premature beat. The fifth complex is an APB. Note the premature P wave on the downslope of the preceding T wave.

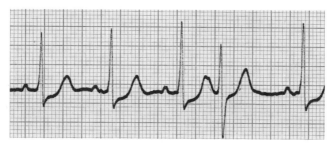

Figure 4–14. Atrial premature beats with aberrant conduction. The fourth complex is an APB. The premature P wave occurs just following the peak of the preceding T wave. The QRS complex is deformed owing to aberrant conduction through the ventricles.

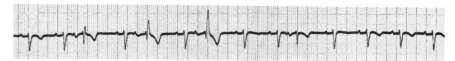

Figure 4–15. Atrial premature beats with aberrant conduction (lead V₁). The third, fifth, and seventh complexes are APB's with varying degrees of aberrant conduction. The tenth complex is also an APB; intraventricular conduction is almost normal.

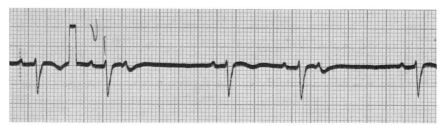

Figure 4–16. Blocked atrial premature beats (lead V₁). Premature P waves are present following the second and fourth QRS complexes. Because the AV node is still refractory to conduction after the preceding sinus beat, the atrial impulse is not conducted to the ventricles. Similarly, the retrograde atrial impulse fails to depolarize the sinus node, which then fires at the usual time. The result is a compensatory pause.

The P wave is usually visible, but different in configuration from the normal sinus P wave because of a different vector; the PR interval is normal. The regularity of the normal sinus rhythm is interrupted by the premature beat, and then sinus rhythm is resumed. The pause after an APB before the next sinus beat usually approximates the sinus P-P interval, measuring from the P wave of the APB to the next sinus P. This is termed a *noncompensatory pause,* and is due to the sinus node "resetting" when it is depolarized by the retrograde impulse from the atrial pacemaker. Occasionally, a full *compensatory pause* occurs; the interval from the P wave of the sinus beat preceding the APB to the succeeding sinus beat is equal to twice the normal sinus P-P interval. This pause occurs when the retrograde atrial impulse fails to depolarize the sinus node, which then fires at the usual time. However, since the atria have just been depolarized by the premature beat, the sinus impulse is not conducted through the atria. The regularity of the underlying sinus rhythm is therefore unaffected.

AV Nodal (Junctional) Premature Beats (NPB, NPC, PNC) *(Fig. 4–17)*

These premature beats arise in the conducting tissues around the AV node and in the bundle of His. The impulse travels antegrade to depolarize the ventricles and retrograde to depolarize the atria and the sinus node.

The QRS complex is usually normal in configuration and duration; however, aberrant conduction may occur.

The P wave may be visible just preceding or just following the QRS complex, or it may occur simultaneously with the QRS complex and be therefore hidden or "buried" in it. The relation of the P wave to the QRS complex depends on the sequence of the antegrade and

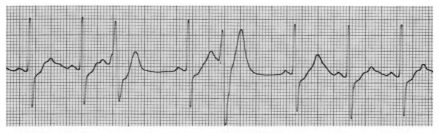

Figure 4–17. Junctional premature beats with aberrant conduction. The third and fifth QRS complexes are junctional premature beats with aberrant conduction and compensatory pauses. No P waves are visible. These beats are very difficult to distinguish from ventricular premature beats.

retrograde conduction—whether the atria are depolarized before the ventricles, or vice versa, or whether both are depolarized simultaneously. The P wave, when visible, is different in configuration from the normal sinus P wave because of its different vector. If the P wave precedes the QRS complex, the PR interval is abnormally short, allowing for differentiation from an APB.

The regularity of the normal sinus rhythm is interrupted by the premature beat; the pause after the premature beat may be noncompensatory, with the sinus pacemaker resetting when it is depolarized by the retrograde atrial depolarization. A fully compensatory pause can occur when the sinus pacemaker is not depolarized by the retrograde impulse.

Ventricular Premature Beats (VPB, VPC, PVC) (Figs. 4–18 to 4–20)

These premature beats may arise anywhere in the conducting tissues of the ventricles—the right and left bundle branches or the ramifications of the Purkinje system.

The QRS complex is wide and distorted and does not resemble the normal supraventricular complex. As a rule, the VPB tends to have more aberrant conduction in the ventricle opposite the one in which they arise, in which the normal conduction pathways are followed to some extent. Thus, VPBs arising in the left ventricle tend to have a right bundle branch block pattern and vice versa.

The P wave may or may not be visible. Since depolarization of the ventricles precedes retrograde depolarization of the atria and the sinus node, the P wave usually follows the QRS complex or is buried in it. Often if the basic rhythm is sinus, the sinus node fires normally and may depolarize the atria before the retrograde impulse from the ventricle passes back through the AV node. In this situation, both impulses may meet in the region of the AV node; and since the tissue through which they have just passed is now refractory, each impulse blocks the further conduction of the impulse from the opposite direction.

If the VPB occurs late in the cycle, after the sinus node has depolarized the atria but before the sinus impulse reaches the ventricle, a *fusion beat* occurs. A fusion beat is characterized by a normally appearing P wave which is "on time," followed by a wide, bizarre QRS complex which comes early as compared to the previous R-R intervals. The PR interval is therefore shorter than expected.

Unlike atrial and junctional premature beats, which usually occur in a setting of normal sinus rhythm, ventricular premature beats often occur in the setting of another arrhythmia.

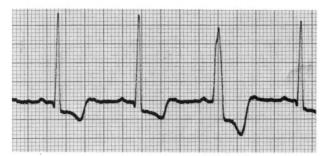

Figure 4–18. Fusion beat. The third complex is a fusion beat. The P wave is "on time" and represents atrial depolarization by a normal sinus impulse. The QRS complex is premature and represents ventricular depolarization partially due to a VPB and partially due to the normal antegrade conduction of the sinus impulse. Note the shorter PR interval.

The rate and rhythm is that of the basic underlying rhythm. If the basic rhythm is sinus and the sinus node is not depolarized by retrograde conduction from the VPB, a fully compensatory pause will occur; this is the most common situation. Occasionally, however, a noncompensatory pause may occur, especially if the underlying sinus rate is slow, allowing retrograde conduction to depolarize the sinus node and "resetting" the sinus node. Rarely, "interpolated" VPBs may occur. In this situation, the VPB occurs between two normal sinus beats, both of which are normally conducted. This can occur when the retrograde conduction from the VPB is blocked by refractory tissue above the ventricles, yet the normal sinus beat following shortly thereafter experiences normal antegrade conduction.

If VPBs occur frequently, they may be seen to all be of the same configuration, and the inference is that they all arise from the same area of pacemaker tissue in the ventricle, in which case they are termed *unifocal.* Alternatively, they may have two or more different configurations, implying different origins and are therefore said to be *multifocal.* The interval from the preceding R wave to the VPB may be constant, in which case "fixed coupling" is said to be present, or the coupling interval may vary.

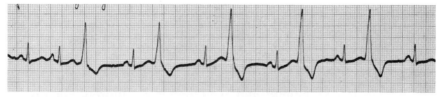

Figure 4–19. Ventricular premature beats in bigeminy. The VPBs are unifocal and show fixed coupling. The second complex may be an APB; note that the P wave is different in configuration from the P waves of the normal sinus beats.

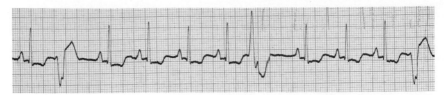

Figure 4-20. Multifocal ventricular premature beats. The second and eleventh beats represent VPBs from the same focus; their configurations and coupling intervals are the same. The seventh beat is a VPB from another focus, with a different configuration and coupling interval. The P wave visible on the ST segment of this beat is "on time": the atria has been depolarized by the normally occurring sinus beat before the retrograde impulse from the VPB has traversed the AV node. The antegrade impulse from the sinus beat is then blocked from reaching the ventricles by the refractory AV node.

In the patient with an acute myocardial infarction, the hazard of developing ventricular tachycardia and subsequent ventricular fibrillation is most marked if the R wave of the VPB falls on the T wave of the preceding beat (*R-on-T phenomenon*) (see Fig. 4–45). VPBs with fixed coupling and a short coupling interval may fall at this dangerous time and are therefore more hazardous than those with a longer coupling interval. Similarly, VPBs with varying coupling intervals and multifocal VPBs may fall in this vulnerable period, and they are also quite hazardous for this type of patient.

Supraventricular Tachycardias

This group of arrhythmias has two features in common: (1) the QRS complex appears normal, although aberrant conduction may occasionally occur; and (2) the atrial rate, as well as the ventricular rate, is greater than 100 per minute.

The arrhythmias included in this group are sinus tachycardia, paroxsymal atrial tachycardia (PAT), atrial tachycardia with block, paroxysmal nodal tachycardia (PNT), atrial flutter, and atrial fibrillation. In addition, in all the arrhythmias except atrial fibrillation and in some instances of atrial flutter, the ventricular response is regular.

Sinus Tachycardia (Fig. 4-21)

In this arrhythmia, the basic sinus pacemaker is accelerated. The P waves are normal in appearance, have a 1:1 relationship to the QRS complex, the PR interval is normal. The rate may be from 100 to 180 per minute, and even higher in children. The rhythm is regular, although a slight variation may occur from beat to beat and from moment to moment.

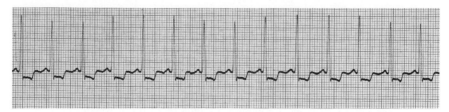

Figure 4-21. Sinus tachycardia at a rate of 115 per minute.

Paroxysmal Atrial Tachycardia (PAT) (Fig. 4-22)

Here the rhythm is due to activation of an ectopic atrial pace-maker. The P waves are usually different in configuration from sinus beats, and often are not readily apparent without the use of specialized leads, because they are buried in the preceding T wave, in which case differentiation from paroxysmal nodal tachycardia is quite difficult. The PR interval is normal and there is a 1:1 relationship of P to QRS. The rate of both atria and ventricles is usually between 180 and 250 per minute and the rhythm is regular.

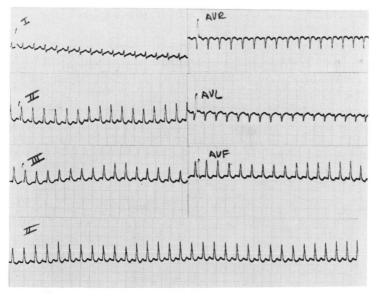

Figure 4-22. Paroxysmal atrial tachycardia at a rate of 250 per minute. The P waves are superimposed on the T waves of the preceding beats.

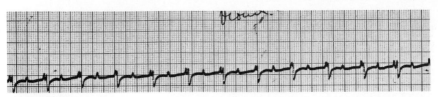

Figure 4-23. Atrial tachycardia with 2:1 block. The atrial rate is 190 per minute and the ventricular rate is 95 per minute. In addition to the P waves apparent between the QRS complexes, P waves immediately precede each QRS complex.

Atrial Tachycardia with Block (Fig. 4-23)

This arrhythmia usually occurs as a manifestation of digitalis toxicity, and, if the patient has been receiving digitalis, it should be so considered until proved otherwise. The P waves are different in configuration from sinus P waves, and, in atrial tachycardia with 2:1 block, only every other one is conducted to the ventricles, resulting in two P waves (one of which may be hidden in the preceding T wave) to every QRS complex. The atrial rate may be slower than that found in paroxysmal atrial tachycardia without block, as low as 120 per minute. With 2:1 block, the ventricular rate is half the atrial rate. The rhythm of the P waves and of the QRS complexes is regular.

Paroxysmal Junctional (Nodal) Tachycardia (Fig. 4-24)

Activation of a rapidly discharging ectopic focus in or near the AV node results in a supraventricular tachycardia in which no P waves are visible because they are buried in the QRS, or the P waves may appear immediately before or after the QRS complex. If the P waves are visible, there is a 1:1 relationship to each QRS complex. The rate is usually between 180 and 250 per minute and the rhythm is regular.

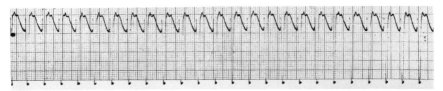

Figure 4-24. Paroxysmal junctional tachycardia. The retrograde P waves appear immediately following each QRS complex.

Atrial Flutter (Figs. 4-25 and 4-26)

Repetitive activation of the atria in a circular fashion is thought to be responsible for this arrhythmia, characterized by a regular rapid depolarization of the atria in which the atrial activity on the electrocardiogram is represented by the characteristic "saw tooth" appearance of the flutter waves (*F waves*). The atrial rate is usually between 250 to 350 per minute. The AV node is unable to conduct such rapid impulses and therefore there is a degree of block—every second, fourth, or sixth impulse is conducted to the ventricles, resulting in a 2:1, 4:1, or 6:1 block, respectively. The ventricular rate is then one half, one fourth, or one sixth of the atrial rate. Rarely, atrial flutter with 3:1 or 5:1 block may occur. The flutter waves are perfectly regular and, if the degree of block is constant, the ventricular rhythm is also regular. Varying degrees of block may occur, however, resulting in an irregularity of the ventricular response.

Atrial Fibrillation (AF) (Fig. 4-27)

When the atria fibrillate, the depolarization wave in the atria is conducted through the atria in a rapid, circular, but disorganized fashion. On the electrocardiogram, this atrial activity is seen as a constant, irregular undulation of the baseline at a rapid rate, often in excess of 350 per minute, and no discrete P waves are visible.

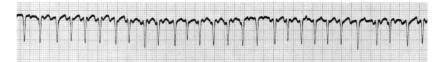

Figure 4-25. Atrial flutter with 2:1 block (lead V_1). The atrial "flutter" waves are regular at 375 per minute, and some are "buried" in the QRS complexes. The ventricular response is somewhat irregular at 188 per minute.

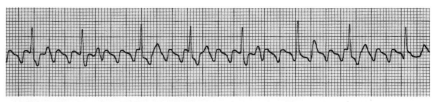

Figure 4-26. Atrial flutter with varying block. The atrial "flutter" waves are regular at 285 per minute. The ventricular response is irregular, the degree of block varying between 3:1 and 4:1.

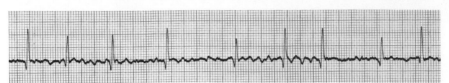

Figure 4–27. Atrial fibrillation with a moderate ventricular response (lead V₁).

The atrial depolarization wave is conducted through the AV node in an irregular fashion, resulting in a grossly irregular ventricular response. The rate of the ventricular response depends on the rapidity with which the atrial depolarization waves are conducted through the AV node, and it may vary from less than 60 to over 200 per minute.

OTHER SUPRAVENTRICULAR ARRHYTHMIAS

In addition to sinus tachycardia, other abnormalities of rhythm which originate in the sinus node may occur. All these arrhythmias are characterized by normal QRS complexes, P waves which have a normal appearance, a 1:1 relationship to the QRS complex, and a normal PR interval.

Sinus Arrhythmia (Fig. 4–28)

Sinus arrhythmia is characterized by irregularity in discharge from the sinus node, with obvious variation in the P-P and R-R intervals. This arrhythmia is often a normal finding, and may be related to respiration. With inspiration, there is a reflex discharge of the vagus nerve, resulting in slowing of the sinus node; with expiration, the vagal influence recedes and the rate speeds. This phenomenon is often striking in children, and in adults most often occurs with slow sinus rates.

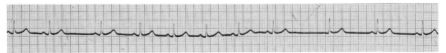

Figure 4–28. Sinus arrhythmia. Note the varying P-P and R-R intervals; the PR interval remains constant. The ninth QRS complex is a junctional escape beat.

Sinus Bradycardia (Fig. 4-29)

Sinus bradycardia is said to exist when the rate of sinus discharge slows below 60 per minute. In all other respects, the rhythm resembles a normal sinus rhythm.

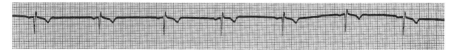

Figure 4-29. Sinus bradycardia at a rate of 40 per minute (lead V_1).

Sinus Arrest and Sinoatrial (SA) Block (Fig. 4-30)

Sinus arrest and sinoatrial block are two arrhythmias occurring in a setting of normal sinus rhythm which cannot be readily differentiated from each other electrocardiographically. Sinus arrest occurs when the sinus node fails to fire at the expected time; SA block occurs when the sinus node fires as expected, but, owing to some abnormality in the tissue surrounding the SA node, the impulse is not conducted out into the atrial conducting tissue. In either case, there is no evidence on the electrocardiogram of a P wave at the expected time, and, after a pause which may often be equal to two P-P intervals, the normal sinus rhythm is resumed.

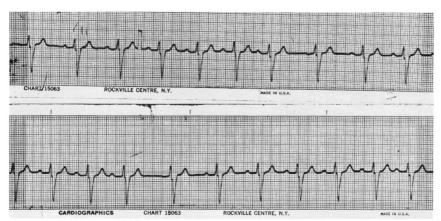

Figure 4-30. Sinoatrial block (continuous strip lead II). Each group of six consecutive normal sinus beats is followed by a pause which is terminated by an atrial escape beat (complexes 1, 8, and 15). This "group beating" and the progressive shortening of consecutive P-P intervals suggest that this is a Wenckebach phenomenon affecting the tissues surrounding the SA node, similar to the Wenckebach phenomenon more commonly seen with AV block. First degree AV block is also present (PR interval of 0.26 seconds).

Wandering Atrial Pacemaker (Fig. 4-31)

Wandering atrial pacemaker occurs when there are multiple pacemakers in the SA node, atria, and AV node, all of which have a tendency to fire at about the same rate. Depending on the moment-to-moment state of various inhibitory factors, one pacemaker will fire a beat and be the dominant pacemaker and then the following beat will be fired by a different pacemaker, which has become dominant. The next beat may come from a third focus. Electrocardiographically, the pacemaker for succeeding beats can be seen to vary between sinus beats, beats which (because of their different P wave configuration and vector) appear to rise in the atria and nodal in junctional beats.

The QRS complex is normal in appearance. P waves will vary in configuration and vector) appear to rise in the atria and nodal in be a 1:1 relationship between the P waves and the QRS complexes, with the exception of junctional beats without visible P waves. The rate is usually normal but may be more rapid. The rhythm of both the P waves and the QRS wave complexes tends to be irregular.

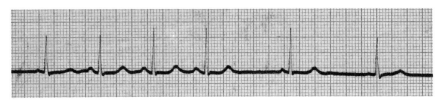

Figure 4-31. Wandering atrial pacemaker. Note the variations in P-P intervals, PR intervals, and P wave configurations.

Nonparoxysmal Nodal Tachycardia (Junctional or Nodal Rhythm) (Fig. 4-32)

Nonparoxysmal nodal tachycardia differs from paroxysmal nodal tachycardia in that it is often associated with digitalis toxicity. It also differs with respect to rate. Although called a tachycardia, the rate is usually between 60 and 100 per minute. The QRS complexes

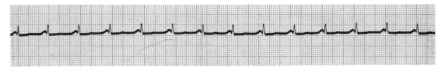

Figure 4-32. Nonparoxysmal nodal tachycardia (nodal rhythm) at a rate of 103 per minute. The P waves immediately precede each QRS complex.

are normal in appearance and duration. P waves may be visible just preceding or just following the QRS complex, in which case they will have an abnormal appearance and vector, or may be buried in the QRS complex. Commonly this arrhythmia is associated with AV dissociation (see later), and then there is no relationship between the QRS complexes and atrial activity. The rhythm of the QRS complexes is quite regular.

Coronary Sinus Rhythm (Fig. 4–33)

Coronary sinus rhythm is an arrhythmia which may be a normal variant and which differs from normal sinus rhythm only in that the P vector is leftward and superior in direction, leading to inverted P waves in leads II, III, and avF. The other features of the rhythm are those of normal sinus rhythm: the QRS complex appears normal, the PR interval is normal, and there is a 1:1 relationship of P waves to QRS complexes. The rate is between 60 and 100 per minute, and the rhythm is basically regular.

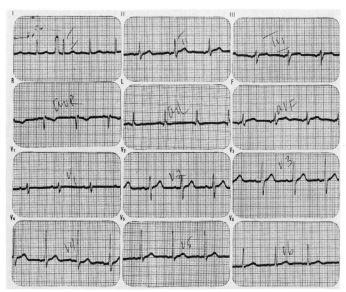

Figure 4–33. Coronary sinus rhythm. The P vector is left and superior, with inverted P waves in leads II, III, and avF.

ESCAPE RHYTHMS

Because of its more rapid rate of spontaneous depolarization, the sinus node is normally the dominant cardiac pacemaker. Lower pacemakers remain dormant because they are depolarized by impulses conducted through them at a rate faster than their own spontaneous rate of depolarization. If, however, the sinus node fails to fire, or if the impulse originating in the sinus node is not conducted below the AV node, then spontaneous depolarization of a lower pacemaker occurs, and this pacemaker assumes dominance, or is said to "escape." Escape may occur intermittently for single beats or more consistently as in complete heart block.

Nodal (Junctional) Escape (Figs. 4–28 and 4–34)

If an impulse fails to traverse the AV node for 1.0 to 1.5 seconds, the pacemaker tissue in the area of the AV node, which normally has an intrinsic spontaneous rate of 45 to 60 beats per minute, will usually fire. The resulting escape beat will have the characteristics of a junctional beat: the QRS complex is normal in configuration and duration. If the escape beat occurs because of failure of conduction of a sinus or atrial beat through the AV node, then the escape beat will be unrelated to the atrial activity. If the escape beat occurs because of failure of the sinus node to fire, the P wave may not be visible, being buried in the QRS complex, or it may immediately precede or follow the QRS complex, in which case it will have an abnormal vector.

Transient failure of the sinus impulse to be generated or conducted may result in a single nodal escape beat, followed by the resumption of the previous rhythm. Complete failure of sinus impulse generation or conduction may result in the nodal pacemaker tissue taking over the dominant pacemaker function of the heart, resulting in a regular rhythm in the range of 45 to 60 beats per minute, with the QRS complexes having a normal appearance and configuration. The P waves may be buried in the QRS complexes or may immediately precede or follow them, or, if the problem is failure of conduction through the AV node, normal appearing P waves may occur without any relationship to the QRS complex.

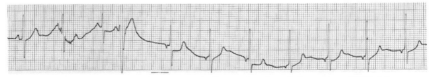

Figure 4–34. Junctional escape rhythm. The fourth beat is a VPB. The pause following this beat allows the junctional pacemaker, which has an intrinsic rate similar to the sinus rate, to assume dominance. In this patient, the rate of the junctional escape rhythm is somewhat more rapid than usually expected.

Ventricular Escape (see Fig. 4–37)

The normal ventricular pacemaker tissue has an intrinsic rate of spontaneous depolarization, resulting in a rate of 45 beats or less per minute. Ventricular escape beats and "idioventricular" rhythm usually occur when there is a lack of conduction of supraventricular beats through the conducting tissues of the ventricles, or when higher pacemakers are depressed because of metabolic disturbances.

Because of this slow rate of spontaneous depolarization, ventricular escape beats usually do not follow the preceding QRS complex by an interval shorter than about 1.5 seconds. The QRS complex is wide and deformed. The P waves that are seen are usually unrelated to the QRS complex, since the underlying disturbance usually affects both antegrade and retrograde conduction below the AV node.

Idioventricular rhythm, in which the slow ventricular pacemaker becomes the dominant pacemaker, is characterized by the wide and deformed QRS complexes occurring at a slow rate. The rhythm tends to be somewhat irregular. Atrial activity is usually either unrelated to the QRS complexes or not identifiable.

ATRIOVENTRICULAR (AV) BLOCK

Abnormally delayed conduction or complete or incomplete failure of conduction of impulses from the atria to the ventricles is referred to as AV block. Abnormalities in AV conduction are common, occurring in settings of myocardial disease, such as acute myocardial infarction or myocarditis; in the elderly with fibrosis of the myocardial skeleton; postoperatively because of trauma to the conducting tissues or to an inflammatory response; due to extension of calcification from calcific aortic stenosis or a calcified mitral annulus; and as a result of metabolic derangements and drugs, particularly digitalis.

It is convenient to divide AV block into increasing degrees of impaired conduction ranging from merely an abnormal prolongation of AV conduction to complete AV block.

First Degree AV Block (see Figs. 4–11, 4–30, and 4–42)

First degree AV block is present when the sole abnormality is a prolongation of the PR interval to greater than 0.20 seconds. The QRS complexes are normal in configuration and duration. The P waves are normal and there is a 1:1 relationship with the QRS complexes. The rate and rhythm are that of the underlying sinus rhythm.

Second Degree AV Block

Second degree AV block is present when some but not all of the sinus impulses are conducted through the ventricles, and this category can be further subdivided into two varieties.

The Wenckebach Phenomenon (Mobitz Type I) (Fig. 4–35). This phenomenon is characteristically composed of recurrent cycles in which there is progressive prolongation of the PR interval until a P wave is not conducted; the cycle is then repeated.

The QRS complex is normal in configuration and duration. The P waves are normal in appearance and their rhythm is regular. The PR interval becomes progressively longer with the maintenance of a 1:1 relationship with the following QRS complex until the dropped beat occurs. The rhythm of the QRS complex is irregular in a characteristic, and at first glance paradoxical, fashion. Although the PR interval lengthens with each succeeding beat, the increment by which this happens becomes less with each succeeding beat, hence the R-R interval becomes progressively *shorter* with each succeeding beat in the cycle until the dropped beat occurs. The R-R interval surrounding the dropped beat is always less than the two preceding R-R intervals. The R-R interval of the cycle preceding the pause is always shorter than that of the cycle following the pause.

Second Degree AV Block (Mobitz Type II).   This type of block differs from the Wenckebach phenomenon in that progressive prolongation of the PR interval does not occur. The P waves are normal and are followed by a QRS complex at a constant PR interval, which may be either normal or prolonged. Then suddenly a dropped beat occurs: the regularly occurring P wave is not followed by a QRS complex. The QRS complexes are normal in configuration and duration; the atrial rate is normal and the atrial rhythm is regular. The ventricular rate and rhythm are the same as the atrial rate and rhythm until a pause occurs. The pause is exactly twice the usual R-R interval.

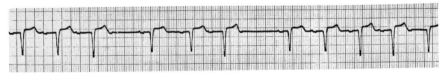

Figure 4–35. Second degree A-V block—Mobitz Type I. The atrial rhythm is sinus in origin at a rate of 80 per minute and is basically regular, although some slight irregularity is present. After three beats with progressively lengthening PR intervals, the fourth P wave is blocked, causing a pause. The cycle is then repeated—a 4:3 Wenckebach phenomenon. The pattern is not repeated in the third cycle, which shows a varying PR interval with each P wave being conducted.

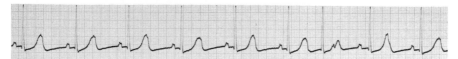

Figure 4–36. 2:1 Atrioventricular block. There are two P waves preceding each QRS complex, one of which occurs at the peak of each T wave and could readily be overlooked. The presence of the second P wave is apparent following the single beat in this series which is conducted with 1:1 conduction and first degree AV block. The QT interval is also prolonged.

Advanced AV Block (Fig. 4–36).   If there are two or more atrial impulses for every conducted QRS complex, advanced AV block is present. A 2:1 AV block, when every other sinus impulse is conducted through the AV node, is the most common form of advanced AV block. The QRS complex is normal in configuration and duration. The P waves are normal in appearance; there are two P waves present for each QRS complex and their relation to the QRS complex is constant. The rhythm of both the atria and the ventricles is regular; the ventricular rate is one half the atrial rate.

Complete AV Block (Fig. 4–37). Complete heart block is present when no atrial activity is conducted to the ventricles; the atria and the ventricles are completely independent of each other. The site of the AV block will determine the location of the lower pacemaker; if the block is located at the AV node, the pacemaker will be just below the node or in the bundle of His, and the QRS complex will have a relatively normal configuration and duration. If the area of the block interrupts the common bundle or both bundle branches, the pacemaker will be more peripheral in one of the ventricles, and the QRS complex will be wide and deformed. The atrial activity is usually normal sinus in origin, although an atrial arrhythmia may be present; in any case, there will not be any relationship between the atrial activity and the QRS complexes. The rate and rhythm of the QRS complexes will reflect the site of the pacemaker—the higher pacemakers with relatively normal QRS complexes will tend to be regular with a rate between 35 and 50. Lower ventricular pacemakers will tend to be slower and somewhat irregular.

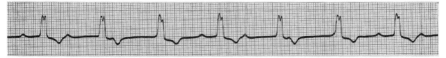

Figure 4–37. Complete atrioventricular block. The atrial rate is 75 per minute. The completely unrelated ventricular escape rhythm has a rate of 44 per minute.

ATRIOVENTRICULAR (AV) DISSOCIATION (Fig. 4–38)

AV dissociation is present when the atrial and ventricular rhythms are independent of each other. Complete heart block can therefore be seen to be a form of AV dissociation; but this latter term is often more narrowly used to indicate a lack of antegrade or retrograde conduction through the AV node without the presence of pathologic AV block.

The phenomenon which allows AV dissociation to occur is termed *interference,* and this specialized type of AV dissociation without AV block is termed *interference dissociation.* The usual setting for interference dissociation is the appearance of an ectopic junctional or ventricular rhythm which is slightly faster than the sinus or atrial rhythm. In this situation, the impulses reaching the AV node retrograde from the ectopic junctional or ventricular focus render the conducting tissue of the lower part of the AV node refractory to conduction of the impulses descending in an antegrade fashion from the atria and prevent their further conduction. Similarly, the penetration of the antegrade impulses into the conducting tissue of the upper AV node renders this tissue refractory to retrograde conduction from below. Hence, there is no conduction either antegrade or retrograde through the AV node—a state of physiological AV block.

The QRS complexes may be normal in configuration and duration if the lower pacemaker is junctional in origin, or wide and deformed if it is ventricular in origin. The configuration of the P wave will depend on the atrial rhythm; there is no relationship between the

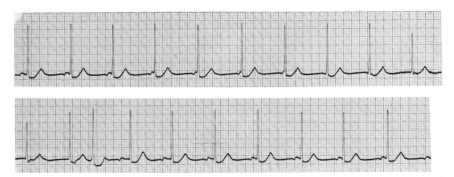

Figure 4–38. Atrioventricular dissociation (continuous strips). A junctional rhythm is present which is slightly faster than the sinus rate, causing interference dissociation. In the upper strip, note the PR interval progressively shortening; the P wave then becomes superimposed on the QRS complex and subsequently emerges following the QRS complex. Thus, the P wave is said to "march through" the QRS complex. The third QRS complex on the lower tracing is a "capture beat"; the P wave following the second QRS complex is conducted antegradely to the ventricles at a prolonged PR interval. The subsequent beats are then conducted antegradely in a normal fashion but with a slight PR prolongation until the faster junctional pacemaker again assumes dominance.

P waves and the QRS complex. The ventricular rate is regular and usually more rapid than the atrial rate; the P waves will be seen to "march through" the QRS complex.

It is apparent that under these conditions the presence or absence of pathologic AV block, in addition to the interference dissociation, cannot be determined. During the course of an arrhythmia such as this, however, occasions usually appear when the relationship of the P waves and the QRS complexes is such that there is a period following a P wave and before the next QRS complex when antegrade conduction could be anticipated to occur if AV conduction were normal. If, in fact, AV conduction is normal, a "capture beat" will occur — the regularity of the QRS complexes will be interrupted by a beat which is early and conducted from the preceding P wave.

INTRAVENTRICULAR BLOCK

Intraventricular block refers to disturbances of conduction at the level of the specialized conduction tissues of the ventricles. Intraventricular block may involve complete block of one of the bundle branches and is so designated — right bundle branch block and left bundle branch block. In bundle branch block, the QRS complex is widened and deformed in a characteristic pattern. Conduction up to the level of the bundle branches is normal, however. If the underlying rhythm is normal sinus, the P waves will be normal in a constant 1:1 relationship to the QRS complexes with a normal PR interval. The rate and rhythm will also be normal. However, bundle branch block may occur in the setting of other arrhythmias.

Right Bundle Branch Block (RBBB)
(Figs. 4–39 and 4–42)

When conduction through the right bundle branch is interrupted, depolarization of the right ventricle is delayed and occurs by different pathways. The result is a widening of the QRS complex to 0.11 seconds or greater due to a prolongation of the late or "terminal" forces which reflect the delayed depolarization of the right ventricle. There is no disturbance in the initial QRS forces, but the prolonged terminal forces are directed to the right and anteriorly. This leads to a deep, wide terminal S wave in lead I and an rsR[1], or simply a broad notched R wave in the anterior precordial leads.

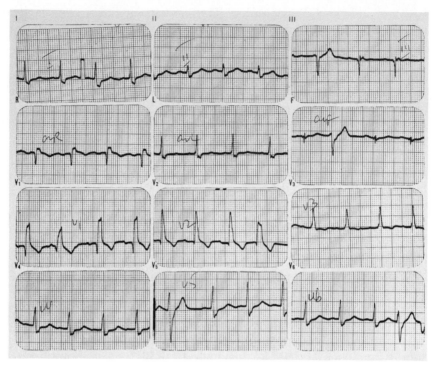

Figure 4-39. Right bundle branch block. The basic rhythm is normal sinus; occasional VPBs are present (leads III, avF, V_2, V_5, and V_6).

Left Bundle Branch Block (LBBB) (Fig. 4-40)

With complete interruption of conduction through the left bundle branch, both initial and terminal QRS forces are affected. Since normally the initial QRS forces are generated by depolarization of the interventricular septum from left to right, these forces are lost with block of the left bundle. Both initial and terminal QRS forces are then leftward and posterior, leading to QRS complexes that are widened to 0.12 seconds or more, with broad R waves in leads I and avL, V_5 and V_6, and an rS or qS deflection over the anterior precordial leads.

The above abnormalities of depolarization also lead to abnormalities of repolarization, and, in left bundle branch block, the ST segment and T wave vectors are opposite in direction to the QRS forces. In right bundle branch block, the ST segment and T wave abnormalities are often less striking, but consist of ST segment and T wave vectors opposite in direction to the abnormal terminal forces.

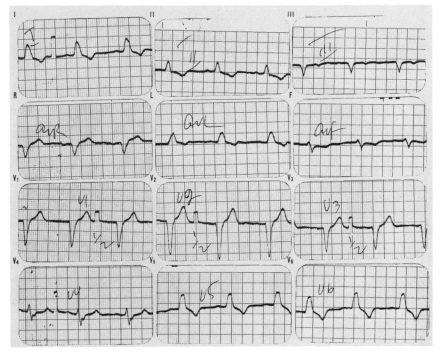

Figure 4–40. Left bundle branch block. (Leads V_1 to V_3 are one half standardization.)

Left Ventricular Hemiblock (Figs. 4–41 and 4–42)

Left ventricular hemiblock refers to a block occurring in one of the two major divisions of the left bundle branch. If the anterior radiation of the left bundle is interrupted, there is a shift in the mean QRS axis leftward and superiorly, with the development of deep terminal S waves in leads II, III, and avF. The QRS duration is usually at the upper limits of normal. This abnormality is referred to as *left anterior hemiblock, marked left axis deviation,* or *superior axis.*

Rarely, block of the posterior radiation of the left bundle may occur, and is then termed *left posterior hemiblock.* Electrocardiographically, it is characterized by a shift of the mean QRS axis to the right, with the appearance of a terminal S wave in lead I, an initial Q wave in lead III, and tall terminal R waves in leads II, III, and avF. The QRS duration may be prolonged to the upper limits of normal.

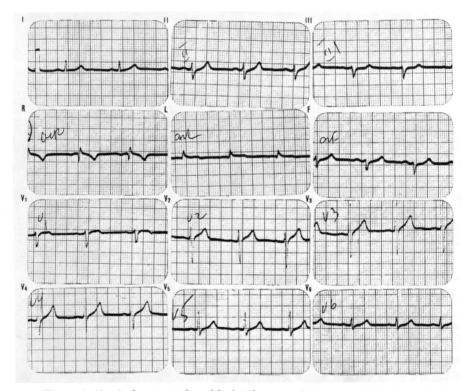

Figure 4–41.   Left anterior hemiblock. The mean QRS axis is shifted superiorly to –45 degrees. Prominent terminal S waves are present in leads II, III, and avF.

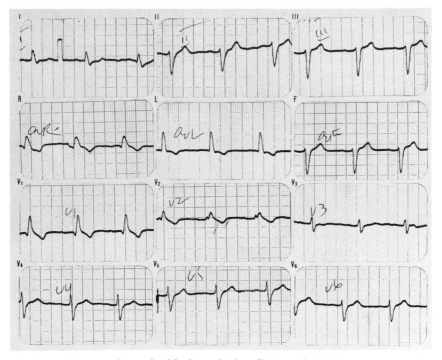

Figure 4–42. Bifascicular block. Right bundle branch block is present, and, in addition, the mean QRS axis is left and superior, indicating that left anterior hemiblock is also present. Conduction of the sinus impulses to the ventricles occurs by the only remaining conduction pathway, or fascicle — the posterior division of the left bundle. First degree AV block is also present (PR interval equals 0.24 seconds).

WOLFF-PARKINSON-WHITE SYNDROME (WPW)
(VENTRICULAR PRE-EXCITATION)

Ventricular pre-excitation, also referred to as the WPW syndrome, is a disturbance of AV conduction in which a secondary pathway exists, in addition to the normal pathway through the AV node. Conduction through this secondary pathway results in a lesser delay in conduction from atria to ventricles than in normal conduction through the AV node. Depolarization of the ventricles then begins and proceeds in an abnormal fashion.

Electrocardiographically, during sinus rhythm there is a short PR interval (less than 0.12 seconds) followed by a ventricular complex of abnormal configuration. The initial portion of the QRS complex is deformed and widened by a slow-rising slurred deflection called a *delta wave*. Repolarization of the ventricles may also be abnormal, resulting in ST segment and T wave abnormalities.

The delta wave represents the initial abnormal activation of the ventricles. The remainder of the QRS complex then is a result of the relative contributions of the abnormally and normally conducted impulses. The electrocardiographic complex often resembles a ventricular fusion beat.

The P waves are normal in configuration during sinus rhythm, and they bear a 1:1 relationship with the QRS complexes. The PR interval, as mentioned, is abnormally short. In sinus rhythm, the rate and rhythm are normal.

In a patient with this syndrome, electrocardiographic complexes typical of pre-excitation may be constantly present, or only intermittently present if conduction alternates between the normal and the abnormal pathway.

The clinical importance of the pre-excitation syndrome is the frequency of supraventricular arrhythmias, particularly atrial fibrillation, in these patients. The contour of the QRS complexes during the arrhythmia is wide and bizarre and the arrhythmia is difficult to distinguish from ventricular tachycardia.

VENTRICULAR TACHYCARDIA (Figs. 4–43 and 4–44)

This arrhythmia, occurring almost always in a setting of serious heart disease, is of special importance because of its grave prognostic implications. Although the arrhythmia may terminate spontaneously, it often accelerates, culminating in ventricular fibrillation in a matter of minutes.

The QRS complexes are wide and deformed, since they are ventricular in origin, and the ST segment and T wave vectors are

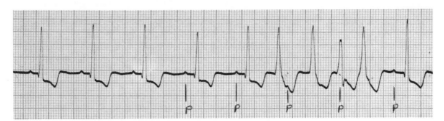

Figure 4-43. Ventricular tachycardia. After five normal sinus beats, four consecutive ventricular ectopic beats are present. The P waves are independent, continuing undisturbed at the basic sinus rate. A normal sinus beat then follows the brief run of ventricular tachycardia.

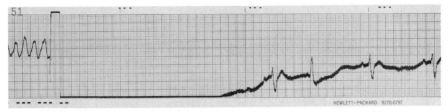

Figure 4-44. Ventricular tachycardia at a rapid rate, terminated by direct current countershock.

often opposite in direction from the mean QRS forces. P waves often cannot be discerned. If they are present, they are usually dissociated from the QRS complexes at an independent and slower rate, although retrograde P waves following each QRS complex may occur. The rate is usually rapid, and the rhythm usually slightly irregular. This arrhythmia must be differentiated from supraventricular tachycardia in the presence of pre-existing intraventricular block, pre-excitation syndrome, or supraventricular tachycardia with aberrant ventricular conduction.

When ventricular tachycardia occurs at a rate in the range of 200 per minute, the electrocardiogram may reveal large continuous waves in which no distinction between the QRS complex and the ST segment and T wave can be made. This is sometimes referred to as *ventricular flutter.*

Ventricular Fibrillation (Fig. 4-45)

If conduction through the ventricular myocardium becomes disorganized and chaotic, the absence of an organized sequence of conduction results in the synergistic contraction of the ventricles being replaced by an uncoordinated quivering. The pumping action of the heart ceases, and the lack of blood flow to the remainder of

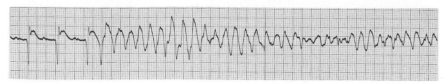

Figure 4-45. Ventricular tachycardia and fibrillation following a VPB which occurs during the T wave of the preceding beat.

the body, especially the brain, causes the syndrome of cardiac arrest. Obviously, the patient cannot survive unless treatment of the arrhythmia is rapidly instituted. The treatment of ventricular fibrillation is electrical defibrillation. If defibrillation cannot be immediately applied, then oxygenation and artificial circulation must be maintained by the principles of cardiopulmonary resuscitation until the means for defibrillation are obtained.

Ventricular fibrillation rarely occurs spontaneously without a pre-existent rhythm disturbance, which is usually ventricular tachycardia or ventricular premature beats falling on the preceding T wave.

Electrocardiographically, ventricular fibrillation is characterized by the replacement of identifiable QRS complexes by irregular undulation of the baseline, varying in amplitude and contour at a rate of 150 to 500 per minute.

ASYSTOLE

Complete cessation of electrical activity in the ventricles is called *ventricular standstill* or *asystole.* The electrocardiogram reveals absence of QRS complexes and a flat baseline which may or may not be interrupted by evidence of atrial activity. As in ventricular fibrillation, no blood is pumped by the heart, and cardiac arrest is soon clinically apparent. Cardiopulmonary resuscitation must be started rapidly and maintained until an effective rhythm is re-established by means of drugs or electrical pacing.

Metabolic and Drug-Induced Electrocardiographic Changes (Figs. 4–46 to 4–48)

POTASSIUM

Hypokalemia, with a decrease in serum potassium concentration to abnormally low levels, leads to an electrocardiographic pattern

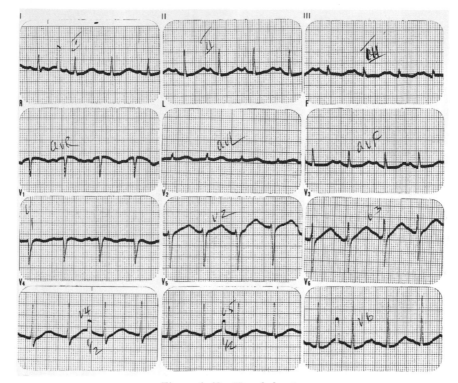

Figure 4-46. Hypokalemia.

characterized by diffuse depression of the ST segments, flattening and widening of the T waves, and prominent U waves (Figs. 4–46 and 4–48D). Owing to the merging of a flat T wave and prominent U wave it is often difficult to measure the actual QT interval. There often appears to be a markedly prolonged QT interval, which is actually a QU interval. In severe hypokalemia, conduction is prolonged, with an increase in the PR interval and an increased amplitude of the P waves.

If the patient is taking digitalis, hypokalemia will exacerbate the cardiovascular manifestations of digitalis toxicity.

Hyperkalemia affects the electrocardiogram, first by causing an increase in the voltage and peaking of the T wave (Fig. 4–48B). With increasing levels of potassium, there is a delay in intraventricular conduction with widening of the QRS complex. The PR interval may then become prolonged with diminution of the amplitude of the P wave (Figs. 4–47 and 4–48C). Progressive QRS widening, loss of identifiable atrial activity on the electrocardiogram, and rhythm disturbances then ensue, terminating in complete AV dissociation, ventricular fibrillation, and asystole, with very high serum potassium concentrations.

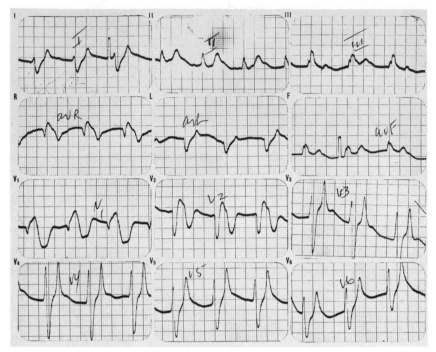

Figure 4-47. Severe hyperkalemia. Atrial activity is not apparent. The QRS complexes are markedly widened, and the T waves are very large and peaked.

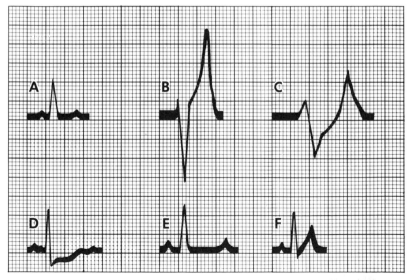

Figure 4-48. Electrolyte disturbances. *A*, Normal ECG. *B* and *C*, Moderate and severe hyperkalemia. *D*, Hypokalemia. *E*, Hypocalcemia. *F*, Hypercalcemia.

CALCIUM

Hypocalcemia is characterized electrocardiographically by prolongation of the QT interval. In contrast to hypokalemia, the QT interval prolongation in hypocalcemia is due to a prolongation of the ST segment, the width of the T wave being normal (Fig. 4–48E). In *hypercalcemia*, the reverse occurs: a shortening of the QT interval due to a shortening of the ST segment (Fig. 4–48F).

DIGITALIS

The administration of digitalis in therapeutic doses usually results in electrocardiographic changes affecting the ST segment and the T wave. Diffuse ST segment depression occurs, associated with a decrease in the amplitude of the T wave and a shortening of the QT interval. These ECG changes are not an index of adequate or excess digitalis dosage.

Toxic doses of digitalis can result in virtually any cardiac arrhythmia, but the more common arrhythmias due to digitalis are the result of prolongation of AV conduction, or an increase in the automaticity of lower pacemakers, or both. Prolongation of AV conduction leads to varying degrees of AV block, ranging from merely a prolongation of the PR interval to second degree heart block, commonly manifested by Wenckebach phenomenon, and rarely to complete heart block. Increased automaticity of lower pacemakers can lead to a variety of arrhythmias. The most frequent are ventricular premature contractions, which are often multifocal and which may lead to ventricular tachycardia or fibrillation. Nonparoxysmal nodal tachycardia may occur, most frequently in a patient who has been in atrial fibrillation. This occurrence can be recognized clinically by the change from a slow irregular ventricular response to a more rapid regular rhythm. Although paroxysmal atrial tachycardia with block can rarely occur in the absence of digitalis administration, its appearance in a patient who is receiving digitalis should be considered evidence of digitalis toxicity until proved otherwise.

MYOCARDIAL DEPRESSANTS (QUINIDINE, PROCAINAMIDE, PROPRANOLOL)

Quinidine and procainamide (Pronestyl) have similar electrophysiologic effects which make them useful in the treatment of cardiac arrhythmias, and they also have similar effects on the electrocardiogram. In therapeutic doses, a prolongation of the QT interval often occurs. As the toxic range is approached, prolongation of both the QRS complex and PR interval may occur. Despite their anti-arrhythmic action, ventricular premature contractions and ventricular tachycardia and fibrillation have been reported to occur as a complication of therapy with these drugs, especially with quinidine.

Propranolol (Inderal) appears to have two modes of action. Firstly, it antagonizes the ability of catecholamines such as epinephrine and isoproterenol to increase the rate of discharge of pacemaker tissue and also antagonizes their effect in increasing the speed of AV conduction. Hence, sinus bradycardia is common in the therapeutic dose range, and conduction through the AV node is slowed, resulting in a decrease of the ventricular rate in atrial flutter and fibrillation. Secondly, propranolol is similar to quinidine in many of its effects, and it may produce similar electrocardiographic changes.

Pericarditis

Inflammation of the pericardium from whatever cause results in involvement of the epicardial surface of the heart, and, to a varying extent, the subepicardial myocardium. The inflammatory response results in ST segment and T wave changes. Since pericarditis is generally a diffuse process, the electrocardiographic abnormalities are also diffuse. Initially, there is generalized ST segment elevation occurring in both the frontal and horizontal planes. As the ST segments return to the baseline over a period of a few days, widespread T wave inversions occur which may persist for months. Abnormalities of the QRS complexes, specifically pathologic Q waves, do not occur.

Bibliography

Goldman, M. J.: Principles of Clinical Electrocardiography. Los Altos, California, Lange Medical Publications, 1967.

Grant, R. P.: Clinical Electrocardiography: The Spatial Vector Approach. New York, McGraw-Hill, Inc., 1957.

Katz, L. N., and Pick, A.: Clinical Electrocardiography: Part I – The Arrhythmias. Philadelphia, Lea & Febiger, 1956.

CHAPTER 5

Diagnostic Techniques

By RICHARD G. SANDERSON, M.D.

Although there are a tremendous number of techniques currently available for making a cardiac diagnosis, most diagnoses can be made with simple tools—the careful and detailed history, the meticulous physical examination, the electrocardiogram, and multiple-view cardiac x-ray films. Special diagnostic procedures (e.g., cardiac catheterization and phonocardiography) may be utilized to confirm diagnoses, to quantify the degree of hemodynamic disability, and to rule out unsuspected associated disease.

This chapter has a dual purpose. Some of the techniques used in history taking and physical examination will be important to the nurse's understanding of disease complexes and her recognition and interpretation of important clinical events in her patients. In addition, it is intended to provide the nurse with a basic overview of some of the diagnostic procedures, so that she may better understand how cardiac diagnoses are confirmed and what her patients will undergo during the procedures.

History Taking and Physical Examination

The groundwork for correct cardiac diagnoses is laid in the techniques of history taking and physical examination. If other accumulated data are at variance with the "history and physical," the latter are likely to be correct and the variant information should be regarded skeptically.

HISTORY TAKING

This is a highly significant and symbolic encounter, since not only can one listen to the patient's symptoms, but one can also evaluate his personality structure and establish a proper relationship with the patient. In relating his symptoms, the patient often colors the discussion with his own attitudes, emotions, and personality traits, allowing the listener to gain further insight into the patient's problems. The circumstances of the patient's social setting are often uncovered in the interview, and his disease complex may be better understood in the context of this setting. For example, some of the initiating causes of a patient's angina pectoris can be found in his relationships with his employer, family, and social circle.

Symptoms

Pain, dyspnea, fatigue, palpitations, edema, syncope, and hemoptysis represent the most frequent cardiovascular complaints.

Pain. The most common pain pattern in cardiac disease is angina pectoris, usually connoting coronary artery disease. Typically, angina pectoris is a pressing or squeezing substernal chest pain that may radiate to the neck and jaw, or to the shoulders, down the arms, and into the fingers. The pain may be brought on by activity, cold, emotional upsets, or large meals, and is usually relieved in a few minutes by rest or sublingual nitroglycerine. If the pain lasts longer than 30 to 60 minutes or is accompanied by sweating, anxiety, and nausea, the more serious events of preinfarction angina or a myocardial infarction should be suspected.

Dissecting aneurysms of the thoracic aorta usually cause excruciating pain, which is sometimes described as "tearing" or "burning." The pain may originate in the anterior chest, particularly with dissections of the ascending aorta, but very often will radiate into the interscapular area. The shifting of this severe pain from one area to another may be related to the progression of the dissection.

The pain of pericarditis is usually sharp in nature and precordial in location. It is not related to exertion, but is usually aggravated by deep breathing, by lying down, or by turning from side to side. Pulmonary embolism also causes pain that is aggravated by deep breathing, but the pain is often located laterally in the area of the ischemic lung.

Dyspnea. This term simply means "shortness of breath." The patient feels that he is unable to "get enough air" and often complains of a choking or smothering sensation. Dyspnea may be present only on exercise (exertional dyspnea, or DOE) and is not necessarily specific for cardiac disease. Dyspnea during recumbency (orthopnea) or dyspnea that interrupts the patient's sleep (paroxysmal nocturnal dyspnea or PND) are particularly characteristic of cardiac disease. A youngster with a ventricular septal defect may become dyspneic while playing with schoolmates, or a bedridden oldster may complain of dyspnea when his thrombophlebitis-originated pulmonary embolism obstructs pulmonary blood flow. Typically, this latter form of the complaint occurs at rest.

Dyspnea should be differentiated from tachypnea (an increase in the rate of breathing, as in anxiety states or pulmonary embolism) and from hyperpnea (an increase in depth and rate of breathing, as seen in Cheyne-Stokes breathing).

Fatigue. Being "tired and listless" and having "no energy to do anything" is a very common cardiac complaint. It is characteristic of patients with mitral insufficiency and in other conditions in which there is marked diminution of cardiac output. The heart is unable to adequately supply oxygen to the body's tissues, particularly during exercise when the oxygen demands are increased.

Palpitations. This symptom is simply an awareness (usually unpleasant) of the heart beat. Palpitations are often experienced with a rapid heart rate, particularly if the rhythm is irregular. Sympathetic nervous system stimulation and cardiac anxiety are common causes.

There often is little or no output of blood from the heart with an ectopic beat, but the next beat has a much greater stroke volume. The patient may become consciously aware of this more forceful contraction. The patient with aortic insufficiency may complain of his head "bobbing" because of the large stroke volume in this disease. The patient with an intracardiac ball-valve prosthesis often can hear his valve "clicking" when he goes to sleep, an abnormal awareness of the heart beat.

Syncope. Syncope is the transient loss of consciousness due to inadequate cerebral blood flow. It is found in patients with aortic stenosis, in tetralogy of Fallot during a "spell," during high-grade atrioventricular block (Stokes-Adams disease), or during a vasovagal attack.

Hemoptysis. Cough accompanied by bloody sputum is termed *hemoptysis* and it may vary in degree from frothy sputum tinged with blood, as in pulmonary edema, to gross bleeding, as exemplified by pulmonary embolism and mitral stenosis. In acute pulmonary edema, the blood comes from pulmonary capillaries which have ruptured because of the high intravascular (high left atrial) pressures. In mitral stenosis, varicosities of the bronchopulmonary veins develop; when the varix ruptures under the high pressures, hemoptysis will result. Massive hemoptysis may signify the rupture of an aortic aneurysm into the tracheobronchial system. Blood-tinged sputum is also seen in severe pulmonary infections, especially tuberculosis and lung abscesses. The nurse should observe not only the color and amount of the bleeding, but also whether the sputum is frothy or purulent.

The uncritical notation of symptoms in a patient's history is insufficient, and their functional significance must be assessed. The patient may be able to continue his busy daily activities despite symptoms, or, on the other hand, he might be confined to bed. In order to quantify the degree of impairment, the following functional classification has been established by the New York Heart Association.

Class I. Patients with cardiac disease but without resulting limitations of physical activity. Ordinary physical activity does not cause undue fatigue, palpitation, dyspnea, or anginal pain.

Class II. Patients with cardiac disease resulting in slight limitation of physical activity. They are comfortable at rest. Ordinary physical activity results in fatigue, palpitation, dyspnea, or anginal pain.

Class III. Patients with cardiac disease resulting in marked limitation of physical activity. They are comfortable at rest. Less than ordinary physical activity causes fatigue, palpitations, dyspnea, or anginal pain.

Class IV. Patients with cardiac disease resulting in inability to carry on any physical activity without discomfort. Symptoms of cardiac insufficiency or of the anginal syndrome may be present even at rest. If any physical activity is undertaken, discomfort is increased.

Past History

Much can be learned about a patient's current cardiac disease by inquiring about past events in his life. German measles during pregnancy might give an historical clue to a child's patent ductus arteriosus, or postnatal cyanosis ("blue baby") may indicate cyanotic congenital heart disease. The definite history of rheumatic fever or even of "nervousness," chorea, sore throats, or "growing pains" (polyarthralgias) may signify a rheumatic etiology of the heart disease. Accidents, injuries, industrial and communicable disease exposures, illnesses, and operations should all be considered as potential clues to the correct diagnosis. Medications (especially cardiac drugs) and the use of tobacco and alcohol should be noted so that their effect on the patient's disease may be properly assessed. The nurse should make a careful notation of each drug the patient is taking and its dosage.

Family History

Additional clues may be gleaned from the family history. Premature deaths from coronary artery disease or hypertension, familial diabetes, congenital heart disease, or rheumatic fever are all highly relevant.

THE PHYSICAL EXAMINATION

In the intensive care of cardiac patients, nurses should be able to evaluate physical findings and form a plan of action that is based on these findings. For example, a nurse who can detect crepitant rales throughout both lung fields will be able to institute oxygen therapy and fluid restriction even before the physician confirms the presence of pulmonary edema and writes the appropriate orders.

The physical examination of the cardiac patient will be arbitrarily divided into four sections: general inspection; inspection and palpation of venous and arterial pulse waves; inspection, palpation, and percussion of the anterior chest; and auscultation.

General Inspection

Many important features of a cardiac patient can be discovered by simple observation. Firstly, consider his appearance. Labored respirations, diaphoresis, and an apprehensive look on the patient's face all indicate that he is in distress. A cyanotic hue of the skin, mucous membranes, or nail beds may be the result of a right-to-left shunt of congenital heart disease, low cardiac output, or poor oxygen uptake by engorged lungs. Bacterial endocarditis is often suspected in patients with splinter hemorrhages under the fingernails and petechial hemorrhages of the lower eyelid. Frothy pink sputum spells pulmonary edema, and massive edema of the extremities usually means right heart failure. Cold, mottled, and cyanotic skin of the extremities usually indicates a very poor cardiac output.

Inspection and Palpation of the Venous and Arterial Pulses

Venous. Observing the neck veins will allow the examiner to study the wave forms of the jugular venous pulsations and to estimate the venous pressure. Indirect lighting, which allows the clearest examination of the venous pulse, can be provided by shining a beam of light tangentially across the skin overlying the vein.

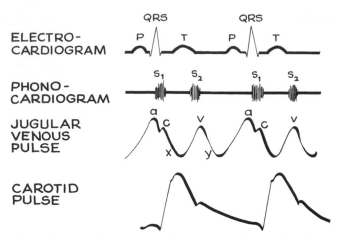

Figure 5-1. Diagram of normal jugular venous and carotid pulses with simultaneous electrocardiogram and phonocardiogram.

Normally, the jugular venous pulse has three positive waves (Fig. 5-1): the a waves caused by atrial contraction, the c waves caused by the transmitted pulsations of the underlying carotid arteries, and the v waves caused by atrial filling. In order to distinguish between a and v waves, *feel* the carotid artery while you *look* at the vein. The a wave just precedes or is coincident with the carotid pulse; the v wave follows it. (The c wave is distinguishable only with a pulse recorder and is not important in bedside examination.)

The a wave is absent in atrial fibrillation since synchronous atrial contraction is lacking. Large a waves are seen when the atrium contracts against increased resistance occasioned by tricuspid stenosis or by elevated right ventricular filling pressures. Giant a waves are seen when the atrium contracts against a closed tricuspid valve (cannon waves), as is seen in complete heart block. Large v waves are evident when there is tricuspid insufficiency, as the ventricular contraction is transmitted through the open valve to the great veins. The descent from the zenith of the v wave is very rapid in tricuspid insufficiency (blood flowing rapidly through the wide-open valve) and is slow in tricuspid stenosis (obstructed blood flow).

Venous pressure may be estimated by observing the height of the blood column in the jugular veins. The external reference or zero point is the junction of the manubrium and the body of the sternum (the sternal angle of Lewis). The patient is flexed at the hips and his upper body is elevated until a point on the neck can be found above which the jugular vein is no longer distended. The vertical distance of this latter point above the zero reference point at the angle of Lewis is an estimate of the central venous pressure. Normally it is not greater than 3 to 4 cm. The level falls with inspiration (as the pressure within the chest falls or becomes more negative) and rises with expiration. When the jugular vein is pulsatile, the summit wave is timed, measured, and specified (e.g., a 10 cm v wave).

Venous pressure can also be measured by a manometer. Through a peripheral vein (antecubital, jugular, cephalic, saphenous), a venous catheter is advanced until its tip rests in the vena cava or in the right atrium. This indwelling central venous line is then connected to a manometer, usually by a three way stopcock in series with an intravenous solution and connecting tubing. The stopcock is turned so that the IV fluid runs up into the manometer. The patient is laid flat and the bottom of the manometer gauge is held at the level of the right atrium (midway through the chest). The stopcock is then turned so that the manometer is connected to the indwelling venous catheter. Patency of the system is assured if respiratory variations are observed. The level of solution in the manometer is then allowed to fall until it reaches a stable level, which is then read as the central venous pressure (CVP) in centimeters of water. A strain gauge transducer could also be connected to the indwelling venous catheter; its oscilloscopic reading would be measured in millimeters of mercury. Millimeters of mercury may be converted to centimeters of water by multiplying by 1.36; for example, 10 mm Hg is the same CVP as 13.6 cm H_2O.

In patients with volume overload, cardiac tamponade, tricuspid stenosis, or right heart failure, the venous pressure will be elevated. Low venous pressures are recorded in hypovolemic states. In constrictive pericarditis, the jugular venous pulsations rise rather than fall with inspiration (Kussmaul's sign), since negative thoracic pressures are not well transmitted to the "constricted" right atrium and right ventricle which are not distensible enough to accommodate the increased venous blood return during inspiration.

Arterial. In all patients, central and peripheral pulses should be carefully examined on both sides of the body. Dissecting aneurysms, arterial thrombosis or embolism, or intrinsic arteriosclerotic disease may weaken or obliterate any one (or more) of these pulses. Normally, the femoral artery pulse and the radial artery pulse are synchronous. These two pulses should be palpated simultaneously, as a delay in the femoral pulse could indicate coarctation of the aorta or severe arteriosclerotic occlusive disease.

The "character" of an arterial pulse is an important observation in the diagnosis of cardiac disease. Small, weak pulses are found in situations of low stroke volume (e.g., aortic stenosis), narrowed pulse pressure (e.g., cardiac tamponade), and increased systemic vascular resistance (e.g., shock states). Hemodynamically significant aortic stenosis causes a pulse with a slow upstroke, an anacrotic wave, and a delayed peak (pulsus parvus and tardus) (see Fig. 5–13 for graphic representation).

Large bounding pulses have an extremely rapid upstroke (a water-hammer pulse), a peak of short duration, and an extremely rapid downstroke (collapsing pulse). These pulses are associated with an increased stroke volume, a wide pulse pressure, and a decreased peripheral resistance; the classic example is the pulse in aortic insufficiency.

Pulsus alternans is a pulse which is perfectly regular in its timing (the ECG shows a regular rhythm) but in which there is a regular alternation of the height of the pulse wave. This abnormality signifies serious left ventricular failure and is thought to be due to an alternation in the length of the left ventricular muscle fibers. A bigeminal pulse has alternating large and small beats, but is caused by regularly occurring premature ventricular or atrial contractions which reduce stroke volume. The electrocardiogram documents the arrhythmia.

In normal persons, the systolic blood pressure may decline 3 to 10 mm Hg during inspiration, but the peripheral pulse is not perceptibly changed. This variation in systolic pressure is thought to be due to the pooling of blood in the lungs (from lung expansion and a more negative intrathoracic pressure), consequently reducing the return of blood to the left heart. A systolic pressure drop greater than 10 mm Hg is termed *pulsus paradoxus* (a misnomer, since it is really an exaggeration of the normal response). Although many conditions may cause this phenomenon, it is particularly important as an aid in diagnosing cardiac tamponade from a pericardial effusion, from compressing blood clots (postoperatively), or from a constricting pericardium.

Inspection and Palpation of the Anterior Chest

The apical area (overlying the cardiac apex) is the site of the greatest number and variety of abnormal pulsations. The apical impulse (the left ventricular thrust) can be felt in normal persons as an early systolic outward movement, brief in duration and of minimal amplitude. It is due to the recoil of the heart as blood is ejected and to the normal, slightly anterior, rotation of the heart with systole. Left ventricular hypertrophy from whatever cause results in an abnormally forceful and sustained outward movement. When the left ventricle is dilated (as in aortic or mitral insufficiency), the apical impulse is diffuse, displaced laterally, and of great force and amplitude but of shorter duration. "Paradoxical" apical pulsations are seen in ischemic heart disease (myocardial infarction and ventricular aneurysms) and are characterized by a sustained outward thrust during all of systole. The normal left parasternal inward retraction is absent as the diseased anterolateral wall of the left ventricle "bulges" outward with the high ventricular pressure.

Auscultation

Probably the most precise part of physical examination of the heart is cardiac auscultation; however, to be optimally informative, this examination must be done with great care. A quiet room without distractions is essential. A systematic sequence of listening is also important, so that less obvious findings will not be overlooked. A nurse must "tune in" a specific area of her attentions (e.g., high-pitched sounds in diastole) and "tune out" any extraneous noises. Both the diaphragm and bell of the stethoscope should be used. The diaphragm brings out the high frequency sounds and attenuates the low frequencies; it should be pressed firmly against the skin. The bell, on the other hand, accentuates the lower range of frequencies; it should be held against the skin with just enough pressure to seal the edges. If the bell piece is applied too firmly, the underlying skin is tautened and acts like a diaphragm.

Heart sounds

FIRST HEART SOUND (S_1). The first heart sound is produced by the almost simultaneous closure of the mitral and tricuspid valves, and the mitral component is normally predominant. The intensity of S_1 often depends upon the thickness of the valves and the rate of rise of ventricular pressure. Mobile but stiff leaflets thickened by rheumatic heart disease may produce a louder than normal S_1; immobile and incompetent leaflets or a weak left ventricle cause a softer S_1.

SECOND HEART SOUND (S_2). The second heart sound is caused by the closure of the semilunar valves (aortic and pulmonic). Normally, these sounds can be heard separately (splitting of the second heart sound). Since the systolic ejection time of the right ventricle is longer than that of the left, pulmonic closure (P_2) follows aortic closure (A_2). During inspiration, the disparity in ejection times is minimized and the two closure sounds tend to approach one another.

Normally, in adults the aortic closure sound is louder and more widely distributed than pulmonic closure. Systemic hypertension increases the intensity of A_2. Pulmonary hypertension intensifies P_2; the right ventricle and pulmonary artery are pushed anteriorly in proximity to the sternum, contributing to the accentuation of P_2. The cardiac nurse should be alert to the appearance of a loud P_2 as it may be one of the early signs of a massive pulmonary embolus.

GALLOP SOUNDS. Heart disease is the most common cause of these diastolic and presystolic sounds. *Gallops* are so termed because the addition of a third sound is auscultatorily reminiscent of a

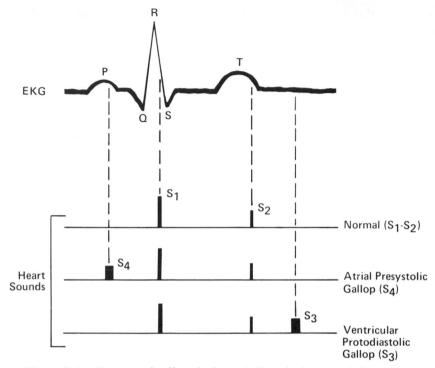

Figure 5–2. Diagram of gallop rhythms. Gallop rhythms result from the exaggeration of the normally inaudible third (S_3) and fourth (S_4) heart sounds. Note the timing of these gallop sounds in relation to the normal first (S_1) and the second (S_2) heart sounds. (From Conn, H. L., Merrill, J. P., and Lauler, D. P.: Modern Concepts in Congestive Failure. Vol. 3. The Therapeutic Series of Hoffman. New York, La Roche, Inc., 1969.)

galloping horse. There are two types of gallop sounds (see Fig. 5–2):

Third Heart Sound (S_3). This low-pitched sound, due to the rapid filling of the ventricle in early diastole, is also known as a ventricular gallop. It is heard in the first part of diastole (protodiastole), usually only .12 to .20 seconds after the aortic valve closure sound (A_2), and can be mimicked by repeating the word "Kentucky." It may be barely audible in healthy children and in young adults. In adults, it is most frequently indicative of myocardial failure or incompetence of the atrioventricular valves (especially mitral incompetence). If an S_3 gallop is heard for the first time early in the course of a myocardial infarction, the nurse should be alerted to the probability of left ventricular failure. Treatment for congestive heart failure is usually started when a ventricular gallop appears.

Fourth Heart Sound (S_4). This sound, heard in late diastole or presystole, is due to the distension of a poorly compliant ventricle by a vigorous atrial contraction. It is also known as an atrial gallop, and can be mimicked by repeating the word "Tennessee." In atrial fibrillation, an S_4 gallop cannot be present as there is no synchronized atrial contraction.

With a slow heart rate, when both the S_3 and S_4 gallops are heard (along with the normal S_1 and S_2), the resultant rhythm is known as *quadruple rhythm.* When both gallop sounds are present with a rapid heart rate, they fuse together in mid-diastole, giving a triple rhythm with a very loud gallop sound—a *summation gallop.*

PERICARDIAL FRICTION RUB. The rubbing together of the roughened surfaces of the epicardium and the pericardial sac causes these scratchy, high-pitched sounds, which have the quality of a creaking leather harness. They may be heard throughout the cardiac cycle or only in systole or diastole. Occasionally, a pericardial friction rub will be heard in the first few days after a myocardial infarction, and probably indicates full-thickness ischemic injury to the ventricular wall.

Heart murmurs. The flow of blood through the normal heart and great vessels does not cause turbulence or eddy formation. However, when the walls of a vessel are uneven, or when there are irregularities of valve surfaces over which blood passes, a murmur will result. Murmurs are classified by their timing (systolic or diastolic), their location and radiation, and their intensity. Systolic murmurs particularly are graded in intensity from Grade I, which is the faintest audible murmur, to Grade VI, which can be heard with the stethoscope just removed from the chest wall. When a murmur increases in intensity after its onset, it is "crescendo"; if it then decreases, it is called a *crescendo-decrescendo murmur* or a *diamond-shaped murmur.* When a phonocardiogram is recorded, the increasing and then decreasing amplitude (intensity) of the murmur resembles the configuration of a diamond, hence a diamond-shaped murmur. Murmurs which span systole and diastole without pause are termed *continuous.* The usual locations of murmurs emanating from the various cardiac valves are shown in Figure 5–3.

MIDSYSTOLIC EJECTION MURMURS. Midsystolic ejection murmurs occur during the period of ventricular ejection, starting in early systole when the semilunar valve opens and ending when blood flow in the aorta (or pulmonary artery) starts to reverse.

Aortic Stenosis (AS). The murmur of aortic stenosis is best heard over the base of the heart, but it may also radiate into the neck or to the ventricular apex. This murmur is not initiated until the left ventricular pressure exceeds central aortic pressure and the aortic valve opens; therefore, it is separated from the mitral valve closure sound (S_1) by a short interval. The murmur increases in intensity until the rapid ejection of blood slows, and then it decreases in inten-

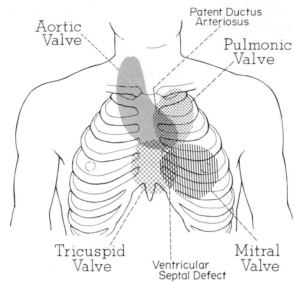

Figure 5-3. Diagram showing the areas in which cardiac valvular murmurs can be most often heard.

sity, stopping before the aortic valve closes—a crescendo-decrescendo (diamond-shaped) murmur. It may be represented graphically as in Figure 5-4.

Coarctation of the Aorta. Coarctation causes an ejection murmur which can be well heard over the entire precordium, but especially well in the back, between the scapulae. It has the same ejection quality, but its peak intensity is reached later in systole because the vascular obstruction is just distal to the left subclavian artery (rather

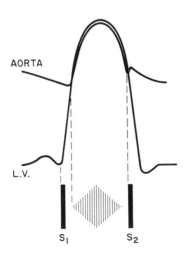

Figure 5-4. Diagram of midsystolic ejection murmurs. (From Leonard, J. J., and Kroetz, F. W.: Examination of the Heart. Part 4. Auscultation. American Heart Association, 1966.)

than at the level of the aortic valve). Since blood flows past the coarctation throughout the cardiac cycle, a continuous murmur is sometimes heard posteriorly, directly over the coarctation.

Pulmonic Stenosis (PS). The murmur of pulmonic stenosis is also an ejection-type murmur, which is heard best over the pulmonic valve area. The murmur may result from obstruction to blood flow at either the pulmonic valve (valvular PS) or the infundibulum of the right ventricle (as in tetralogy of Fallot). A pulmonic ejection murmur can also be caused by increased blood flow across the valve — a *pulmonic flow murmur,* a relative stenosis. This increased blood flow may be limited to the pulmonary circulation, as in an atrial septal defect, or it may be general with an overall increase in cardiac output, as in hyperthyroidism, anemia, and pregnancy.

SYSTOLIC REGURGITANT MURMURS. These murmurs are caused by the backward flow of blood from a chamber of higher pressure to one of lower pressure (mitral and tricuspid insufficiency, ventricular septal defect). The murmur usually begins with the first heart sound and continues up to and through the aortic closure sound, i.e., pan-systolic (throughout systole). After the second heart sound, ventricular pressures remain higher than atrial pressure and regurgitation continues until the pressure in the ventricle becomes lower than the atrium. Figure 5–5 diagrammatically depicts these relationships. Often there are exceptions to the expected pansystolic behavior of regurgitant murmurs. For example, mitral insufficiency from a "floppy valve" may not occur until midsystole when the redundant leaflet prolapses into the atrium.

Mitral Insufficiency (MI). The murmur of mitral insufficiency is usually blowing in character and is heard best at the apex. Typi-

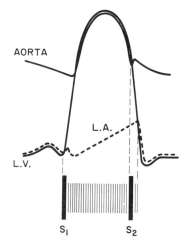

Figure 5–5. Diagram of pansystolic regurgitant murmurs. (From Leonard, J. J., and Kroetz, F. W.: Examination of the Heart. Part 4. Auscultation. American Heart Association, 1966.)

cally it radiates well into the axilla, but there are exceptions. For example, in mitral insufficiency due to a ruptured papillary muscle, chordae tendineae, or leaflet perforation, the murmur may be "scratchy" and well heard along the left sternal border, under the clavicles, and even over the carotid arteries. A rapid filling sound, heard in early diastole (S₃), is a common accompaniment of the murmur.

Tricuspid Insufficiency (TI). This murmur is heard well along the left sternal border at the xiphoid and sometimes to the right of the sternum or out toward the apex. It does not radiate to the axilla. The murmur of tricuspid insufficiency often has a "close-to-the-ear" quality, since the tricuspid valve lies just beneath the sternum. With inspiration, right ventricular stroke volume increases, intensifying the murmur. This respiratory variation is an important feature in differentiating tricuspid from mitral insufficiency, particularly when both are heard at the apex, since the mitral murmur tends to soften on inspiration. In congestive heart failure, dilatation of the right ventricle causes a functional insufficiency of the tricuspid valve. The nurse may observe the disappearance of the tricuspid insufficiency murmur when the congestive heart failure is brought under control.

Ventricular Septal Defect (VSD). The murmur of a ventricular septal defect is heard just beside the sternal border in the fourth, fifth, and sixth intercostal spaces; it is accompanied by a forceful systolic thrill, and radiates rightwardly across the chest. Although it is a pansystolic (holosystolic) murmur, it often has midsystolic accentuation. It does not radiate to the axilla, nor are there respiratory variations, thereby differentiating it from mitral or tricuspid insufficiency.

The sudden appearance of a systolic regurgitant murmur in a patient with a myocardial infarction should alert the nurse to the probability of subsequent severe and fulminant congestive heart failure. The coronary ischemia can cause rupture of a papillary muscle or chordae tendineae, or a perforation of the interventricular septum; in these instances, a rapidly deteriorating course ensues.

DIASTOLIC MURMURS AT THE MITRAL AND TRICUSPID VALVES. These filling murmurs, which are caused by a normal flow of blood across diseased atrioventricular valves, or by increased flow across normal valves, have a rumbling quality, hence the name *diastolic rumble*. Since diastolic filling of the ventricle occurs at relatively low pressures, rumbles are low in frequency and are best heard with the stethoscope bell. Ventricular filling is most rapid in early diastole (rapid-filling phase) and in late diastole (or presystole) when the atrial contraction adds its filling impact; rumbles are best heard at these times in the cardiac cycle.

Mitral Stenosis (MS). This murmur is often heard in a very localized area just inside the apical impulse, and auscultation is facilitated with the patient lying on his left side. Presystolic accentuation of the murmur results from atrial systole (and might be thought of as an *atrial systolic ejection murmur*), and it terminates in a prominent first heart sound. In very severe cases, when cardiac output is markedly reduced and blood flow over the mitral valve is also decreased, the murmur cannot be heard—the "dumb" or "silent" mitral.

Tricuspid Stenosis (TS). This murmur has the same auscultatory characteristics as mitral stenosis, but is best heard over the lower half of the sternum.

Diastolic Flow Murmurs. In ventricular septal defects and in patent ductus arteriosus, there is a significant increase in the amount of blood flowing to the lungs and returning to the left heart. The resultant increase in blood flow across the mitral valve during early diastole causes a rumbling mitral murmur which is very short and is often confused with a rapid-filling sound (S_3). A similar murmur may be heard less constantly over the tricuspid valve in patients with atrial septal defects.

EARLY DIASTOLIC MURMURS OF AORTIC AND PULMONIC VALVES. *Aortic Insufficiency (AI).* This murmur typically resembles the high-pitched sound of rushing water and often requires careful concentration on the diastolic timing in order to appreciate its presence. When the murmur is soft, its intensity can be accentuated by having the patient in the sitting position, leaning somewhat forward and holding his breath in deep expiration. Listen for the sound of a distant waterfall, or of a soft wind rustling leaves. The murmur of aortic insufficiency is best heard along the lower left sternal border. When the left ventricle relaxes in early diastole, a large gradient from the aorta to the left ventricle is immediately established, and the peak intensity of the aortic insufficiency murmur is correspondingly immediate. Subsequently, there is a progressive reduction in the aorta to left ventricle gradient, giving the murmur its characteristic decrescendo quality.

In patients with bacterial endocarditis, the development of a murmur of aortic insufficiency may be an ominous sign. Perforation of one (or more) of the cusps of the aortic valve by the inflammatory process (see Fig. 1–34) may lead to rapid cardiac decompensation; the nurse should be alert to this possibility.

Pulmonic Insufficiency. Most valvular pulmonary insufficiency murmurs are due to pulmonary hypertension, but may also result from bacterial endocarditis or postsurgical changes. This murmur has the same quality, location, and radiation as aortic valvular insufficiency, and differentiation of the two murmurs by auscultation alone is difficult.

In summary of this section, the physical findings sometimes seen in acute myocardial infarction will be reviewed. The cardiac nurse should be alert to these abnormalities. A large majority of patients with myocardial infarction, however, do not show any significant cardiac abnormalities.

When a large area of ventricle is infarcted, it cannot contribute effectively to ventricular contraction. During systole, this area fails to contract and, in fact, bulges outwardly with the high ventricular pressure. This sustained outward thrust can often be palpated on the chest wall, usually at the cardiac apex. If a ventricular aneurysm develops at the infarction site, this paradoxical apical pulsation is very easily appreciated.

Abnormal rubs, sounds, and murmurs are sometimes heard at varying stages in the course of a myocardial infarction. If the ischemic process involves the full ventricular wall thickness, the roughened epicardial surface may rub against the pericardial sac, causing a pericardial friction rub over the infarcted area. This rub may be heard in either systole or diastole, or both.

Should the infarction cause enough hemodynamic impairment to precipitate left ventricular overload, the ejection time of that chamber will be prolonged. A delay in the closure of the aortic valve ensues. Then with inspiration, the ejection time of the left and right ventricles is nearly equal and aortic valve closure (A_2) and pulmonic valve closure (P_2) are simultaneous or unsplit. With expiration, the right ventricular ejection period is less than the left, and P_2 will precede A_2, a situation exactly opposite the normal physiologic splitting of the second heart sounds (a paradoxical splitting). The appearance of a ventricular gallop (S_3) or atrial gallop (S_4) usually indicates ventricular failure.

The appearance of pansystolic murmurs somewhat later in the course of a myocardial infarction usually is an ominous sign. Ventricular dilatation from congestive failure can cause dilatation of the annulus of either the mitral or tricuspid valves, or both, with resultant mitral or tricuspid insufficiency. If the failure can be controlled, the ventricular dilatation usually disappears, as do these murmurs.

Of greater consequence is the rupture of a papillary muscle or chordae tendineae; both these pathologic lesions produce a murmur of mitral insufficiency. The clinical course is often one of rapid deterioration, as the heart cannot tolerate the combined burden of the infarction and the hemodynamic deficit imposed by the regurgitant mitral valve. Perforation of the interventricular septum, an uncommon result of septal infarction, produces a similar systolic murmur heard best in the VSD area. The clinical "dysfunction" of the papillary muscle complex is the result of ischemic degeneration (but not rupture) of the papillary muscle. During early systole, mitral competence is maintained (i.e., no murmur). As ventricular ejection progresses, the mitral valve becomes incompetent part way through systole, resulting in a diamond-shaped ejection murmur of mitral insufficiency. The clinical course of the syndrome of papillary muscle dysfunction is usually not fulminant, but may be quite debilitating.

If the cardiac nurse is alert to the diagnostic and therapeutic corollaries of these pathologic sequences, she will be much more effective in the care of her patients.

X-ray Films

The chest roentgenogram, or x-ray film, is essential in the diagnosis of patients with cardiac disease. Not only can certain anatomic abnormalities be clearly identified by x-ray films, but physiologic alterations can also be inferred. X-ray film techniques include routine "plain" films of a cardiac series, portable chest films, fluoroscopy, and angiography (angiocardiography, aortography, and selective coronary arteriography).

ROUTINE CHEST FILMS

The silhouette of the heart, its chambers, and great vessels can be seen on an x-ray film because the radiographic density of the heart (muscle and blood) is different from surrounding structures like lung (air), pericardial fat, and the esophagus when filled with barium. Routine chest films are taken with the patient erect and in deep inspiration. The patient's anterior chest is in contact with the x-ray plate and the x-ray beam originates 6 feet behind the patient (a 6 foot posteroanterior [PA] film). Significant changes in the size and contour of the heart are apparent if the film is taken at a different phase of respiration, if the tube distance is varied, if the patient is supine, or if the x-ray beam passes from front to back (anteroposterior [AP] film). The other projectional views composing a cardiac series delineate specific portions of the cardiac contour by projecting them in profile against the radiolucent lung as the body is rotated. These additional views are the lateral, the right anterior oblique, and the left anterior oblique views. Right and left oblique refer to the portion of the anterior chest that is placed against the x-ray film. Figure 5–6 portrays diagrammatically and graphically these relationships.

When fluid accumulates in the lungs or pleural cavities, it can be detected easily because it is dense while the air-filled lungs are lucent. Pulmonary edema often causes fluffy densities around the root of the lung, in a batwing distribution. Pleural effusions usually obscure the sharp costophrenic angles and sometimes the diaphragmatic shadows, curving upward on the lateral and posterior portions of the chest wall. The septa between pulmonary lobes are normally

(Text continued on page 216.)

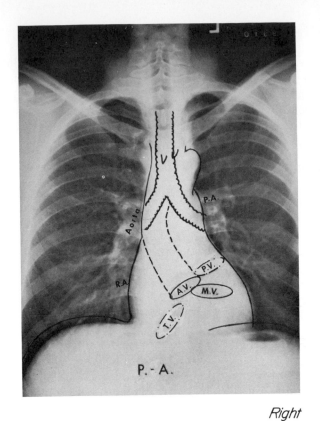

Right

PA

STERNUM

Figure 5–6. Schematic diagram of the chest showing the projections of the routine "cardiac series." The dark arrow in this diagram and in the following diagrams indicates the direction of the x-ray beam.

(Illustration continues on following pages.)

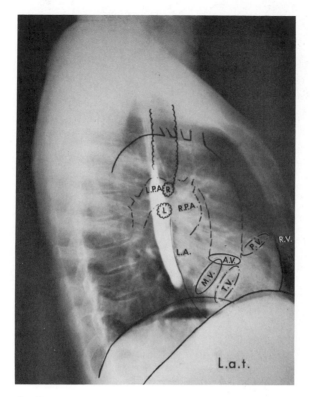

Left

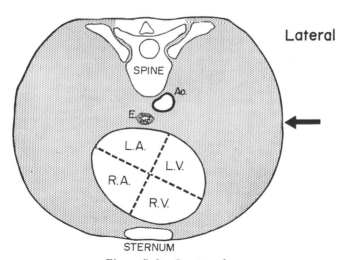

Figure 5–6. *Continued.*

Right

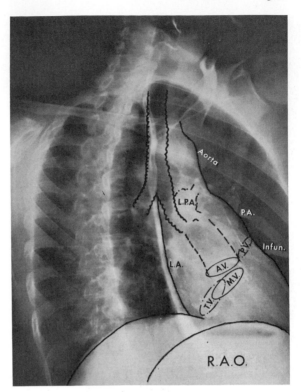

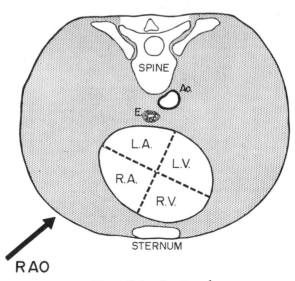

Figure 5–6. Continued.

Left

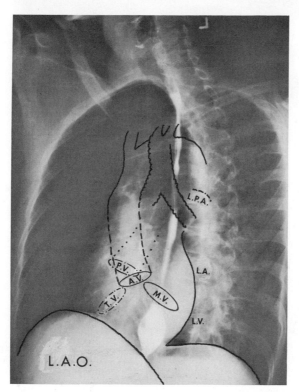

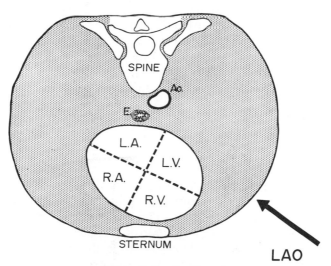

Figure 5–6. *Continued.*

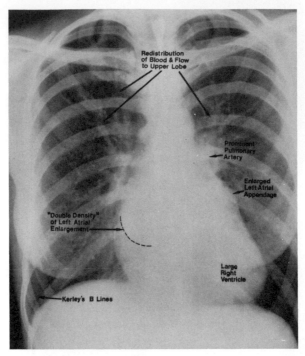

Figure 5–7.   Chest film of mitral stenosis. Note the prominence of the pulmonary artery and the left atrial appendage causing the straightened left heart border. Left atrial enlargement is also seen as "double density" on the right side of the heart.

free of fluid and are radiographically invisible. Fluid accumulating in these septa causes linear radiographic densities, a significant event requiring etiologic clarification. Patients with tight mitral stenosis or left heart failure often exhibit Kerley's B lines, indicating pulmonary venous hypertension (Fig. 5–7). These lines are short, flat, horizontal radiodensities usually seen in the periphery of the lower lobes; they represent edema fluid in the interlobular septa.

FLUOROSCOPY

Fluoroscopy is a technique in which heart, lung, and vessel movements are viewed on a luminescent x-ray film screen in a darkened room. Modern image amplifiers and television display of the projected image have increased the clarity of the views. The specific contribution of fluoroscopy derives from this motion analysis of the intrathoracic structures—the heart beating, the lungs expanding, the diaphragm moving, and so forth. Fluoroscopy is also very useful in the placement and positioning of an intravenous pacemaking electrode.

ANGIOGRAPHY

Angiography is an invaluable tool in cardiac diagnosis and has greatly extended the understanding of heart and blood vessel pathology. Iodinated water-soluble compounds that are opaque to the x-ray beam (called *contrast agents*) are injected into the circulation at appropriate sites. Rapidly changing films or movies (*cineangiograms*) record the dynamics of the passage of the contrast agent through the vascular tree, starting at the site of injection.

Angiocardiograms are recorded when the contrast agent is injected into a cardiac chamber. This technique is particularly useful for analyzing valvular lesions (e.g., valvular stenosis), valvular insufficiency, intracardiac shunts, and the patterns of ventricular contraction (Fig. 5–8).

Movie film recording of these angiographic studies (*cineangiography*) is particularly valuable, because the film can be viewed at both rapid and slow speeds, and detailed and unlimited review of the component cardiac action is possible. Cine techniques are particularly valuable in demonstrating the narrowing or obstructions of coronary arteries.

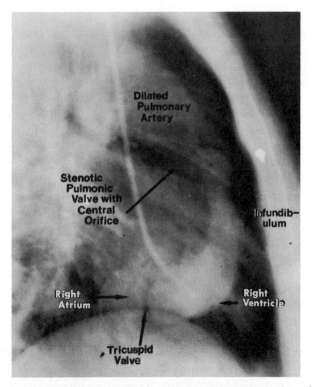

Figure 5–8. Angiocardiogram of valvular pulmonic stenosis, lateral view. The catheter is in the hypertrophied right ventricle. Note the reflux of contract agent back into the right atrium, the "doming" of the stenotic pulmonic valve with its small central orifice, and the poststenotic dilatation of the pulmonary artery.

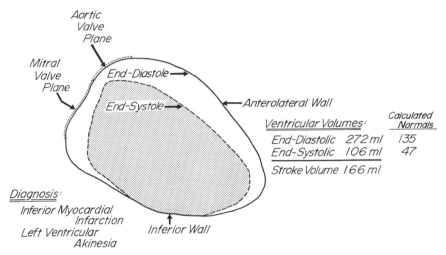

Figure 5-9.   Left ventricular volume measurement by angiocardiographic methods in left ventricular akinesia. Note the lack of motion of the interior wall of the heart between end-systole and end-diastole.

Angiocardiography is also used to determine left ventricular volumes. Contrast agent is injected into the left ventricle and the contraction of the ventricle is recorded on movie film or rapidly changed films. The end-systolic and end-diastolic surface areas of the left ventricular shadow are viewed in two planes. Making appropriate corrections for magnification, the volume and shape of the left ventricle can be determined by assuming that the ventricle has an elliptical shape and by using the geometric equation for the volume of an ellipse (Fig. 5-9).

Aortography involves the injection of a bolus of contrast agent into the aorta through a long (80 to 100 cm) radiopaque catheter. The catheter is introduced via the brachial or femoral artery and guided in a retrograde direction to the selected site under fluoroscopic control. Abnormalities in the aorta and its major branches are often best seen by filming the opacified vessel serially with a rapid film-changing device. Static anatomic detail rather than dynamics of motion is the desired end result (Fig. 5-10).

Newer techniques and arterial catheter design have allowed the selective cannulation of relatively small caliber arteries. The injection of contrast material into such an artery usually provides excellent detail of its pathologic anatomy. For example, the segmental obstructions of the individual coronary arteries can be nicely visualized (by either cine or rapid-changing film techniques) by delivering contrast agent into a coronary artery through a catheter that has been positioned in its orifice (selective coronary arteriography).

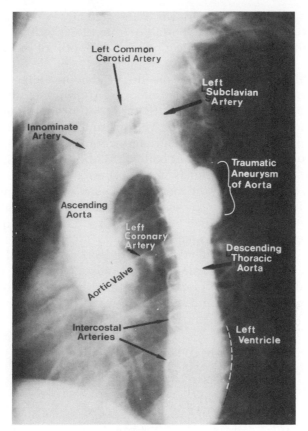

Figure 5–10. Aortogram of traumatic aneurysm of the thoracic aorta, left anterior oblique projection.

PORTABLE CHEST FILMS

In patients with myocardial infarctions or in the postoperative care of cardiac surgery patients, repeated portable chest films are valuable in following the patient's progress. Portable film technique is quite different from the standard procedure for the 6 foot PA films taken in the x-ray film department. Portable chest films are usually taken at a shorter tube distance (40 to 45 inches) in the AP direction with the x-ray film placed posteriorly, and often with the patient supine. It is important to consider these differences in technique when viewing portable films because the heart and great vessels assume a different size and configuration. In the AP projection, the anteriorly situated heart is further from the x-ray film than in the PA projection and therefore casts a larger "shadow" on the x-ray film. Changes in heart size cannot be accurately compared on AP and PA projections. Reliable comparisons of the size of the heart and mediastinum between sequential portable films are possible only when similar tube distances, projections, and depth of inspiration are achieved.

Portable films can also be useful in showing lobar or platelike atelectasis, hemothorax, or pneumothorax. Appropriate treatment with more aggressive pulmonary toilette, diuretics, or inotropic drugs, and with thoracentesis is instituted. The presence of a large gastric air bubble below the left hemidiaphragm requires aspiration by nasogastric intubation. A significant collection of blood clots in the mediastinum or around the heart is usually seen as a localized widening or bulging of the heart or the mediastinal shadows. If this mediastinal widening is accompanied by excessive blood loss through the chest tubes or by signs of cardiac tamponade, reoperation is indicated to remove the offending clots.

Other findings which may be noted on portable films are the endotracheal tube, epicardial pacing wires, valvular prostheses, mediastinal and pleural drainage catheters, the sternal closure wires, and the electrocardiogram leads (Fig. 5–11).

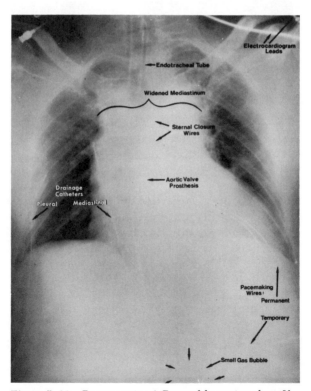

Figure 5–11. Postoperative A-P portable supine chest film.

Cardiac Catheterization

Although the passage of a long slender catheter into the heart was first accomplished 40 years ago, the sophisticated diagnostic technique of cardiac catheterization has made its most rapid developmental strides in the past 10 to 15 years. At the present time, nearly every type of anatomic intracardiac abnormality can be detected by appropriate catheterization techniques.

TECHNIQUES

In concept, catheterization of the right side of the heart is a simple procedure. A slender plastic catheter is inserted into a peripheral vein (femoral, antecubital) and is advanced through the venous system into the right atrium. The catheter may then be manipulated under fluoroscopic control through the tricuspid valve into the right ventricle, through the pulmonic valve into the main pulmonary artery, and then through the pulmonary vessels until it becomes wedged in a very small peripheral branch (the pulmonary capillary wedge [PCW] position). In this wedge position, it obstructs arterial blood flow but can record pressure oscillations transmitted from the pulmonary veins and the left atrium, thus reflecting indirectly the pulmonary venous or left atrial pressures.

Catheterization of the left side of the heart is not quite so simple. Retrograde entry into the left ventricle can be accomplished by advancing a catheter from a peripheral arterial puncture site (femoral, brachial, axillary) into the ascending aorta, and then through the aortic valve into the left ventricle. The left ventricle may also be entered by percutaneous puncture through the chest wall. This is a somewhat more hazardous technique, but is particularly useful in patients who have undergone aortic valve replacement in whom it is unwise to pass a catheter through the prosthesis, or in patients whose aortic valves are so stenotic that the catheter cannot be advanced through them.

The left atrium, however, can seldom be reached by these techniques. More commonly, *trans-septal puncture* is used to gain access to the left atrium; a long, terminally curved, catheter-sheathed needle is advanced from the femoral vein into the right atrium and the mid or lower third of the atrial septum is engaged by rotating the curved needle posteromedially. Pressure is then exerted on the needle against the septum. Perforation of the septum and entry into the left atrium is confirmed by the appearance of a left atrial pressure trace on the monitoring oscilloscope. After drawing a sample of blood from this new site to ensure that there is a high oxygen saturation (i.e., left atrial blood), the catheter itself is advanced over the needle into the left atrium. The needle is withdrawn and the catheter can then be advanced past the mitral valve into the left ventricle.

DATA COLLECTION

When cardiac catheters are passed through the venous or arterial system back into the various chambers of the heart, pressure measurements and blood oxygen measurements can be made. As the catheter has end holes or side holes, blood for oxygen analysis may be withdrawn from the various cardiac chambers through the catheter system. Pressures from the heart are recorded by attaching the catheter to a strain gauge transducer with its connecting amplifier and recording device. Further, radiopaque contrast agents or indicator dyes can be injected through the catheters for the purpose of angiocardiography and cardiac output determinations (see below).

Pressure Measurements

Pressure measurements are valuable in diagnosing intracardiac pathology and in evaluating the degree of hemodynamic abnormality. The shape of the pressure wave forms may help determine the type of valvular pathology (i.e., stenosis or insufficiency). Elevation of the mean pressures in cardiac chambers and the great vessels is indicative of the severity of the pathologic physiology involved. For example, the severity of mitral stenosis can be assessed by determining the mean left atrial pressure, the right ventricular pressure, and the mean pulmonary artery pressure if the cardiac output is also measured.

Atrial pressures. Normally, right atrial pressure varies from 0 to 5 mm Hg, left atrial pressure from 5 to 10 mm Hg. With an intact atrial septum, the mean pressures of the two atria should differ by 3 to 5 mm Hg, but in atrial septal defects the atria have the same pressure. Elevated mean atrial pressures occur with stenosis (or insufficiency) of the atrioventricular valves, ventricular failure, or with constrictive pericarditis. In mitral or tricuspid insufficiency, ventricular blood refluxes back through the valve, causing high atrial pressures during ventricular contraction.

If blood flow across the mitral valve were obstructed by a stenotic orifice, left atrial pressure would not fall promptly during diastole. The left atrial pressure will thereby be higher than the left ventricular pressure early in diastole. This pressure differential is called a *gradient* across the valve. At the beginning of ventricular diastole, the gradient

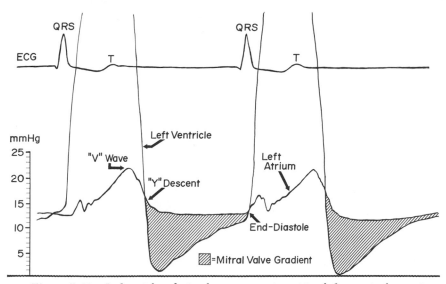

Figure 5–12. Left atrial and simultaneous equisensitive left ventricular tracings in mitral stenosis. Note the shallow slope of the "y" descent indicating valvular stenosis. The gradient in early diastole far exceeds the end-diastolic gradient.

is high but then decreases progressively to the point of end-diastole when ventricular pressure starts to rise (Fig. 5–12).

Ventricular pressures. The left ventricle normally has a systolic pressure of 120 mm Hg and a diastolic pressure of 10 mm Hg or less. Corresponding normal pressures for the right ventricle are 25 mm Hg and 0 to 5 mm Hg, respectively.

Elevation of peak ventricular pressures are caused by obstruction of the outlet valves (aortic and pulmonic stenosis) and by increased resistance in the distal vascular bed (systemic hypertension and pulmonary hypertension of whatever cause). When there is decreased ventricular compliance (as in ventricular hypertrophy or constrictive pericarditis) or when the end-diastolic volume is increased (as in congestive failure, aortic insufficiency, and mitral insufficiency), the pressure at the end of diastole may be elevated (an elevated end-diastolic pressure).

Pressures in the great vessels (aorta and pulmonary artery). The systolic pressures in the great vessels are normally the same as the ventricles from which they arise, 120 mm Hg in the aorta and 25 mm Hg in the pulmonary artery. The diastolic pressure depends upon the resistance of the distal circuit. The systemic arterioles are quite resistive and the normal aortic diastolic pressure descends only to 80 mm Hg, whereas the diastolic pressure in the pulmonary artery will drop to about 10 mm Hg, reflecting the low resistance in that circuit.

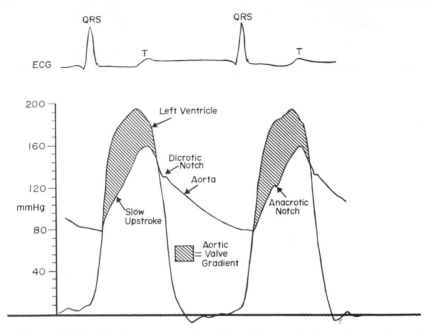

Figure 5–13. Simultaneous, equisensitive left ventricular and central aortic pressure tracings in aortic stenosis. Note the shallow slope of the aortic upstroke and the prominent anacrotic notch (both indicating valvular stenosis) and the gradient across the valve (cross-hatched area).

Elevated pulmonary artery pressures are found in patients with increased pulmonary blood flow (e.g., atrial and ventricular septal defects, patent ductus arteriosus), increased pulmonary arteriolar resistance (e.g., chronic lung disease, pulmonary embolism), and elevated pulmonary capillary (wedge) pressures (e.g., mitral stenosis, left ventricular failure). Low pulmonary artery pressures are seen in patients with proximal obstruction to pulmonary blood flow (e.g., infundibular stenosis, pulmonic valvular stenosis). Elevated aortic pressures are seen in systemic hypertension and aortic insufficiency. Low aortic systolic pressure is seen in aortic outlet obstruction — subaortic stenosis, aortic valvular stenosis, or supravalvular stenosis. The rate of rise of the aortic pulse tracing is also very slow in aortic stenosis owing to the slow ejection of blood from the ventricle. Valvular obstruction is quantitated by the gradient between the ventricle and the aorta when the cardiac output is known (cross-hatched area in Figure 5–13).

Low aortic diastolic pressure is evident in aortic insufficiency, which also causes the dicrotic notch to appear further down the descending limb of the aortic pulse trace.

Blood Oxygen Measurements

Samples of blood can easily be withdrawn from the cardiac catheters at various sites along their passage path and can subsequently be analyzed for their oxygen content.

Normal blood oxygen contents and saturations at different sampling sites are listed in Table 5–1.

The inferior vena caval blood has a higher oxygen saturation because of renal arteriovenous shunting. The coronary sinus oxygen saturation is extremely low because of the very high rate of oxygen extraction by cardiac muscle. The high oxygen saturation of the left-sided samples reflects the oxygen uptake of blood passing through the lungs.

These oxygen determinations provide useful information for localizing the site of a left-to-right shunt, for oxygenated blood entering the right side of the heart will immediately cause an oxygen step-up at that site. For example, oxygen contents of 15 vol per cent in the inferior vena cava and 19 vol per cent in the right atrium indicate the presence of atrial septal defect. Right-to-left shunts are detected by finding a less than normal oxygen saturation (95 per cent saturation) in the left-sided samples in the absence of lung disease. In a patent ductus arteriosus, oxygen content will be normal in the cavae, right atrium, and right ventricle but elevated in the pulmonary artery sample.

Since optimum mixing of blood from the cavae, coronary sinus, and Thebesian veins is normally achieved by the time it reaches the pulmonary artery, sampling from this site gives the most representative sample for oxygen content of mixed venous blood. In the absence of right-to-left shunts, oxygen content as found in the left atrial, left ventricular, or peripheral arterial sites are all representative of arterial oxygen content. The difference of oxygen content between the mixed venous and arterial samples is called the *arteriovenous oxygen difference* (the AVO_2 difference). Normally, this AVO_2 difference ranges between 3.5 and 4.5 ml of oxygen per 100 ml of

TABLE 5–1.   Normal Blood Oxygen Contents and Saturations

Sampling Site	O₂ Content (Vol per cent)	O₂ Saturation
Superior vena cava	14 (± 1)	70%
Inferior vena cava	16 (±1)	80%
Right atrium, right ventricle, and pulmonary artery	15 (± 1)	75%
Coronary sinus		20%
Left atrium, left ventricle, and peripheral arteries	18.9 to 19.3	94 to 96%

blood. Higher values indicate that greater amounts of oxygen are being extracted by the peripheral tissues and infer that blood is circulating more slowly through those tissues (lower cardiac output than normal), allowing greater oxygen extraction. This measurement correlates very well with changes in cardiac output and also with the severity of the patient's symptoms.

Determination of Cardiac Output

The amount of blood the heart propels forward is called the *cardiac output.* The determination of cardiac output is an important technique in cardiac catheterization because it quantitates the patient's hemodynamic impairment. A low cardiac output indicates that the heart, because of congenital or acquired disease, is unable to provide the tissues with an adequate blood supply, particularly in times of increased need (stress, exercise). Cardiac output is measured in liters of blood per minute in a normal-sized adult. The normal cardiac output is 6 liters per minute.

Relating cardiac output to body size provides more easily comparable values in determining the severity of a patient's heart disease. Therefore, the body surface area (as measured in square meters) is used to establish this relationship, which is known as the *cardiac index.* If a patient had a body surface area of 2 square meters (M²), the normal cardiac index would be half the cardiac output, $\dfrac{6 \text{ L/min}}{2 \text{ M}^2}$, 3 L/M²/min. The range of normal cardiac index is 2.6 to 4.0 L/M²/min. Cardiac output may be determined by either the Fick method or by dye dilution techniques.

Fick method. In 1870, Fick wrote, "The total uptake or release of a substance by an organ is the product of the blood flow to the organ and of the arteriovenous concentrations of the substance." In the case of oxygen, oxygen consumption equals the cardiac output times the AVO₂ difference. Therefore,

$$\text{Cardiac output} = \frac{\text{oxygen consumption (ml/min)}}{\text{arteriovenous O}_2 \text{ difference (ml/100 ml blood)}}$$

Oxygen consumption is determined by the collection and oxygen analysis of expired air under steady-state conditions. Normal oxygen consumption is 240 to 300 ml per min. From the previous section, we know that the mixed venous oxygen content is about 15 ml per 100 ml and the arterial blood is 19 ml per 100 ml. Applying these values to the Fick equation, normal resting cardiac output =

$$\frac{240 \text{ ml/min}}{19\text{--}15 \text{ ml/100 ml}} = \frac{240 \text{ ml/min}}{4 \text{ ml/100 ml}} = 6000 \text{ ml/min}$$

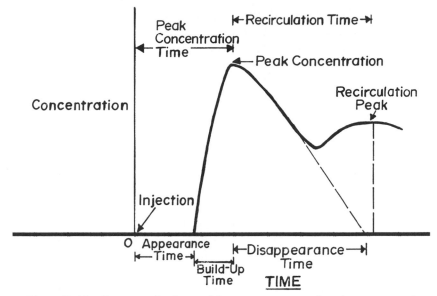

Figure 5–14. Diagram of indicator dilution curve, normal cardiac output without shunting.

Indicator dilution method. This sophisticated method is based upon the measurement of the concentration and dispersal of a dye which is injected centrally (e.g., pulmonary artery) and sampled at a peripheral arterial site (e.g., brachial artery). The arterial sample is continuously withdrawn through a sensing photoelectric cell (densitometer) by a constant flow pump. A time-concentration curve (dye-dilution curve) of the indicator is recorded from the densitometer,

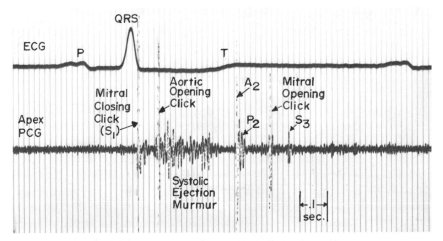

Figure 5–15. Phonocardiogram of double valve replacement. Note the systolic outflow murmur of the aortic prosthesis, and the opening and closing clicks of both the aortic and mitral prostheses. The S_3 indicates rapid ventricular filling.

which produces a "signal" that is proportional to the changing indicator concentration in the blood flowing through it (Fig. 5–14).

The cardiac output is computed from the known dose of the injected indicator and the area of the time-concentration curve. Characteristic curves are inscribed by low (or high) cardiac output, right-to-left shunts, and left-to-right shunts.

Phonocardiogram (PCG)

In phonocardiography, heart sounds are translated into electrical energy by a microphone and are recorded. The recorder must be equipped with an amplifier designed for the purpose. Usually an electrocardiogram and an indirect carotid pulse wave are recorded simultaneously for reference purposes in the timing of heart sounds. This technique is valuable for demonstrating those heart sounds and murmurs which approach the limits of audibility with the ordinary stethoscope. Its most valuable application is its precision in timing multiple sound events and in relating them to each other and to the electrocardiogram or carotid pulse (Fig. 5–15).

COMPLICATIONS

Cardiac catheterization is not an altogether innocuous procedure. Being aware of the possible complications of the procedure, the cardiac nurse should look closely for signs of these complications.

In the cardiac catheterization laboratory, the patient is required to lie flat on a hard x-ray table for one to four hours. Sometimes he is required to perform vigorous exercise so that chamber pressures and cardiac output can be measured under these stressful conditions. After puncture of an artery or a vein, the cardiac catheters often remain in the vessel for prolonged periods.

As a result of these manipulations, the patient is tired, hungry, and often complains of a backache or of pain in the arterial puncture site. Supportive treatment to make the patient more comfortable is a prime consideration. He would greatly benefit from a comforting word, a hot meal, a back rub, or some medication for his pain.

Whether the femoral, brachial, or axillary artery is used as the site of arterial puncture, a pressure dressing is usually applied over the site to help prevent additional bleeding from the artery. The nurse should periodically look at the tissue around the pressure dressing to make sure the area is not becoming swollen or ecchymotic. Significant swelling or discoloration should be brought to the physician's attention.

The arterial catheter occasionally causes thrombosis at the

cannulation site, sometimes with distal propagation of the clot. Should the patient complain of numbness, tingling, or coldness of the extremity, or should the nurse note the loss of a peripheral pulse or observe pallor or cyanosis, the physician should be immediately notified. Commonly, the loss of the peripheral pulse is due to arterial spasm secondary to the cannulation of the artery, and may be only transitory. If the pulse does not return in a few hours, investigative arteriography and surgical removal of the clot may be necessary; heparinization may help prevent distal thrombosis.

Arrhythmias, especially premature ventricular contractions, are very common during the passage of the catheters through the cardiac chambers or during the injection of the radio-opaque contrast agents into the ventricles. Usually, the arrhythmias have subsided by the time the patient returns to the ward, but occasionally they may persist. The cardiac nurse should observe closely for arrhythmias (feeling the pulse, listening to the apical beat) and be prepared to monitor the patient's electrocardiogram.

Rarely, a cardiac catheter will perforate through the wall of the heart, causing bleeding into the pericardial sac, resulting in cardiac tamponade. This complication can happen during direct left ventricular puncture, trans-septal catheterization, or even with a simple right heart catheterization. This serious event should be watched for closely. If the patient develops distended neck veins, a narrowing pulse pressure, pulsus paradoxus, or the signs of low cardiac output, the physician should be notified immediately. Pericardiocentesis or open thoracotomy may be necessary to reverse the severe hemodynamic consequences of this complication.

Bibliography

HISTORY TAKING AND PHYSICAL EXAMINATION

Benchimol, A., and Tippit, H. C.: The clinical value of the jugular and hepatic pulses. Progr. Cardiovasc. Dis. *10*:159–186, 1967.

Bristow, J. D., and Metcalfe, J.: Physical signs in congestive heart failure. Progr. Cardiovasc. Dis. *10*:236–245, 1967.

Criteria Committee of the New York Heart Association, Inc.: Diseases of the Heart and Blood Vessels (Nomenclature and Criteria for Diagnosis). 6th ed. Boston, Little Brown and Company, 1964.

Dunphy, J. E., and Botsford, T. W.: Physical Examination of the Surgical Patient. Philadelphia, W. B. Saunders Company, 1964.

Examination of the heart: Part One—History taking; Part Two—Inspection and palpation of venous and arterial pulses; Part Three—Inspection and palpation of the anterior chest; and Part Four—Auscultation. American Heart Association, 1965–1966.

Fyler, D. C., Gallagher, M. E., and Nadas, A. S.: Auscultation in the evaluation of children with heart disease. Progr. Cardiovasc. Dis. *10*:363–384, 1968.

Hultgren, H. H., Hancock, E. W., and Cohn, R. E.: Auscultation in mitral and tricuspid valvular disease. Progr. Cardiovasc. Surg. *10*:298–322, 1968.

Hurst, W. J., and Logue, R. B.: Examination of the cardiovascular system: Section A— History and physical examination, The Heart. New York, McGraw-Hill Book Company, 1966.

Marx, H. J., and Yu, P. N.: Clinical examination of the arterial pulse. Progr. Cardiovasc. Dis. *10*:207–235, 1967.

Mounsey, J. P. D.: Inspection and palpation of the cardiac impulse. Progr. Cardiovasc. Dis. *10*:187–206, 1967.

Perloff, J. C.: Clinical recognition of aortic stenosis. Progr. Cardiovasc. Dis. *10*:323–352, 1968.

X-RAY FILMS

Felson, B., Weinstein, A. S., and Spitz, H. B.: Principles of Chest Roentgenology, A Programed Text. Philadelphia, W. B. Saunders Company, 1965.

Hurst, J. W., and Logue, R. B.: The Heart. New York, McGraw-Hill Book Company, 1966.

Lester, R. G.: Radiologic concepts in the evaluation of heart disease, I and II. Mod. Conc. Cardiovasc. Dis. 37:113–118, 1968 and 38:7–12, 1969.

CARDIAC CATHETERIZATION

Hurst, M. J., and Logue, R. B.: The Heart. New York, McGraw-Hill Book Company, 1966.

Kory, K. C., Tsagaris, T. J., and Bustamante, R. A.: A Primer of Cardiac Catheterization. Springfield, Illinois, Charles C Thomas, Publisher, 1965.

CHAPTER 6

Respiratory Care

By ARTHUR N. THOMAS, M.D.

Introduction

IMPORTANCE OF PULMONARY CARE IN CARDIAC PATIENTS

Circulation of blood provides oxygen and nutrients and permits removal of carbon dioxide and metabolic wastes. Optimal function of this system is of crucial importance to cardiac patients, because the total blood flow or cardiac output may already be functioning at nearly 100 per cent capacity. Almost all normal blood flow is utilized to provide oxygen, but only 1/20 as much blood flow is required for carbon dioxide removal, 1/100 for provision of nutrients, and 1/200 for removal of metabolic wastes. The heart provides this oxygen delivery system, including the supply for itself. Not only is the heart especially susceptible to reduced blood flow, but hypoxia and acidosis caused by poor circulation can further compromise an already weakened heart.

SPECIAL NEEDS OF CARDIAC PATIENTS

Cardiac patients have special susceptibility to respiratory failure and recovery from a cardiac illness is often determined by the adequacy of pulmonary care. Pulmonary complications occur in cardiac patients because of both direct and indirect pulmonary effects of heart disease and impaired circulation. There is often a fragile

231

MECHANISMS OF HYPOXIA

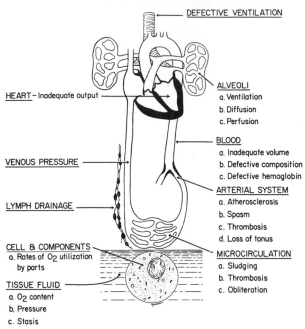

DEFECTIVE VENTILATION

HEART – Inadequate output

VENOUS PRESSURE

LYMPH DRAINAGE

CELL & COMPONENTS
a. Rates of O_2 utilization
   by parts

TISSUE FLUID
a. O_2 content
b. Pressure
c. Stasis

ALVEOLI
a. Ventilation
b. Diffusion
c. Perfusion

BLOOD
a. Inadequate volume
b. Defective composition
c. Defective hemoglobin

ARTERIAL SYSTEM
a. Atherosclerosis
b. Spasm
c. Thrombosis
d. Loss of tonus

MICROCIRCULATION
a. Sludging
b. Thrombosis
c. Obliteration

Figure 6–1. Oxygen demands of the cell. The diagram illustrates numerous factors which may influence the amount of oxygen delivered to the cell and its component parts. (From Hardy, J. D.: Tissue hypoxia in surgical practice. Amer. J. Surg. *106*:476, 1963.)

metabolic balance which is incapable of increased performance and intolerant of less than ideal conditions. Fortunately, good pulmonary care minimizes pulmonary deterioration.

Respiration is effected by the status of the lungs, circulation, metabolism, and health of every body cell. The essence of the respiratory system is illustrated by a schematic diagram showing the needs of a single cell (Fig. 6–1). There are three main phases of respiration — gaseous, blood, and tissue.

When the cellular environment is not maintained, chemical changes occur. When a cell membrane is injured, potassium leaks out and sodium enters, cellular swelling occurs, and intracellular enzymes and protein breakdown products are released. Adjacent cells can be injured and further propagate this phenomenon. Absorption of cell breakdown products into the blood stream can decrease myocardial pumping ability, depress the muscular tone and patency of the vascular system, and perpetuate a vicious cycle which is potentially irreversible; if it is not interrupted it will surely lead to the patient's death.

Hypoxemia means inadequate blood oxygenation; hypoxia means inadequate tissue oxygenation. Anoxemia and anoxia literally mean *no* oxygenation; the terms are often used loosely as the equivalent of hypoxemia and hypoxia. Hypoxia is exceedingly common. Deficient oxygenation also promotes hypercarbia, acidosis, and electrolyte changes. These changes present an immediate danger to the cardiac patient, because cardiac arrhythmias may occur and mechanical performance of the heart may be impaired, leading to circulatory failure and death.

SPECIAL NEEDS FOR PULMONARY CARE IN CARDIAC SURGERY PATIENTS

Multiple factors set the stage for respiratory problems in cardiac surgery patients. The *pulmonary status* is often abnormal. Long-

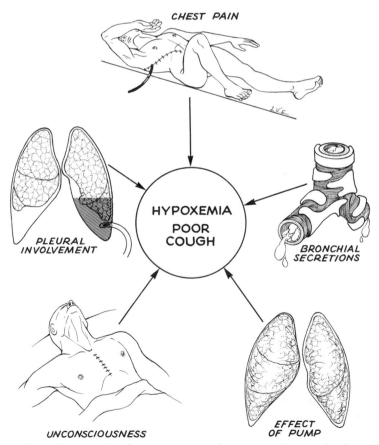

Figure 6–2. Postoperative factors promoting hypoxemia. See text for discussion.

standing changes, such as those associated with decreased compliance, congestion, pulmonary vascular changes (related to abnormal pressures, or to pulmonary emboli or thrombosis) can all predispose to pulmonary complications and failure. Cardiac patients undergoing surgery may have their pulmonary status further compromised because of the following factors (Fig. 6–2).

Consciousness is decreased by anesthesia, hypothermia, and extracorporeal circulation. The patient's respiratory excursions are limited by *chest pain* from the incision, leading to reduced *ability to cough,* and further suppressed by narcotics for analgesia. There is a high incidence of *pleural involvement* from hemothorax or atelectasis attendant to cardiac surgery. *Secretions* are likely to be thick and voluminous. Under these conditions, secretions are poorly cleared, causing airway blockage, and this leads also to a greater susceptibility to infection. Extracorporeal circulation causes special effects upon lung: decreased pulmonary function includes problems of diffusion, reduced compliance, and increased airway resistance; pathologic changes in the lung include interstitial hemorrhage, endothelial thickening, and surfactant depletion (see later).

The Respiratory Apparatus

ANATOMY OF THE RESPIRATORY TRACT

The anatomy of the respiratory tree begins with the mouth or nose and includes the pharynx, larynx, trachea, bronchi, and smaller airways down to the alveoli in which gas exchange occurs (Fig. 6–3). There are two main parts of the airway system: the conduction system in which essentially no gas is exchanged, and the alveoli in which a large amount of gas is exchanged. The conduction system includes the trachea, the right and left mainstem bronchi, and a sequence of smaller and smaller bronchial subdivisions, after 20 or 30 divisions of which the alveoli are reached. About 300 million alveoli, with a network of capillaries, form the gas exchange units. Each alveolus has a diameter of about 75 to 300 μ (1 μ equals .001 mm). The alveolar wall is less than 0.1 μ thick. The capillaries supplying the alveoli are also about 0.1 μ thick. The total surface area for gas exchange is about 70 square meters, or 40 times the entire surface area of the body. The lining of the airways is highly specialized. It is lined by cells that have a whiplike projection into the lumen called cilia. The movement of the cilia is important in propelling secretions and foreign

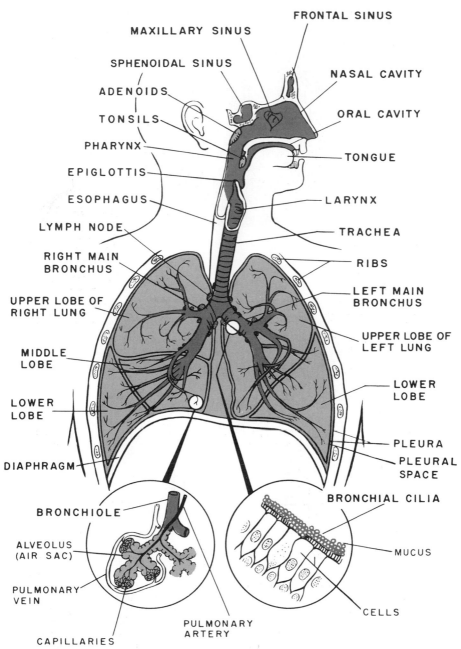

Figure 6–3. Anatomy of the respiratory tract. See text for discussion. (From Secor, J.: Patient Care in Respiratory Problems. Philadelphia, W. B. Saunders Company, 1969.)

STATIC LUNG VOLUMES

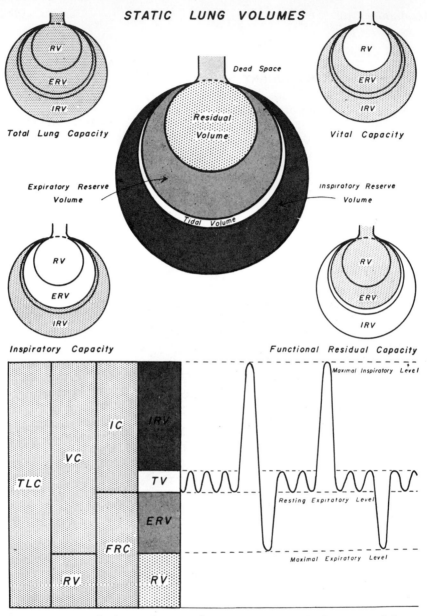

Figure 6–4. The lung volumes and capacities. *Above*, the large central diagram illustrates the four primary lung volumes and approximate magnitude. The outermost line indicates the greatest size to which the lung can expand; the innermost circle (residual volume), the volume that remains after all air has been voluntarily squeezed out of the lungs. Surrounding the central diagram are smaller diagrams; shaded areas in these represent the four lung capacities. The volume of dead space gas is included in residual volume, functional residual capacity, and total lung capacity when these are measured by routine techniques. *Below*, lung volumes as they appear on a spirographic tracing; shading in the vertical bar next to the tracing corresponds to that in the central diagram above. (From THE LUNG: CLINICAL PHYSIOLOGY AND PULMONARY FUNCTION TESTS, 2nd edition by Julius H. Comroe, Jr., et al. Copyright © 1962, Year Book Medical Publishers, Inc. Used by permission.)

236

material into the major airways so that they can be cleared by coughing. Cilia are very delicate and may be inactivated by infection, lack of humidification, or oxygen concentrations greater than 20 per cent. Another specialized function of the respiratory epithelium is the secretion of surfactant. This chemical substance promotes the expansion of alveoli and it may be decreased in the same situations which cause depressed ciliary action.

ANATOMY AND TERMINOLOGY OF AIR SPACES

During inspiration and expiration, the patient moves a certain volume of air, which can be subdivided into four static lung volumes and four capacities (Fig. 6–4 and Table 6–1).

The resting end-expiratory position is used here as a baseline, because it varies less than the end-inspiratory position. Some of these volumes and capacities require special methods for measurement.

The vital capacity (VC) can be measured at the bedside and is a good index of the reserve which is required for deep breathing, coughing, and clearing of secretions. The functional residual capacity (FRC) becomes important in concept when we discuss atelectasis and certain methods of assisted ventilation, such as continuous positive pressure breathing (CPPB).

TABLE 6–1. *The Lung Volumes and Capacities**

A. VOLUMES. There are four primary volumes which do not overlap:
  1. *Tidal Volume,* or the depth of breathing, is the volume of gas inspired or expired during each respiratory cycle. Tidal volume reflects the "depth of breathing."
  2. *Inspiratory Reserve Volume* is the maximal amount of gas that can be inspired from the end-inspiratory position.
  3. *Expiratory Reserve Volume* is the maximal volume of gas that can be expired from the end-expiratory position.
  4. *Residual Volume* is the volume of gas remaining in the lungs at the end of a maximal expiration.
B. CAPACITIES. There are four capacities, each of which includes two or more of the primary volumes:
  1. *Total Lung Capacity* is the amount of gas contained in the lung at the end of a maximal inspiration.
  2. *Vital Capacity* is the maximal volume of gas that can be expelled from the lungs by forceful effort following a maximal inspiration.
  3. *Inspiratory Capacity* is the maximal volume of gas that can be inspired from the resting expiratory level.
  4. *Functional Residual Capacity* is the volume of gas remaining in the lungs at the resting expiratory level.

*(From THE LUNG: CLINICAL PHYSIOLOGY AND PULMONARY FUNCTION TESTS, 2nd edition by Julius H. Comroe, Jr., et al. Copyright © 1962, Year Book Medical Publishers, Inc. Used by permission.)

Normal Respiratory Physiology

NORMAL VENTILATION

The mechanism by which air is delivered to the alveoli is the process of *alveolar ventilation*—the gaseous phase of respiration. Alveolar ventilation is the component of respiration most vulnerable to failure. Clinical problems of ventilation are far more frequent than those of either the blood or tissue phases of respiration.

During *inspiration*, the thorax is expanded by contraction of the intercostal muscles, the diaphragm, and the accessory muscles of respiration (Fig. 6–5). The pressure within the chest cavity becomes negative in respect to the "outside" atmospheric pressure; i.e., it is subatmospheric. Intra-alveolar gas pressure also becomes subatmospheric, and fresh air rushes into the airway and alveoli. At the end of inspiration, the pressure inside and the pressure outside the lung are essentially equalized. *Expiration* is normally a relatively

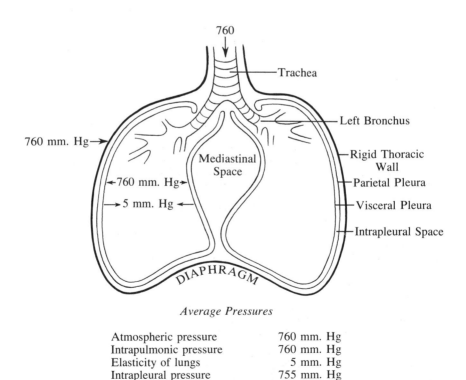

Average Pressures

Atmospheric pressure	760 mm. Hg
Intrapulmonic pressure	760 mm. Hg
Elasticity of lungs	5 mm. Hg
Intrapleural pressure	755 mm. Hg

Figure 6–5.   Schematic diagram of the chest at rest. See text for discussion. (From Secor, J.: Patient Care in Respiratory Problems. Philadelphia, W. B. Saunders Company, 1969.)

passive process. Air is expelled from the lungs by a lowering of the rib cage and the intrinsic elastic recoil of the lungs and does not normally require any effort.

THE PARTIAL PRESSURE CONCEPT

The purpose of respiration is to deliver to tissue about 250 ml of oxygen (O_2) and to remove about 200 ml of carbon dioxide (CO_2) per minute. The status of respiration is indicated by the changes of the gas content and the pH of venous and arterial blood. Some laws of the physics of gases are of considerable clinical importance.

Blood gas tensions or pressures are used frequently in most intensive care units in this country and are closely related to atmospheric pressure. The atmospheric pressure is determined by the weight of the gas that surrounds us, or ambient pressure, and this is equal to about 14.7 pounds per square inch (psi) or 760 mm Hg (Fig. 6–6).

At a very high altitude, such as in a space flight, the outside of a space capsule is exposed to a zero atmospheric pressure. As one descends to levels encountered in high altitude flying, or in mountainous areas, atmospheric pressure then becomes measurable, although pressures are reduced. At sea level, the atmospheric pressure is said to be equal to one atmosphere absolute pressure (1 ATA). One atmosphere of pressure is equivalent to 14.7 psi, 760 mm Hg, or 33 feet of sea water. Medical terminology for *gas tensions* is usually in mm Hg absolute pressure, gas pressure at sea level being 760 mm Hg, dependent upon daily fluctuations of barometric pressure. Arterial and venous pressures are measured as "gauge pressures," which are one atmosphere (or 760 mm Hg) greater than the equivalent absolute pressure.

The most frequent clinical gas measurements are the partial pressures of oxygen (P_{O_2}) and carbon dioxide (P_{CO_2}). The partial pressure of a gas is described by *Dalton's Law,* which states that in a mixed gas (composed of more than one gas) the pressure exerted by each gas is independent of the other gases and the partial pressure of each gas is proportional to the concentration (percentage) of the gas contained in the mixture. The total pressure of the gas mixture is the sum of the separate pressures of each of the gases. The same principle applies to gases dissolved in liquids, if not chemically combined. The partial pressure of mixed gas is then determined by the concentration (in per cent) multiplied by the total absolute pressure (760 mm Hg at sea level). For example, the air we breathe is approximately 21 per cent (20.94 per cent) oxygen. At sea level, when the barometric pressure is 760 mm Hg, the partial pressure of oxygen (P_{O_2}) of dry air is 21 per cent $\times$ 760 mm Hg, or 159 mm Hg.

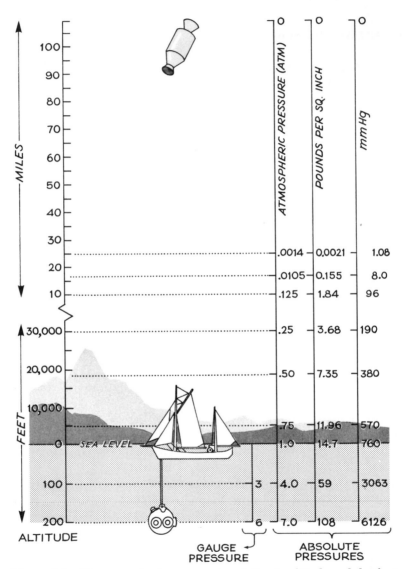

Figure 6-6. The atmospheric pressure in relation to altitude and depth at sea. Equivalent pressures in atmospheres, pounds per square inch, and in millimeters of mercury are listed for comparison.

However, humidity or water vapor tension (P_{H_2O}) also acts as a gas. In normal breathing, water vapor is fully saturated and comprises 6.2 per cent of the inspired gas at a body temperature of 37.5°C. The partial pressure of the water vapor is then 6.2 per cent × 760 mm Hg, or 47 mm Hg. Thus, at sea level, a humidified gas fully saturated with water vapor can have a maximum partial pressure of 713 mm Hg (760 mm Hg − 47 mm Hg). When humidified air is breathed (inspired air), the partial pressure of oxygen of the inspired gas ($P_{I_{O_2}}$) is 0.2094 × 713, or 149 mm Hg. The $P_{I_{O_2}}$ of 100 per cent oxygen would be 760 − 47, or 713 mm Hg.

THE ALVEOLAR VENTILATION CONCEPT

How Gases are Mixed in the Lungs

Gas exchange occurs mainly in the alveoli and is negligible in the remainder of the respiratory tract. During inspiration, fresh air is mixed with the air in the lungs which remains from the previous breath, which has been changed in composition from that of the inspired air. First it was humidified, then it gave up some oxygen in the alveoli in exchange for some carbon dioxide. Mixture of gases in the alveoli results in a partial pressure of oxygen of about 104 mm Hg and this equilibrates with the pulmonary venous side of the circulation. The partial pressure of CO_2 (P_{CO_2}) in the alveoli is 40 mm Hg. The exchange of oxygen and carbon dioxide occurs rapidly and is fully equilibrated with the blood in pulmonary capillaries. In normal young people one can assume that the gas tensions in the alveolus (P_{O_2} and P_{CO_2}) are essentially equal to that of the pulmonary capillaries and hence to that of the pulmonary venous and the systemic arterial blood.

If fresh air doesn't reach the alveoli, such as in breath holding, O_2 uptake and CO_2 elimination are stopped. The arterial blood is then said to be hypoxemic (low in oxygen) and hypercarbic (high in carbon dioxide).

The clinical counterpart of breath holding is apnea ("no breathing") and unless corrected, the consequences are rapid clinical deterioration. More commonly, the level of ventilation is intermediate between normal ventilation and apnea. If this reduced level of ventilation is inadequate, the patient has *hypoventilation*. If ventilation is excessive, this is called *hyperventilation*. As previously pointed out, gas exchange does not occur in the larger air passages, but only within the alveoli; therefore, the amount of alveolar ventilation is the best indication of the adequacy of ventilation.

The exact alveolar mixing process is quite variable from time to time, since not all alveoli are used with every breath. The alveolar P_{O_2} ($P_{A_{O_2}}$) is determined largely by the amount of CO_2 being liberated from the blood vessels while oxygen is being taken in. Normally, the amount of oxygen taken in per minute by the lungs is 250 ml; at the same time, 200 ml of CO_2 are released. The respiratory exchange ratio (R) of CO_2/O_2 is then normally about 0.8. The normal gas tensions in the airway are determined as follows:

P_{O_2} dry air = .2094 × 760 mm Hg = 159 mm Hg

P_{O_2} water vapor = .62 × 760 mm Hg = 47 mm Hg

Inspired P_{O_2} breathing 100 per cent O_2 = 760 mm Hg − 47 mm Hg = 713 mm Hg

Inspired P_{O_2} breathing room air = .2094 × 713 mm Hg = 147 mm Hg

Alveolar P_{O_2} breathing room air = 104 mm Hg ⎫ Same as pulmo-
Alveolar P_{CO_2} breathing room air = 40 mm Hg ⎬ nary venous
and systemic
arterial values

The Physiologic Dead Space

The *anatomic dead space* is the internal volume of the series of tubes that connect the ambient atmosphere to the alveoli; gas exchange does not occur in the anatomic dead space. The *alveolar dead space* is the portion of the tidal volume ventilating alveoli that are not functioning normally in gas exchange (i.e., reduced or absent blood flow to a ventilated alveolus). The *physiologic dead space* (total dead space) is composed of the anatomic and alveolar dead spaces. The dead space concept is best thought of as any portion of the tidal volume that does not contribute to arterializing venous blood in the lungs, or that is ineffective in removing carbon dioxide (Fig. 6–7).

Alveolar Ventilation

The volume of *alveolar ventilation* is the most important component of the tidal volume. The dead space volume is a component of the residual volume. Since the dead space volume is more or less constant for an individual at a particular time, the effective ventilation of alveoli will be related to the tidal volume. The ratio of the tidal volume to the dead space volume determines the rate of alveolar respiration. Carbon dioxide removal from the body is essentially proportional to alveolar ventilation. For practical purposes, hypercarbia (excess retention of CO_2) is always caused by inadequate

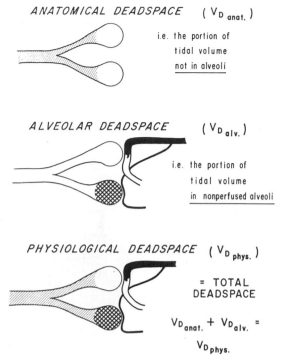

ANATOMICAL DEADSPACE ($V_{D\ anat.}$)

i.e. the portion of
tidal volume
not in alveoli

ALVEOLAR DEADSPACE ($V_{D\ alv.}$)

i.e. the portion of
tidal volume
in nonperfused alveoli

PHYSIOLOGICAL DEADSPACE ($V_{D\ phys.}$)

= TOTAL
DEADSPACE

$V_{D\ anat.} + V_{D\ alv.} = V_{D\ phys.}$

Figure 6–7. Subdivisions of the physiologic dead space. (From Bendixen, H. H. et al.: Respiratory Care. St. Louis, C. V. Mosby Company, 1965.)

alveolar ventilation. Normally, an individual breathes about 15 times per minute and a tidal volume of 400 cc per breath, or a total minute volume of 6 liters. The volume of dead space in man is about 1 cc per pound of body weight. If a person weighed 150 pounds, the respiratory dead space would be about 150 ml. If each breath was 400 ml and 150 ml would not reach the alveoli, then 250 ml does reach the alveoli and alveolar ventilation is thus 250 ml per breath. Assuming that a respiratory rate of 15 maintains his P_{CO_2} within normal levels, he requires 15×250 ml, or 3750 ml per min of alveolar ventilation to adequately remove carbon dioxide. If he either spontaneously ventilates or is artificially ventilated less than this (hypoventilation), carbon dioxide will not be adequately removed, his blood levels of carbon dioxide will rise, and he will be hypercarbic. If, on the other hand, he overbreathes (hyperventilation), an excess of carbon dioxide will be removed and he will then be hypocarbic. The metabolic sequelae of ventilation abnormalities have a profound effect on body pH, electrolytes, and circulatory status and will be discussed later in this chapter.

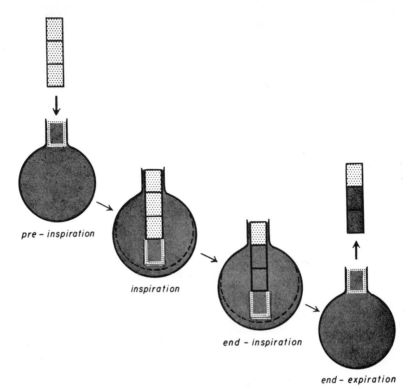

Figure 6–8. Alveolar ventilation. Each block represents 150 ml of gas. Dotted blocks represent inspired air; shaded blocks represent alveolar gas. During inspiration, 150 ml of dead space gas plus 300 ml of inspired air enter the alveoli (dotted lines indicate the pre-inspiratory lung volume). Almost instantly the inspired air mixes with alveolar gas and becomes part of it (end-inspiration). During expiration, 450 ml of gas leaves the alveoli; 150 ml remains in the respiratory dead space and 300 ml leaves as expired gas along with 150 ml of dead space gas. (From THE LUNG: CLINICAL PHYSIOLOGY AND PULMONARY FUNCTION TESTS, 2nd edition by Julius H. Comroe, Jr., et al. Copyright © 1962, Year Book Medical Publishers, Inc. Used by permission.)

Using Figure 6–8 as a schematic representation of alveolar ventilation, milliliters of gas breathed will be substituted for the shaded units in the illustration. For example, a normal tidal volume might be 450 ml, a normal dead space 150 ml. When a breath of 450 ml is taken, 150 ml of air that was in the dead space returns back into the alveoli. The gas in the anatomic dead space has already been equilibrated with the capillaries in the alveoli from the previous breath. An additional 300 ml of fresh gas mixes with this. When the person breathes out, or expires, the 450 ml of gas in the alveoli comes out — 300 ml to the air around us, 150 ml remaining in the airway as before.

Breathing Patterns

By creating a negative (subatmospheric) pressure within the airway, air will rush into the lungs. This inward movement of air is produced by a descent of the diaphragm and by the contraction of the intercostal muscles. The movement of the diaphragm downward as much as 10 cm causes an increase of pressure within the abdomen. The resistance to this movement is greater if abdominal movement is restricted, such as when the abdomen is distended or is tense from other causes. A paralyzed diaphragm further limits the influx of air.

The contraction of intercostal muscles narrows the space between the ribs and tends to lift the chest wall upward; because the ribs are angled downward, elevation increases the anterior-posterior diameter of the chest. The most important accessory muscles of respiration are the sternocleidomastoid muscles and scalene muscles. They ordinarily do not contract with quiet breathing.

Expiration is usually passive unless increased ventilation is required. Under these circumstances, the abdominal wall muscles may contract, helping force the diaphragm upward.

The common patterns of breathing are listed as follows:

Eupnea: Normal breathing—repeated rhythmic inspiratory-expiratory cycles without inspiratory or expiratory pause; inspiration is active and expiration passive.

Hyperpnea: Increased breathing; usually refers to increased tidal volume with or without increased frequency.

Polypnea, tachypnea: Increased frequency of breathing.

Hyperventilation: Increased alveolar ventilation in relation to metabolic rate (i.e., alveolar $P_{CO_2} < 40$ mm Hg).

Hypoventilation: Decreased alveolar ventilation in relation to metabolic rate (i.e., alveolar $P_{CO_2} > 40$ mm Hg).

Apnea: Cessation of respiration in the resting expiratory position.

Apneusis: Cessation of respiration in the inspiratory position.

Apneustic breathing: Apneusis interrupted periodically by expiration; may be rhythmic.

Gasping: Spasmodic inspiratory effort, usually maximal, brief, and terminating abruptly; may be rhythmic or irregular.

Cheyne-Stokes respiration: Cycles of gradually increasing tidal volume, followed by gradually decreasing tidal volume.

Biot's respiration: Originally described in patients with meningitis by Biot (Lyon Med. 23:517, 561, 1876) as irregular respiration with pauses; today, it refers to sequences of uniformly deep gasps, apnea, then deep gasps.

Kussmaul breathing: Deep rapid ventilation or "air hunger" seen in patients with diabetic acidosis.   (From Comroe, 1965).

TRACHEA DURING NORMAL BREATHING

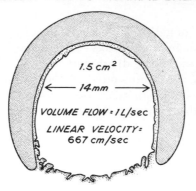

TRACHEA DURING COUGH

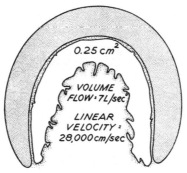

Figure 6–9. Tracheal air velocity during cough. The positive intrathoracic pressure inverts the noncartilaginous part of the intrathoracic trachea and decreases its cross-sectional area to one sixth of normal. This, added to a sevenfold increase in flow rate increases the linear velocity 42-fold. (From THE LUNG: CLINICAL PHYSIOLOGY AND PULMONARY FUNCTION TESTS, 2nd edition by Julius H. Comroe, Jr., et al. Copyright © 1962, Year Book Medical Publishers, Inc. Used by permission.)

Coughing is a special type of forced expiration which involves the abdominal musculature. A cough is initiated by closing the glottis, then the muscles of expiration contract, raising intrathoracic and intrapulmonary pressures. The glottis opens abruptly, suddenly releasing the large pressure build-up to the atmosphere, and a rapid flow rate of air is achieved. Because there is a high positive intrathoracic pressure and intrapulmonary pressure prior to the opening of the glottis, there is inversion of the membranous or noncartilaginous part of the major airways to one sixth of its normal area (Fig. 6–9). The flow rate of gas from pressure increases are about seven-fold.

The combined effects of the increased pressure and narrowing of the airways gives a 42-fold increase in linear velocity. The linear velocity achieved is about 500 miles per hour. Coughing is the essential force that dislodges foreign material or mucus from the airway. If for some reason the glottis cannot be closed (such as when an endotracheal tube is present), the coughing mechanism is far less effective.

RESPIRATORY REFLEXES

Ventilation and respiration are controlled by a system that senses three primary chemical changes: decreased blood P_{O_2}, increased blood P_{CO_2}, and decreased blood pH. The respiratory center is located in the medulla of the brain.

Inadequate oxygen in the arterial blood (hypoxemia) is detected by chemoreceptors in the aorta and the external carotid artery. The respiratory drive from hypoxemia alone is less in normal individuals than in chronically hypoxemic individuals, such as those with emphysema. In patients with chronic lung disease, oxygen administration can remove the hypoxemic stimulus to respiration, markedly decrease respiratory rate and alveolar ventilation, and lead to CO_2 retention at dangerous levels, even to "CO_2 narcosis."

The normal respiratory center in the brain is very sensitive to changes in arterial P_{CO_2}. Hypoventilation causes CO_2 retention and usually stimulates an increased alveolar ventilation. However, if patients are depressed by narcotics, anesthetics, or severe hypoxemia, they may be unresponsive to this mechanism. It must also be remembered that even if *respiratory reflexes* are adequate, attempts to improve ventilation may be ineffective in postoperative patients because they may have mechanical limitations of the lung or chest wall resulting from surgery. Acidosis (decrease of blood pH) can also stimulate an increase of ventilation; both the medullary and chemoreceptor pathways are involved. Kussmaul-type breathing, seen in diabetic acidosis, is an example of how acidosis stimulates hyperventilation.

Respiration is also influenced by *protective reflexes*, such as the cough reflex, which is an upper respiratory reflex to irritants that cause glottic closure and bronchial constriction. Swallowing also causes reflex glottic closure and prevents aspiration of food. *Stretch reflexes* (or Hering-Brewer reflexes) limit inflation volume of the lungs to a certain degree of stretch. A body *temperature increase* will reflexly stimulate respiration.

THE BLOOD PHASE

We have discussed the gaseous phase of respiration and must now consider how gas is exchanged between the blood and the inspired air. Reviewing briefly, the *gaseous phase* includes the inspired air as it passes through respiratory passages to the alveolar membrane. The alveolar-capillary membrane separates the gaseous phase from the *blood phase* in which oxygen is combined with hemoglobin and dissolved in plasma, then pumped to the cells by the cardiac action. The *tissue phase* involves the release of oxygen to the cells in exchange for carbon dioxide.

Diffusion and the Alveolar-capillary Membrane

The alveolus is the key gas exchange unit, and the process by which gas from the alveolus enters the blood stream is called *diffusion*. The rate of diffusion is remarkably rapid, so that in the 0.75 second required for blood to pass through a pulmonary capillary, the exchange of oxygen for carbon dioxide is accomplished.

The thin division between the air phase and the blood phase is called the *alveolar capillary membrane*. The alveolar capillary membrane is composed of two membranes separated by a thin layer of interstitial fluid (Fig. 6–10).

Diffusion of oxygen from the alveolus to the red blood cell is dependent on the alveolar surface area. This surface area is proportional to body size and is diminished with age, increased with increased lung volume, exercise, and hypoxemia, and changes with position. Primary diseases that involve the alveolar-capillary membrane may cause an *alveolar-capillary block* to diffusion. Pulmonary fibrosis, sarcoidosis, berylliosis, asbestosis, and scleroderma are some diseases associated with an alveolar-capillary block. Emphysema is the most common cause of a decreased diffusion, but this is related to a decreased surface area of alveoli, resulting from obliteration of alveoli and capillaries. Diffusion is rarely measured at the bedside and is seldom the primary problem in postoperative patients.

Blood Oxygen — Transport System and Carrying Capacity

Blood carries oxygen to tissue in two forms: (1) physical solution in the aqueous portions of blood as dissolved oxygen, and (2) in chemical combination with hemoglobin (HbO_2).

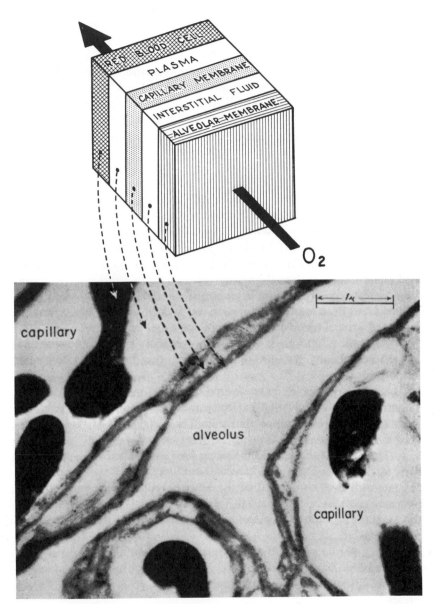

Figure 6-10. Schematic representation and electron microscopic picture of alveolar capillary membrane. Note its relation to the alveolus on one side and to the red blood cell in the pulmonary capillary on the other side. (From THE LUNG: CLINICAL PHYSIOLOGY AND PULMONARY FUNCTION TESTS, 2nd edition by Julius H. Comroe, Jr., et al. Copyright © 1962, Year Book Medical Publishers, Inc. Used by permission.)

The amount of either the dissolved or chemical forms of oxygen is proportional to the P_{O_2}.

Henry's Law. Henry's Law of gas solubility states that the volume of dissolved oxygen in physical solution is directly proportional to the P_{O_2}. The amount of dissolved gas also varies with the temperature of the liquid; cooling increases the amount of gas dissolved, and fever decreases the amount dissolved. The solubility of oxygen is different for different liquids. Oxygen solubility in blood is defined by the *Bunsen solubility coefficient*, which is 0.234 ml O_2 per ml blood per 760 mm Hg at 0°C. When breathing air, blood contains only about 0.29 ml of dissolved (not chemically combined) oxygen per 100 ml blood. The amount of dissolved oxygen bears a linear relationship to P_{O_2}.

Oxygen hemoglobin dissociation curve. Hemoglobin has a remarkable ability to chemically combine with oxygen. One gram of hemoglobin can combine with 1.34 ml of oxygen. If a normal amount of hemoglobin is present in blood (about 15 gm per 100 ml), then the oxygen carried by hemoglobin is 15 × 1.34, or 20.3 ml per 100 ml blood. The relationship between P_{O_2} and the amount of oxygen chemically combined with hemoglobin is not linear or a straight line as it is for dissolved oxygen, but is an S-shaped curve (Fig. 6–11).

The slope of the curve is very steep between 10 and 50 mm Hg of P_{O_2} and relatively flat between 70 and 100 mm Hg. At P_{O_2} values greater than 100 mm Hg, essentially no further HbO_2 combination occurs. The nature of the O_2Hb dissociation curve is fortunate. A 20 per cent decrease of P_{O_2} from 100 to 80 mm Hg causes only a 5 per cent change in the amount of oxygen combined with hemoglobin. However, when blood passes through tissues (average P_{O_2} of 40 mm Hg), hemoglobin can give up large quantities of oxygen for metabolic utilization.

Per cent saturation (of hemoglobin). When all hemoglobin is combined with oxygen (oxyhemoglobin state; HbO_2), it is said to be fully or 100 per cent *saturated*. When hemoglobin is not combined with oxygen, it is said to be in the reduced form, or unsaturated (Hb). The per cent of hemoglobin saturation or "per cent saturation" is an expression of the ratios of hemoglobin oxygen to the total amount of hemoglobin. Normally, oxygenated blood is about 97.1 per cent saturated.

Oxygen-carrying capacity. The *oxygen-carrying capacity* is the *total possible amount* of oxygen in blood in both the dissolved and the HbO_2 forms. Normally, the oxygen-carrying capacity is the sum of the 0.29 ml (dissolved O_2) and the 20.3 ml (hemoglobin-bound O_2); the total is 20.6 ml O_2 per 100 ml blood. As can be seen from Figure 6–12, the oxygen-carrying capacity is dependent not only

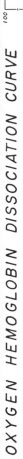

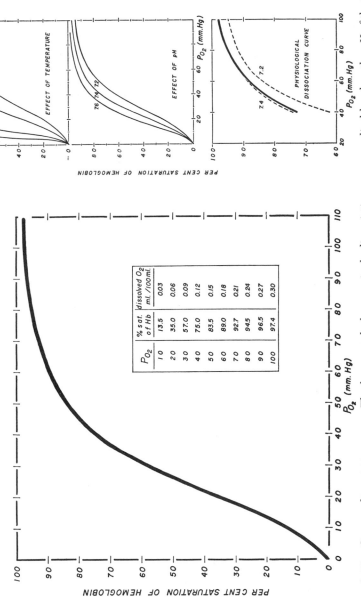

Figure 6–11. Oxygen dissociation curve. The large graph shows a single dissociation curve, applicable when the pH of the blood is 7.4 and the temperature is 37°C. The blood O₂ tension and saturation in patients with CO₂ retention, acidosis, alkalosis, fever, or hypothermia will not fit this curve, because the curve "shifts" to the right or left when temperature, pH, or P$_{CO_2}$ is changed. Effects on the O₂ hemoglobin dissociation curve of change in temperature (*upper right*) and in pH (*middle right*) are shown in the smaller graphs. A small change in blood pH occurs regularly in the body; e.g., when mixed venous blood passes through the pulmonary capillaries, P$_{CO_2}$ decreases from 46 to 40 mm Hg and pH rises from 7.37 to 7.40. During this time, blood changes from a pH 7.37 dissociation curve to a pH 7.40 curve; an approximate "physiological" dissociation curve (*solid line, bottom right*) has been drawn to describe this change. (From THE LUNG: CLINICAL PHYSIOLOGY AND PULMONARY FUNCTION TESTS, 2nd edition by Julius H. Comroe, Jr., et al. Copyright © 1962, Year Book Medical Publishers, Inc. Used by permission.)

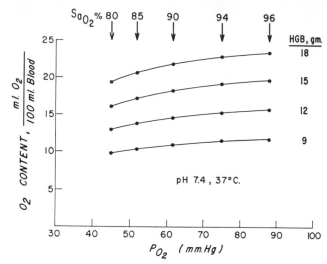

Figure 6–12.   Oxygen-carrying capacity of blood. The oxygen-carrying capacity of blood is dependent on an adequate hemoglobin content and a sufficiently high arterial oxygen tension. (From Bendixen, H. H., et al.: Respiratory care. St. Louis, C. V. Mosby Company, 1965.)

upon the arterial oxygen tension, but also upon the amount of circulating hemoglobin.

Oxygen content.   The *oxygen content of blood* is the *actual amount* of oxygen contained (ml oxygen per 100 cc of blood or volumes per cent) as measured in the patient and is always somewhat less than the oxygen carrying capacity unless enriched oxygen mixtures (mixtures with oxygen concentrations greater than air) are breathed.

It should be apparent that the blood might be normally oxygenated, but because of severe anemia still be incapable of carrying a normal amount of oxygen. It can also be seen (see Fig. 6–11) that blood pH and temperature affect the HbO_2 dissociation curve.

The Carbon Dioxide Transport System

Inspired air contains insignificant amounts of CO_2 (0.04 per cent); thus, the CO_2 equilibrating between the alveoli and blood is almost all derived from tissue metabolism. Carbon dioxide diffuses from tissue cells into the capillary bed and is carried in the venous blood to the alveoli by both physical solution and by chemical combination. In the alveoli, CO_2 diffuses across the alveolar-capillary membrane

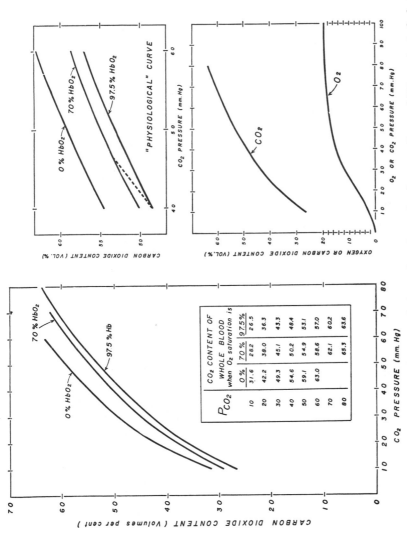

Figure 6–13. CO₂ dissociation curve. The large graph shows the relationship between P_{CO_2} and CO_2 content of whole blood; this varies with changes in saturation of hemoglobin with O₂. *Above right*, a greatly magnified portion of the large graph shows the change that occurs as mixed venous blood (70 per cent HbO₂, P_{CO_2}, 46 mm Hg) passes through the pulmonary capillaries and becomes arterial blood (97.5 per cent HbO₂, P_{CO_2}, 40 mm Hg). The dashed line is a hypothetical transition between the two curves. *Below right*, O₂ and CO₂ dissociation curves plotted on the same scale to show the important point that the O₂ curve has a very steep and a very flat portion and that the CO₂ curve does not. (From THE LUNG: CLINICAL PHYSIOLOGY AND PULMONARY FUNCTION TESTS, 2nd edition by Julius H. Comroe, Jr., et al. Copyright © 1962, Year Book Medical Publishers, Inc. Used by permission.)

until equilibrated with the alveolar gas and then is expelled in the expired gas.

Carbon dioxide transport occurs from chemical reactions both in the plasma and within the red blood cell. In plasma, CO_2 reacts with water to form bicarbonate and hydrogen ions or it may react with amino groups to form carbamino compounds.

However, most CO_2 transport occurs by chemical reactions within the red blood cell. Chemical reactions of CO_2 within the red blood cell are of three types: dissolved CO_2, formation of carbamino compounds, and formation of H^+ and HCO_3^- ions. The latter process is rapidly accomplished because of the existence of concentrated amounts of a specific enzyme, carbonic anhydrase, which is located primarily within the red blood cells. The action of carbonic anhydrase is facilitated by a reduction of HbO_2 to Hb. Therefore, when oxygen is given up by the red cell to the tissues, the process facilitates the taking up of CO_2 by the red cell.

In the lung, the process is reversed; i.e., CO_2 is released from its chemical combinations, diffuses very rapidly across the alveolar membrane, and is breathed out in the expired air. Although plasma contains about 75 per cent of the total CO_2 contained in blood, it is the portion within the red blood cells (facilitated by the carbonic anhydrase system) that provides the most CO_2 exchange in the lung. The amount of CO_2 in blood is related to the P_{CO_2}, but unlike the S-shaped oxygen dissociation curve, the relationship between P_{CO_2} and CO_2 content is almost linear (Fig. 6–13).

Carbon dioxide diffuses about 20 times more rapidly in water and plasma than does oxygen. In patients, it is extremely unusual to have gradients of CO_2 diffusion across the alveolar membrane. For practical purposes, in people with normal lungs the alveolar P_{CO_2} is equal to the arterial P_{CO_2}. In pulmonary embolism, however, there may be an alveolar to arterial CO_2 gradient, because pulmonary vascular occlusion causes blood containing CO_2 to be shunted within the lung and not to be exposed to alveolar ventilation. Diamox is a diuretic that inhibits the carbonic anhydrase enzyme. It can reduce the efficiency of CO_2 transfer in the alveolus if given in large doses.

The mixed venous P_{CO_2} is usually about 6 mm Hg higher than arterial P_{CO_2} (46.5 mm Hg versus 41 mm Hg). If the P_{CO_2} in a sample of gas taken at the end of expiration exceeds 50 mm Hg, it is almost certain that blood P_{CO_2} is also abnormally high. Regulation of ventilation in patients receiving assisted ventilation is determined by the arterial P_{CO_2}. Whenever the lungs are incapable of adequately removing CO_2, there is almost certainly a problem with oxygenation as well, unless the patient is breathing enriched oxygen mixtures.

By way of summary of these O_2 and CO_2 considerations, the following table of normal values is presented.

TABLE 6–2. *Mean Values for Blood O_2, CO_2, and pH in Healthy Young Men**

	ARTERIAL BLOOD	MIXED VENOUS BLOOD
1. O_2 pressure (mm Hg)	95	40
2. Dissolved O_2 (ml O_2/100 ml WB†)	0.29	0.12
3. O_2 content (ml O_2/100 ml WB)	20.3	15.5
4. O_2 combined with Hb (ml O_2/100 ml WB)	20.0	15.4
5. O_2 capacity of Hb (ml O_2/100 ml WB)	20.6	20.6
6. Per cent saturation of Hb with O_2	97.1	75.0
7. Total CO_2 (ml CO_2/100 ml WB)	49.0	53.1
(mM/L)	21.9	23.8
8. Plasma CO_2/100 ml plasma)	59.6	63.8
(a) Dissolved CO_2 (ml CO_2/100 ml)	2.84	3.2
(b) Combined CO_2 (ml CO_2/100 ml)	56.8	60.5
(c) Combined CO_2/dissolved CO_2	20/1	18.9/1
(d) CO_2 pressure (mm Hg)	41	46.5
9. Plasma pH	7.4	7.376

*(From PHYSIOLOGY OF RESPIRATION by Julius H. Comroe. Copyright © 1965, Year Book Medical Publishers. After Albritton, E. C. (ed.): Standard Values in Blood. Philadelphia, W. B. Saunders Company, 1952.)
†WB = whole blood.

THE LUNG REGULATION OF pH

A normal arterial pH is 7.38 to 7.42. Whenever arterial pH falls below this range, it is called *acidosis*; if greater than 7.42, *alkalosis* is present. If the pH abnormality is due to changes in CO_2 tension, it is either respiratory acidosis or respiratory alkalosis. If the pH abnormality results from the accumulation or depletion of fixed acids, it is called metabolic acidosis or metabolic alkalosis. pH measurements of blood are commonly used in assessing a patient's respiratory and cardiac status. The importance of the lungs in regulation of pH and acid-base balance is sometimes underestimated. Normally, the kidney excretes 50 to 100 mEq per day of fixed acids, while the lungs excrete 13,000 mEq per day of carbonic acid.

The level of the arterial P_{CO_2} is a balance between the rate of tissue CO_2 production and clearance to the air by alveoli. When CO_2 is not cleared adequately, it promotes acidosis by permitting hydrogen ion (H^+) to accumulate in the body fluids. This process is expressed by the following formula:

$$CO_2 + H_2O \underset{\text{anhydrase}}{\overset{\text{carbonic}}{\rightleftarrows}} H_2CO_3 \rightleftarrows H^+ + HCO_3^-$$

The normal relationships of this reaction are described by the classic Henderson-Hasselbach equation:

$$pH = pK + \log \frac{(HCO_3^-)}{(CO_2)}$$

The pK is a constant which is equal to 6.1. Values for HCO_3^- and CO_2 were given in Table 6–2. The log value for the normal ratio of $\dfrac{HCO_3^-}{CO_2}$ is 1.3; therefore, pH = 6.1 + 1.3 = 7.40. This ratio is normally 20:1. If CO_2 accumulates in the blood, the denominator increases and the log $\dfrac{HCO_3^-}{CO_2}$ will be less, pH will fall, and, as defined, a pH less than 7.38 is acidosis. Since the decrease of pH is caused by CO_2 retention, it is a respiratory acidosis. The opposite (respiratory alkalosis) occurs when ventilation is excessive and low arterial CO_2 levels occur.

The pH is kept at a normal level by a delicate mechanism controlling alveolar ventilation. Whenever the arterial P_{CO_2} rises, the medullary respiratory center of the brain is stimulated, alveolar ventilation is increased, and P_{CO_2} returns to normal. As with other respiratory control mechanisms, sedation, analgesia, anesthesia, and so forth interfere with its sensitivity.

INTERRELATIONSHIPS OF P_{O_2}, P_{CO_2} AND pH

The Effect of Hypoventilation

Respiratory function must be thought of in terms of satisfactory tissue oxygen exchange, not in relation to the chest x-ray appearance or the shape of the thorax. The best indications that respiration fails to meet tissue requirements are abnormalities of the blood P_{CO_2}, P_{O_2}, and pH. These measurements are best obtained simultaneously from arterial blood or mixed venous blood. Table 6–3 illustrates changes in arterial measurements when alveolar ventilation is normal, increased, or decreased.

Use of Nomograms for Clinical Assessment

Clinically, the interrelationships between pH, CO_2, and metabolic status can be interpreted better by plotting the measurements of a nomogram such as the Siggaard-Andersen Alignment Nomogram or the Siggaard-Andersen Curve Nomogram. The Siggaard-Andersen

TABLE 6–3. *Effect of Normal, Increased, and Decreased*
Alveolar Ventilation on Arterial Blood*

TYPE OF VENTILATION	ALVEOLAR VENTILA-TION L/min	ALVEOLAR AND ARTERIAL GAS TENSIONS* O_2 mm Hg	CO_2 mm Hg	ARTERIAL BLOOD GAS CONTENTS O_2 % Sat.	CO_2 mM/L	ARTERIAL pH Units
Hypoventilation	2.50	67	69	88.5	27.2	7.24
Normal	4.27	104	40	97.4	21.9	7.40
Hyperventilation	7.50	122	23	98.8	17.5	7.56

*(From THE LUNG: CLINICAL PHYSIOLOGY AND PULMONARY FUNCTION TESTS, 2nd edition by Julius H. Comroe, Jr., et al. Copyright © 1962, Year Book Medical Publishers, Inc. Used by permission.)

†In each case, respiratory exchange ratio of 0.8 and oxygen consumption of 250 ml/per min are assumed.

Alignment Nomogram (Fig. 6–14) requires measurement of arterial P_{CO_2} and pH. The values are marked on the appropriate columns (point A equals P_{CO_2}, point B equals pH) and a line drawn to connect them. A minor adjustment is made for hemoglobin level. The metabolic status is determined by the amount of base excess and a positive base excess value indicates metabolic alkalosis, a negative value indicates metabolic acidosis. For example, a patient whose blood pH is 7.54 and who has a P_{CO_2} of 42 mm Hg has a base excess of +12 which indicates that his system has excessive alkali equivalent to 12 mEq per liter of body water.

   The Siggaard-Andersen Curve Nomogram (Fig. 6–15) uses a different method to obtain the same information when arterial P_{CO_2} has not been measured. The patient's arterial blood sample is divided and equilibrated with two CO_2-containing gas mixtures, usually 4 per cent (point C) and 8 per cent CO_2 (point B). The pH of the original sample (point A) is measured and after equilibration with each gas, the three pH values are plotted on the nomogram and connected by drawing a line through them (dotted line in Fig. 6–15). The patient's P_{CO_2} is determined by sighting across the horizontal intersect from the patient's blood pH (60 mm Hg in the illustration). In Figure 6–15, the dotted line represents a respiratory problem in which ventilation is inadequate, but metabolic status is normal, pH is 7.30, and P_{CO_2} is increased to 60 mm Hg. The base excess is 0.7. By definition then, the patient is acidotic (pH less than 7.38) and it is respiratory in origin (metabolic status is normal). To correct this abnormality, arterial P_{CO_2} needs to be reduced and this is accomplished by increasing alveolar ventilation. Arterial P_{O_2} under these circumstances would almost certainly be reduced and if the situation were allowed to persist, metabolic acidosis secondary to hypoxia would likely complicate the picture.

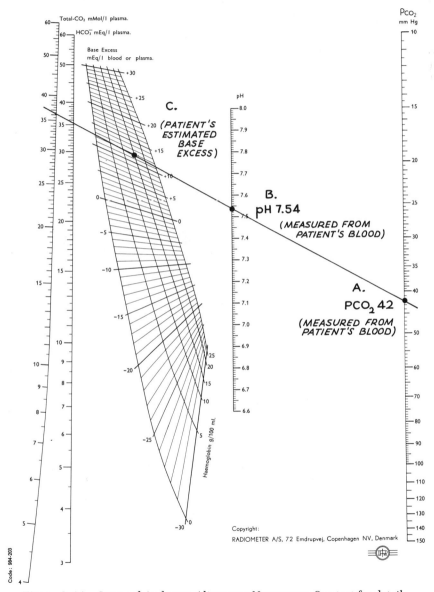

Figure 6–14. Siggaard-Andersen Alignment Nomogram. See text for details.

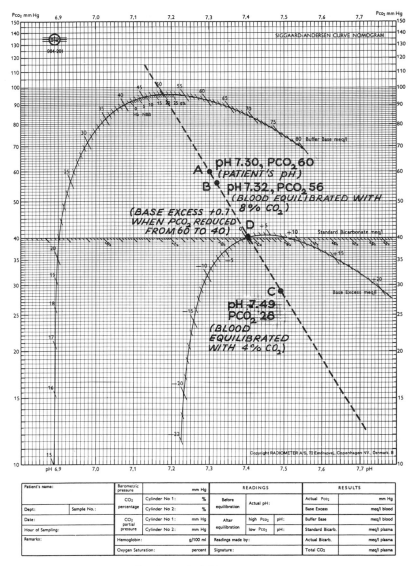

Figure 6–15. Siggaard-Andersen Curve Nomogram. See text for details.

The Astrup nomogram can be used to indicate the effect of ventilation on the respiratory component of the acid-base status by sighting vertically up and down the line obtained from the blood determinations. A change of ventilation does not move the location of the line or its slope. In our example (dotted line in Fig. 6–15), if ventilation is increased and arterial P_{CO_2} is reduced to 40 mm Hg, the pH would again be 7.42 (point D).

THE OXYGEN DELIVERY SYSTEM

The delivery of adequate oxygen to the tissues depends upon three factors: (1) an adequate P_{O_2} of the blood to fully saturate hemoglobin, (2) adequate hemoglobin in the blood to provide the required oxygen carrying capacity, and (3) adequate circulation of blood to deliver the oxygen to the tissue.

Tissue oxygenation, which is really the goal in respiration, is a dynamic process involving several levels of interaction. Figure 6–16 is a schematic overview of the problem. The blood oxygenation phase has previously been discussed in some detail. Basically, this figure depicts two pumps and two capillary beds, and blood fills the entire system. The oxygenator, the pumps, and the blood oxygen content

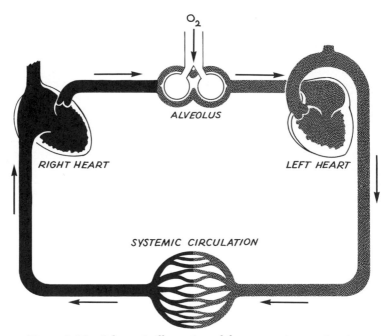

Figure 6–16. Schematic illustration of the oxygen transport system.

are all essential components. Fully oxygenated blood will not be enough if the pump system is not capable of transporting the oxygen to where it will be used. In some situations, even normal capabilities will be inadequate if tissue demands for oxygen are abnormally large. The demand for oxygen is continuous.

The normal adult requirement of 250 ml O_2 per min is accomplished by pumping about 5 liters of blood per minute. Therefore, the difference in oxygen content between the arterial and venous blood (the A-VO$_2$ difference) is 250 ml per min divided by 5000 ml per min equals 5 ml O_2 per 100 ml blood. The elimination of about 200 ml per min of CO_2 must simultaneously be accomplished by adequate alveolar ventilation and the same amount (5 liters) of blood flow to the lungs.

In normal people, there may be a great cardiopulmonary reserve function, particularly in those who are physically fit, e.g., athletes. An extremely well trained athlete can have the capacity to increase oxygen consumption from 250 cc per min to about 6000 cc per min, or a 24-fold increase. This capacity is limited by the cardiovascular delivery system more than by ventilatory restriction. Minute ventilation (amount of exchange per minute) can be increased from 6 L per min at rest to a maximum of about 54 L per min, or a ninefold increase. However, the capacity of a normal individual to increase cardiac output is from a normal of 5 L per min to a maximum of 15 L per min, only a threefold increase.

Increased oxygen requirements occur in fever, sepsis, shivering, restlessness, or combativeness. Compensatory mechanisms to meet these requirements are to increase cardiac output and to widen the A-VO$_2$ difference. Since the ratio of CO_2 production to O_2 consumption is relatively constant, increased oxygen requirements usually mean an increase of CO_2 elimination and, therefore, an increase of alveolar ventilation is required, which is done by increasing the depth and rate of breathing.

Unfortunately, a cardiac patient is not always able to maintain all these functions even at normal levels. For example, if his maximum cardiac output is only 3 L per min, the A-VO$_2$ difference must then increase to about 8.5 ml per 100 cc in order to supply 250 ml per min of oxygen. Anemia is another example in which adjustments are required. If the hemoglobin is decreased by one third to 10 gm, the oxygen-carrying capacity of the blood is also decreased by one third. To deliver the same amount of oxygen per minute, cardiac output would have to increase by one third, or the arteriovenous oxygen difference must increase proportionately. In cardiac patients, adjustments like this are not desirable and may cause clinical problems.

The *oxygen reserve* is defined as the difference between the nor-

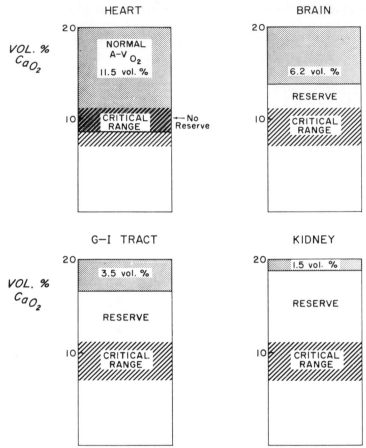

Figure 6-17. Oxygen reserves of vital organs. $C_{a_{O_2}}$ is the content of oxygen in pulmonary venous and systemic arterial blood. Individual tissues vary greatly in their oxygen uptake. The overall arteriovenous oxygen content difference (normal value equals 5 ml of oxygen per 100 ml of blood) is not representative of the oxygen reserve in vital tissues. Oxygen reserve is defined as the difference between the normal oxygen content of venous blood leaving that tissue and the oxygen content at the critical range of oxygen tensions, below which oxygen can no longer be transferred from blood to tissue. (From Bendixen, H. H., and Laver, M. B.: Clin. Pharmacol. Ther. 6:510, 1965.)

mal oxygen content of venous blood leaving an organ and the lowest oxygen content at which that particular organ will accept oxygen transfer. When oxygen tension in blood is below this level, oxygen is not transferred from the blood to the tissues.

It must be remembered that when normal oxygen consumption is said to be about 5 ml O_2 per 100 ml blood flow, this is only an average figure for the entire body. Unfortunately, it does not apply to specific vital organs, such as the heart or brain that have a much higher oxygen requirement. When the blood oxygen tension is at a level that prevents oxygen transfer to the cells of that organ, it is said to be in the "critical range of oxygen tension." This range occurs when hemoglobin is approximately 50 per cent saturated (P_{O_2} 27 mm Hg). Figure 6–17 depicts normal A-VO$_2$ differences for vital organs.

It can be seen that the heart normally extracts a maximum amount of oxygen from blood; its normal A-VO$_2$ difference is 11.5 vol per cent and there is no oxygen reserve. In fact, the circulation to the heart is almost always in the critical range. It is apparent that a cardiac patient must be adequately oxygenated and the demand for increased cardiac output minimized. There are progressively greater oxygen reserves for the brain, the gastrointestinal tract, and the kidneys.

TISSUE EXCHANGE UNITS

The distance separating each capillary from another capillary determines the distance required for diffusion of gases and metabolic products. When capillaries are widely separated from each other, the ability of this tissue or organ to provide itself increased amounts of oxygen is limited. This situation often exists in cardiac enlargement or hypertrophy. Although there is an increase of muscle mass, there is not an equivalent increase in numbers of capillaries. The net effect is to increase the distance between capillaries. With this increased distance for diffusion of oxygen, the relative effectiveness of the oxygen delivery system is limited.

Disturbances of Normal Pulmonary Function

HOW THE GAS EXCHANGE UNITS WORK

Normal Pulmonary Circulation

The gas exchange units or alveoli have two main functioning components: ventilation of the air side of the alveolar capillary membrane and pulmonary circulation of the blood side. The pulmonary capillaries contain a surface area for gas exchange of 70 square meters. The blood volume in the pulmonary circulation is about 900 ml, but of this amount only 75 per cent is in the capillaries at any one time. The capillaries are normally not all open at once.

Perfusion of the pulmonary capillaries is dependent upon the "driving pressure," which is the mean pressure difference between the arterial and venous sides of the pulmonary circulation. The driving pressure of the lungs is normally only 9 mm Hg. This low driving pressure permits the normal colloidal osmotic pressure outside of the capillaries (normally 25 to 30 mm Hg) to return fluid from the alveoli to the blood. The pressure difference between the inside and the outside of the capillaries is only about 6 mm Hg. However, in patients with pulmonary congestion due to congestive failure, mitral stenosis, and so on, the mean capillary pressure may rise and this transcapillary pressure may be increased from a normal of 6 mm Hg to 25 mm Hg, or more. At this level it approaches the osmotic pressure (25 to 30 mm Hg) of the tissue outside of the capillary and may cause pulmonary edema.

The low pulmonary perfusion pressures explain the effects of position on pulmonary function. A normal man standing upright may have 30 cm distance in height between the capillaries of the lung near the diaphragm and those at the apex of the lung. The pulmonary circulation pressure to the apices is then lower than that near the diaphragm. Similarly, there is a greater perfusion pressure in the posterior portions of the lung when the patient is lying supine. These dependent portions of the lung, therefore, have a higher transmural pressure, which promotes fluid leaving the capillaries and causing pulmonary edema. Pulmonary edema and congestive changes in cardiac patients have long been recognized to follow this dependent pattern.

Alveolar Gas Mixing and Diffusion

When we breathe, the inspired gas mixes very rapidly with the dead space gas (alveolar gas residual from the previous breath). The alveoli are small enough so that equilibration of the gases (admixing of gases within an alveolus) is rapidly accomplished (0.002 sec). When the gas enters the alveolar wall, *Henry's Law* for solubility of gases in solution applies and the solubility is proportional to its partial pressure. Carbon dioxide is about 21 times more soluble in water than is oxygen. For this reason, diffusion of gas in the alveoli is mainly a problem of oxygen diffusion. Carbon dioxide diffusion problems do not occur in the absence of severe oxygenation problems.

Oxygen diffusion can be abnormal when (1) the alveolar wall is thickened; (2) the capillary membrane is thickened; (3) the two membranes are separated by interstitial edema, fluid, exudate, or fibrous tissue; (4) the lining of the alveolus is covered by edema or fluid

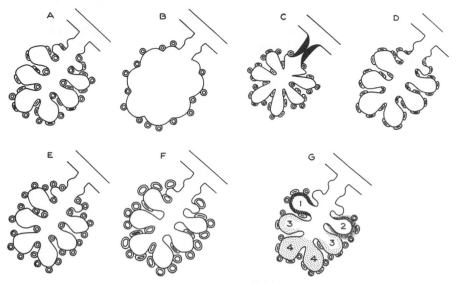

Figure 6–18. Area for gas exchange. *A*, Normal arrangement of alveoli clustered about an alveolar duct; about half of the alveolar capillaries are open and half are closed. *B*, Destruction of alveolar septa and of about half of the total available number of capillaries. *C*, Obstruction of bronchiole and decreased area for gas exchange with no decrease in potential alveolocapillary contact surface. *D*, Obstruction of the pulmonary circulation; no alveolocapillary blood flow. *E*, Increase in the number of open capillaries, as might occur in exercise. *F*, Capillary enlargement, as might occur in chronic mitral stenosis. *G*, Longer paths for diffusion due to (1) thickening of alveolar epithelium, (2) tissue separating alveolar capillary from alveolar epithelium, (3) beginning pulmonary edema, and (4) nonventilated alveoli filled with edema fluid or exudate. (From PHYSIOLOGY OF RESPIRATION, by Julius H. Comroe, Jr., et al. Copyright © 1965, Year Book Medical Publishers, Inc. Used by permission.)

exudate; and (5) capillary diameter is greatly increased from engorgement, e.g., from mitral stenosis (Fig. 6–18).

The Interrelation of Ventilation and Perfusion

The efficiency of respiration depends upon the relationship of ventilation and perfusion of each gas exchange unit. The ideal or maximally efficient lung would distribute the inspired gas equally throughout all 300 million alveoli and this would be matched by equal perfusion of the pulmonary capillaries for each of these alveoli. Actually this never occurs, as all alveoli are not normally ventilated equally, and some not at all. The extent of variations in alveolar ventilation is referred to as uniform or nonuniform in distribution. Pulmonary capillary blood flow is also subject to variations. An ideal uniformly perfused lung would have identical P_{O_2} and P_{CO_2} concen-

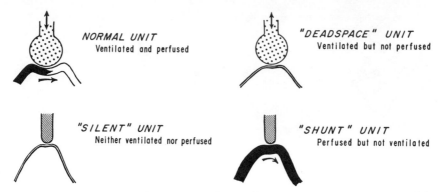

NORMAL UNIT
Ventilated and perfused

"DEADSPACE" UNIT
Ventilated but not perfused

"SILENT" UNIT
Neither ventilated nor perfused

"SHUNT" UNIT
Perfused but not ventilated

Figure 6–19. Gas exchange units. Gas exchange units may exist in any of the illustrated states, in the normal as well as the diseased lung. (From Bendixen, H. H., et al.: Respiratory Care. St. Louis, C. V. Mosby Company, 1965.)

trations in blood leaving each capillary. The four main categories of alveolar ventilation and capillary perfusion relationships are illustrated schematically in Figure 6–19. Gravity also plays an important role in determining which areas of the lung are perfused, and ventilation-perfusion relationships in a particular area of lung will change in relation to the position of the patient (Fig. 6–20). The importance

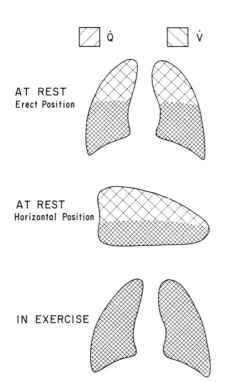

$\dot{Q}$ $\dot{V}$

AT REST
Erect Position

AT REST
Horizontal Position

IN EXERCISE

Figure 6–20. Effect of gravity on ventilation. This drawing shows, and exaggerates, the influence of gravity and physical activity on the distribution of ventilation and perfusion in the lung. At rest, the dependent part of the lung receives most of the pulmonary capillary blood flow as well as the larger part of the tidal volume. Only in exercise is the entire lung put to full use. (From Bendixen, H. H., et al.: Respiratory Care. St. Louis, C. V. Mosby Company, 1965.)

of the relationship of alveolar ventilation (V_A) to perfusion $(\dot{Q})$ is of particular importance in cardiac patients, because variations in the amount of perfusion are even greater in situations in which cardiac output is low. Dramatic improvement of oxygenation can occur in these patients if position is changed so that nonedematous and well ventilated areas of lung are dependent and hence maximally perfused. Exercise and high cardiac output tend to minimize the effect of position.

PHYSIOLOGIC DISTURBANCES OF RESPIRATION IN CARDIAC PATIENTS

Cardiac patients manifest disturbances of pulmonary function with almost predictable frequency. The most common causes of respiratory failures are (1) *increased physiologic shunt*, (2) *increased physiologic dead space*, (3) *increased work of breathing*, and (4) *decreased oxygen transport in blood*. Each of these disturbances may be present alone, but more frequently they occur together.

Increased Physiologic Shunting

Shunting of blood refers to the passage of blood from the venous (right) side of the circulation to the arterial (left) side of the circulation without benefit of pulmonary blood gas exchange (Fig. 6–21). The total physiologic shunt $(Q_{s_{phys}})$ is determined by a constant anatomic portion $(\dot{Q}_{s_{anat}})$ that is related to the normal bronchial, pleural, and Thebesian venous circulation and usually comprises about 3 per cent of the cardiac output. A far more important and variable shunt occurs at the pulmonary capillary level $(Q_{s_{cap}})$. The most frequent cause of this shunt is atelectasis; uneven distribution of ventilation and perfusion, or diffusion gradients, may also be responsible. In atelectasis, it is not uncommon for 30 to 40 per cent of the cardiac output to be shunted (i.e., returned from the venous to the arterial circulation without gas exchange).

Increased Physiologic Dead Space

Alveolar ventilation is reduced when dead space volume is large in proportion to the tidal volume. One of the ways to decrease dead space volume is to bypass the upper air passages by performing a tracheostomy. The pattern of breathing can be important in deter-

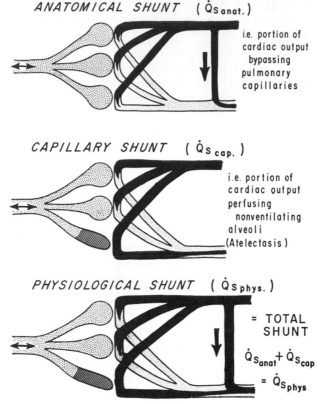

Figure 6-21. Subdivisions of the physiological shunt. (From Bendixen, H. H., et al.: Respiratory Care. St. Louis, C. V. Mosby Company, 1965.)

mining the volume of the dead space relative to the tidal volume (Fig. 6–22). It can be seen that rapid shallow respiration causes even a normal dead space volume to be of significance and can cause a serious decrease in ventilation.

Increased Work of Breathing

The work of breathing is the amount of work or energy required to drive the muscles of respiration. Normally, the amount of oxygen required to support this system is about 2 per cent of the total oxygen requirement. The work of breathing is an important concept when considering the patient's capability of adequately breathing or ventilating for himself. It is also an important factor in the decision of whether or not ventilator assistance of respiration is required. Decreased compliance of the lung and increased airway resistance are two common causes of increased work of breathing (Fig. 6–23).

BREATHING PATTERNS & DEAD SPACE

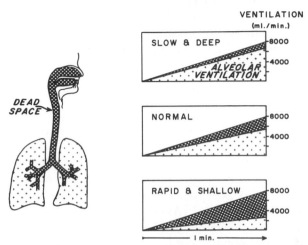

Figure 6-22. Dead space ventilation as related to tidal volume. Note the wide variations in the amount of dead space air moved with the different breathing patterns. (From Kinney, J. M., and Wells, R. E., Jr.: Problems of ventilation after injury and shock. J. Trauma 2:370–385, 1962.)

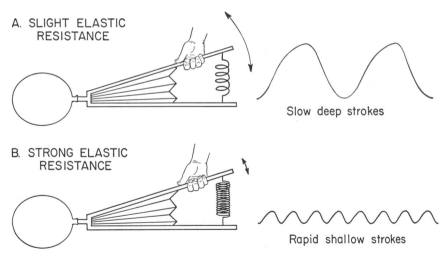

Figure 6-23. Work of breathing. Note that a compliant lung (A) can be easily ventilated by slow deep strokes, while a "stiff" lung (B) requires rapid shallow strokes. (From Rushmer, R. F.: Cardiovascular Dynamics. 3rd ed. Philadelphia, W. B. Saunders Company, 1970.)

Changes in Pulmonary Compliance

Lung compliance is a measurement that indicates if the lungs are "stiff" or resistant to expansion. Compliance is a mechanical characteristic of the lung and indicates the change in volume when a unit pressure difference across the lung is developed by the muscles of respiration. In patients receiving ventilator therapy, it is measured by the ratio of tidal volume change to change in airway pressure. (The symbol Δ means "change in."

$$C_L = \frac{V_T}{\Delta P}$$

C_L = lung compliance in ml per cm H_2O

V_T = tidal volume

ΔP = airway pressure change measured directly from the ventilator

In patients receiving prolonged artificial ventilation, the tidal volume and the peak positive airway pressure can easily be measured and compliance calculated. Average normal values for pulmonary compliance are in the range of 35 to 45 ml per cm H_2O.

A *fall* in pulmonary compliance (i.e., reduced expansion or

TABLE 6–4. *Factors that Influence Oxygen Transport**

Factors	Requirements
A. Gas Phase	
1. Inspired air	P_{O_2} normal or as high as necessary
2. Airways	Unobstructed by secretions, collapsing bronchi offering low resistance
3. Lungs	Normal volumes, capacities, and compliance
4. Alveolar ventilation	Tidal volume adjusted to maintain arterial P_{CO_2} normal; evenly distributed so that ventilation perfusion relationship is normal
B. Blood Phase	
1. Arterial P_{O_2}	Sufficient to fully utilize oxygen-carrying capacity of blood
2. Arterial O_2 content	Normal hemoglobin content and P_{O_2}
3. Cardiac output	Normal blood volume, peripheral resistance, appropriate distribution, and capacity of heart as a pump
4. Pulmonary circulation	Normal volume and distribution of ventilated alveoli being normally perfused
5. Chemical environment	Normal pH, temperature, buffer, and electrolyte content
C. Tissue Phase	
Capillaries and tissue	Normal membrane permeability, tissue requirements not excessive, microcirculation adequately perfused

*(From Bendixen et al.: Respiratory Care. St. Louis, The C. V. Mosby Company, 1965.)

more pressure required to maintain the same expansion) is associated with pulmonary complications, such as atelectasis, pneumonia, and pulmonary edema (processes also associated with intrapulmonary arteriovenous shunts).

Decreased Oxygen Transport

Adequate oxygen transport depends upon all three phases of respiration and is summarized in Table 6–4.

PHYSIOLOGIC RESPONSES TO INADEQUATE OXYGENATION

The Oxygen Stores

The human body has no significant oxygen stores beyond those held in the gas volume of the lungs and those combined with circulating hemoglobin. These stores amount to only about 1.5 liters O_2 in the average adult and hence can provide normal tissue demands (average of 250 ml O_2 per min) for only a few minutes. The normal balance between supply and demand renders the organs with high oxygen requirements the most vulnerable (heart, brain).

Oxygen Supply and Demand

Normal resting demand for oxygen is related to size, sex, and age and can be predicted within ±15 per cent from standard tables of basal metabolic rate. The demands for oxygen relative to the supply can also be important. Oxygen demand is *decreased* by fasting, paralysis (e.g., with curare, sedation, anesthesia), hypothermia, and peripheral vasoconstriction (seldom desirable). Oxygen demands are *increased* by (1) muscular contraction, shivering, and combativeness; exercise can temporarily increase oxygen requirement to 10 times the normal value. (2) Fever will increase oxygen consumption approximately 7 per cent per degree Fahrenheit, because the metabolic rate is accelerated. (3) Sepsis increases oxygen requirements by causing fever, but also because bacteria and inflammatory responses consume oxygen; (4) any factor which increases the work of breathing will increase oxygen demands. Normal people can increase the work of breathing during heavy work or exercise from 2 per cent of their energy requirements to 5 or 10 per cent. However, if secretions obstruct the airways or the lung compliance is reduced, the energy

cost of breathing can become 20 to 25 per cent of the total requirement. Patients who are critically ill are often unable to meet these
demands, i.e., their oxygen transport system potential is decreased
at the same time as the oxygen demand is increased.

Physiologic Response to Hypoxemia

Hypoxemia is a powerful sympathetic stimulator and causes the
cardiac rate to increase, which may lead to an increase of cardiac
output. Hypoxemia also causes vasoconstriction (selective) and this,
combined with the associated increased cardiac output, is likely to
increase the blood pressure. Therefore, hypertension and tachycardia
are early signs of hypoxemia. This circulatory compensation occurs
because sympathetic activity can be mobilized. Figure 6–24 illustrates
these considerations. The oxygenation of the arterial blood (point a) is
reduced (moved down to the left on the oxyhemoglobin dissociation
curve). However, because the cardiac output has increased to 10 liters

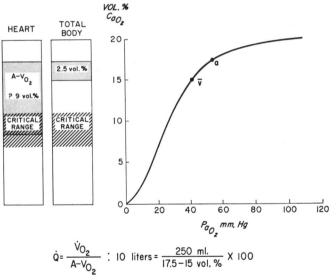

$$\dot{Q} = \frac{\dot{V}_{O_2}}{A\text{-}V_{O_2}} \quad : \quad 10 \text{ liters} = \frac{250 \text{ ml.}}{17.5\text{-}15 \text{ vol. \%}} \times 100$$

Figure 6–24.   Hypoxemia with circulatory compensation. In moderately severe
hypoxia, circulatory compensation consists of an increased cardiac output. The arterial
point is moved to the left on the dissociation curve, but the increased cardiac output
makes it possible for the mixed venous point to remain unchanged. For the heart, an
increased coronary flow is assumed to allow a decreased oxygen uptake, per 100 ml
of blood, thus keeping the venous point unchanged. The clinical signs are tachycardia
and mild hypertension. (From Bendixen, H. H., and Laver, M. B.: Clin. Pharmacol. Ther.
6:510, 1965.)

(from a normal of 6 L per min), the amount of oxygen remaining in venous blood (point v) is unchanged, but arteriovenous oxygen difference is less than normal, both in the heart and for the total body.

Cardiac patients who have severe disease or drug requirements, or who are debilitated or recovering from an operation may be unable to make this response. In the absence of sympathetic activation, this lack of circulatory compensation for hypoxemia leads to further failure of cardiac function (Fig. 6–25). It can be seen that oxygenation of both the arterial and venous blood is reduced (shifted to the left). Under these circumstances, the total body may have some oxygen reserve, but because the heart does not, oxygen demand has exceeded supply and the cardiac response to this myocardial hypoxia will be manifest by bradycardia, hypotension, and a falling cardiac output. The end result of this sequence will be death if prompt therapy is not given.

Patient factors that reduce circulatory compensation to hypoxia are cardiopulmonary disease, increasing age, obesity, anemia, hypovolemia, acidosis, fever, and drugs and medications such as antiadrenergic agents, sedatives, analgesics, and anesthetics. In addition, postoperative cardiac patients often have other mechanical or restrictive factors related to their operation which limit their compensation.

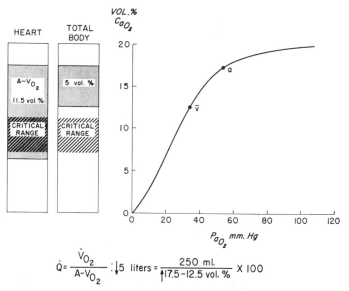

$$\dot{Q} = \frac{\dot{V}_{O_2}}{A - V_{O_2}} : |5 \text{ liters} = \frac{250 \text{ ml.}}{\uparrow 17.5 - 12.5 \text{ vol. }\%} \times 100$$

Figure 6–25. Hypoxemia without circulatory compensation. In the presence of the same degree of hypoxia as shown in Figure 6–24, but in the absence of circulatory compensation, not only the arterial point but also the mixed venous point will move to the left on the dissociation curve. For the total body, a modest oxygen reserve remains in spite of the hypoxia. For the heart, the lack of increase in coronary flow makes the demand for oxygen exceed the supply; the result is myocardial tissue hypoxia with bradycardia, hypotension, and a reduced cardiac output. (From Bendixen, H. H., and Laver, M. B.: Clin. Pharmacol. Ther. 6:510, 1965.)

Consequences of Uncompensated Hypoxemia

Adaptation to inadequate oxygen supply. The tissue supply of oxygen is often protected by compensations provided by other portions of the oxygen transport mechanism when failure of one component occurs. The ability to do this is of course within limits; in cardiac patients the limits are extremely narrow. Tissue hypoxia of a mild-to-moderate degree will stimulate ventilation and cardiac output, whereas severe hypoxia will often cause a fall in cardiac output. A reduced cardiac output, in turn, causes a decreased capillary blood flow, which is followed by an increased arteriovenous extraction of oxygen. Because the heart has the highest arteriovenous oxygen difference of any tissue, it would undoubtedly be the first organ to suffer in hypoxemia were it not for its ability to selectively increase coronary blood flow. Depending upon reserves, moderate hypoxemia then will cause coronary vasodilatation, in addition to tachycardia and hypertension. Uncompensated hypoxemia leads to bradycardia, arrhythmias, hypotension, and metabolic changes.

Some of the effects of hypoxemia upon the central nervous system are mental confusion, restlessness, and paranoia. It should be remembered that a restless, combative patient, particularly in the postoperative period, may not need analgesia for pain but requires better oxygenation.

Metabolic deterioration caused by inadequate oxygenation. When tissue is poorly oxygenated, function is impaired and metabolic consequences ensue. These changes occur promptly. When circulation is interrupted for only a few minutes, as in cardiac arrest, profound acidosis can occur. Even more dramatically, transient hypoxemia of one or two minutes, such as may occur with ventilator adjustment or nasotracheal suction, may precipitate cardiac arrhythmias from which patients cannot be resuscitated. The management of oxygen therapy has therefore been referred to as the "oxygen tightrope," and we must be mindful of this sensitive balance that is required to sustain critically ill patients.

Tissues respond to local decreases of oxygen supply by changing the metabolic pathways from an aerobic (with O_2) to an anaerobic (without O_2) metabolism. Reserve energy stores within cells are utilized, e.g., phosphate bond energy in the form of ATP and creatine phosphate. Anaerobic metabolism prevents the immediate death of a cell, but a price is paid. Anaerobic metabolism can produce new ATP by conversion of glucose to lactate, but this results in the accumulation of acid byproducts—a metabolic acidosis. Cardiac function and response to drugs may be further decreased by acidosis and just when cardiac compensation is needed most it is lacking. A vicious cycle of progressive deterioration ensues.

Pulmonary Assessment

SOME FACTORS PREDISPOSING TO PULMONARY FAILURE

Postoperative pulmonary complications are not events that always occur as a matter of chance like roulette numbers. Development of pneumonia postoperatively is not the result of just an unfortunate bit of luck. Most often, the degree of risk can be quite accurately assessed preoperatively and measures can be established to prevent pulmonary complications. The following list (from Bendixen et al., 1965) outlines some of the more common factors that predispose to pulmonary complications.

1. The Patient
   a. Smoking
   b. Previous pulmonary disease or symptoms
   c. Age
   d. Obesity
   e. Cardiopulmonary disease
   f. Anemia
   g. Hypovolemia
   h. Acidosis
   i. Trauma
2. Restrictive Factors
   a. Pain
   b. Abnormal positions
   c. Casts and bandages
   d. Abdominal distension
3. Depressive Factors
   a. Narcotics
   b. Sedatives
   c. Anesthetics
   d. Muscle relaxants
4. Special Factors
   a. Vasoconstrictor drugs
   b. Positive pressure ventilation (with improper pattern)
5. Increased Oxygen Requirements
   a. Fever
   b. Burns
   c. Hyperthyroidism

These factors are red flags of warning in the preoperative phase. They may also be indications of the need to improve pulmonary function preoperatively. Patients should be instructed to stop smoking. Two or three weeks are required for depressed ciliary function to return, for secretions to decrease, and for bronchospasm to be relieved. A past history of pulmonary disease is of special importance and in patients who smoke it is particularly well correlated with the incidence of pulmonary complications. Preoperative physiotherapy directed at improving breathing and the ability to cough correctly is important. Preoperative training in the use of a respirator is also important to prevent postoperative atelectasis and to eliminate patients' anxieties about the apparatus.

MEASUREMENT OF PULMONARY FUNCTION

The objective assessment of the patient's breathing apparatus is extremely valuable in the preoperative phase as a baseline for later evaluation, improvement with treatment, choice of operative procedure, and selection of anesthesia for operation. In the postoperative phase, function studies help to evaluate the progress of recovery and to identify areas of pulmonary deterioration.

The functions of the lung include (1) the exchange of oxygen and carbon dioxide between the atmosphere and the blood, (2) a blood reservoir within the circulation, having both resistance and capacitance, (3) excretion of water vapor and drugs such as ethanol or gaseous anesthetics, (4) temperature regulation, (5) detoxification and metabolic degradation, (6) secretion of substances such as histamine and thromboplastin, (7) cleansing and filtering of air of such substances as carbon and silica, and (8) filtering blood of fibrin, blood clots, or other emboli. These functions and their evaluation are summarized in Table 6–5.

The normal values for pulmonary function tests are listed in Table 6–6.

The more preoperative information that one has the better, but practical considerations lead us to assess particular areas of function or concern or to perform screening tests that measure many functions. Blood gases, vital capacity, timed vital capacity, maximum breathing capacity, and maximum expiration flow rate are felt by many to be reliable parameters. Cardiac catheterization preoperatively usually includes hemodynamic assessment of the pulmonary circulation. The vital capacity and tidal volume are easily measured at the bedside using a device such as the Wright respirometer. Peak inspiratory pressure is measured on many standard respirators. Simple functional tests, such as the *stairway test*, (a patient's ability to climb two flights of stairs without excessive dyspnea) are felt by some to be the most reliable of screening tests. Measurements of the mechanics of breathing necessitate a patient's maximum effort to be reliable.

TABLE 6-5. *Classification of Pulmonary Function Tests**

	Office	Hospital Laboratory
I. LUNG VOLUMES	LAB Vital capacity, tidal volume, expiratory reserve volume, inspiratory capacity.	Residual volume, functional residual capacity, total lung capacity, RV/TLC ratio.
II. RESPIRATORY GAS EXCHANGE		
1. Ventilation	PE Lateral chest and diaphragm excursion; diffuse wheezing; cyanosis. X-ray Inspiratory-expiratory films; fluoroscopy. LAB Rate, tidal volume, minute volume.	Volume expired per min per M^2; ventilatory response to inhalation of O_2 and CO_2; end expired CO_2 (CO_2 meter); arterial P_{CO_2}, O_2 sat.
2. Distribution—Gas	PE Nonuniform chest expansion, percussion note, breath sounds; wheezing, rhonchi; cyanosis. X-ray Nonuniform lung expansion, hyperinflation, bullae, localized air trapping on inspiratory-expiratory films.	Dead space ventilation; alveolar ventilation; N_2 washout on O_2 breathing; helium distribution test; bronchospirometry; single breath N_2 washout on O_2 breathing.
3. Diffusion	PE Tachypnea—rest and exercise; cyanosis during exercise; crackling basal rales. X-ray Diffuse infiltration.	Arterial O_2 sat. and P_{CO_2} at rest, on exercise, during O_2 breathing. Alveolar-arterial P_{O_2} gradient. Diffusion capacity for O_2 or CO_2.
4. Distribution—Blood	PE Cyanosis at rest, not relieved by 100 per cent oxygen. X-ray Nonuniform pulmonary vascular markings. LAB Hct.	Arterial O_2 sat. during O_2 breathing (anatomic R-L shunt); pulmonary angiography.
5. Circulation	PE RV heave, incr. P2, enlarged tender liver, warm extremities. X-ray Enlarged RV outflow tract, pulmonary conus. LAB Clockwise rotation, RVH by ECG.	Cardiac catheterization (pressures, flows, resistances, O_2 content); pulmonary angiography.
III. MECHANICS OF BREATHING	LAB MBC, spirogram timed vital capacity; maximal inspiratory-expiratory flow rates (all before and after bronchodilators).	Pulmonary compliance; total pulmonary resistance.

TABLE 6–6. *Normal Values for Pulmonary Function Tests**

These are values for a healthy, resting, recumbent young male (1.7 M² surface area), unless other conditions are specified. They are presented merely to give approximate figures. These values may change with position, age, size, sex, and altitude; there is variability among members of a homogeneous group under standard conditions.

I. LUNG VOLUMES (BTPS)
Inspiratory capacity	3600 ml
Expiratory reserve volume	1200 ml
Vital capacity	4800 ml
Residual volume (RV)	1200 ml
Functional residual capacity	2400 ml
Total lung capacity (TLC)	6000 ml
RV/TLC × 100	20%

II. RESPIRATORY GAS EXCHANGE
1. Ventilation (BTPS)
Tidal volume	500 ml
Frequency	12 respirations/min
Minute volume	6000 ml/min
Respiratory dead space	150 ml
Alveolar ventilation	4200 ml/min

2. Distribution of Inspired Gas
Single-breath test (% increase N_2 for 500 ml expired alveolar gas)	$< 1.5\%$ N_2
Pulmonary nitrogen emptying rate (7 min test)	$< 2.5\%$ N_2
Helium closed circuit (mixing efficiency related to perfect mixing)	76%

ALVEOLAR VENTILATION/PULMONARY CAPILLARY BLOOD FLOW
Alveolar ventilation (L/min)/blood flow (L/min)	0.8
Physiologic shunt/cardiac output × 100	$< 7\%$
Physiologic dead space/tidal volume × 100	$< 30\%$

PULMONARY CIRCULATION
Pulmonary capillary blood flow	5400 ml/min
Pulmonary artery pressure	25/8 mm Hg
Pulmonary capillary blood volume	60–100 ml
Pulmonary capillary blood pressure	8 mm Hg

ALVEOLAR GAS
Oxygen partial pressure	104 mm Hg
CO_2 partial pressure	40 mm Hg

*(From THE LUNG: CLINICAL PHYSIOLOGY AND PULMONARY FUNCTION TESTS, 2nd edition by Julius H. Comroe, Jr., et al. Copyright © 1962, Year Book Medical Publishers, Inc. Used by permission.)

(Table continued on opposite page.)

TABLE 6–6.   *Normal Values for Pulmonary Function Tests* (Continued)

DIFFUSION AND GAS EXCHANGE

O_2 consumption (STPD).. 250 ml/min
CO_2 output (STPD).. 200 ml/min
Respiratory exchange ratio, R (CO_2 output/O_2 uptake)...... 0.8
Diffusing capacity, O_2 (STPD)..................................... 20 ml O_2/min/mm Hg
Diffusing capacity, CO (steady state) (STPD).................. 17 ml CO/min/mm Hg
Diffusing capacity, CO (Single-breath) (STPD) .... 17 ml CO/min/mm Hg
Fractional CO uptake (in %)....................................... 53%
Maximal diffusing capacity (exercise) (STPD)................. 60 ml/min/mm Hg

ARTERIAL BLOOD

O_2 saturation (% saturation of Hb with O_2) 97.1%
O_2 tension .... 95 mm Hg
CO_2 tension... 40 mm Hg
Alveolar-arterial P_{O_2} difference .... 9 mm Hg
Alveolar-arterial P_{O_2} difference (12–14% O_2)........... 10 mm Hg
Alveolar-arterial P_{O_2} difference (100% O_2)............... 35 mm Hg
O_2 saturation (100% O_2) .... 100% (+1.91 − 2.00 ml
                                                                  dissolved O_2/100 ml blood
pH 7.40

III. MECHANICS OF BREATHING
Maximal breathing capacity (BTPS) .... 125–170 L/min
Timed vital capacity... 83% in 1 sec; 97% in 3 sec
Maximal expiratory flow rate (for 1 liter) (ATPS)...... 500 L/min
Maximal inspiratory flow rate (for 1 liter) (ATPS) ... 400 L/min
Compliance of lungs and thorax .... 0.1 L/cm H_2O
Compliance of lungs .... 0.2 L/cm H_2O
Airway resistance .... 1.6 cm H_2O/liter/sec
Work of quiet breathing .... 0.5 kgm/min
Maximal work of breathing .... 10 kgM/breath
Maximal inspiratory and expiratory pressures .... 60–100 mm Hg

STPD = 0°C, 760 mm Hg, dry
BTPS = body temperature and pressure saturated with water vapor
ATPS = ambient temperature and pressure saturated with water vapor

BLOOD SAMPLING TECHNIQUES

Both arterial and venous blood may be used for gas analysis. Arterial samples are obtained by needle puncture or from indwelling catheters of the femoral, brachial, or radial arteries. Samples are obtained in a 5 or 10 ml syringe wetted with heparin solution. When blood is obtained from indwelling arterial catheters, the catheter line must be adequately flushed with fresh arterial blood so that the analysis reflects the arterial system at that moment. Blood withdrawn for flushing can be returned through the catheter. When the sample is obtained, any air in the syringe is expelled. To maintain the sample in an anaerobic condition, the syringe is capped, the needle is stuck into a cork, and the disposable needle is bent. Gas and pH values will change unless analysis is done promptly. If a delay is required, the syringe with the blood sample should be stored in ice.

When blood samples are obtained by arterial puncture, it is best to maintain pressure over the puncture site for 5 or 10 minutes to prevent hematoma formation. Whenever arterial blood samples are obtained, a note should be made of the $P_{I_{O_2}}$ (inspired oxygen tension), since the effectiveness of oxygenation cannot be assessed unless the oxygen tensions in both the alveoli and the arterial blood are known. When mixed venous blood is analyzed, it is best to obtain this from a central venous pressure catheter (optimally in the pulmonary artery) using similar sampling techniques.

The inspired P_{O_2} gas analysis sample can be obtained from the ventilating apparatus by needle aspiration as close as possible to the point of delivery to the patient. It must be obtained after the point of connection of the vaporizer and the aspiration timed to be withdrawn just as the inspiratory phase of respiration ends.

CLINICAL DIAGNOSIS OF HYPOXEMIA

The classic descriptions of symptoms and signs of hypoxemia or hypercapnia included restlessness, confusion, delirium, impaired motor function, dizziness, tremor, unconsciousness, hypotension or hypertension, tachycardia, arrhythmias, perspiration, warm or cold extremities, cyanosis, and tachypnea. These symptoms and signs fit into categories of (1) altered mental status, (2) changes of the hemodynamics of circulation, (3) autonomic nervous system manifestations, or (4) cyanosis. The first three are quite nonspecific and are relatively unreliable guides to hypoxemia or pulmonary failure. They do, however, serve as reminders to consider this possibility in patients who present these findings.

Before blood gases were commonly available, cyanosis was thought to be the most reliable index of hypoxemia. Cyanosis, manifested by blueness of the lips, nail beds, and mucosal surfaces, is present when the absolute amount of reduced hemoglobin is 5.0 grams or more. It does not adequately indicate the absolute degree of hemoglobin desaturation. For example, patients with polycythemia (excessive available hemoglobin) may have cyanosis even though tissue oxygen supply is normal; on the other hand, a severely anemic patient may not have enough circulating hemoglobin to demonstrate cyanosis, although he may be severely hypoxemic. Furthermore, the visual acuity of the observer affects the ability to detect the color changes of cyanosis, so that it is often unrecognized until the arterial oxygen saturation has dropped to very low levels.

The threshold for appearance of cyanosis is also dependent upon the local blood flow and cardiac output. If oxygen requirements do not change, then the amount of oxygen extracted from blood and thus the amount of reduced hemoglobin will be proportional to the blood flow. Figure 6–26 illustrates the effect of flow on the amount

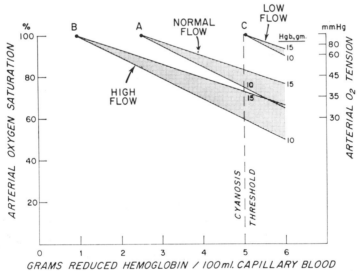

Figure 6–26. Effect of flow upon reduced hemoglobin. The cyanosis is assumed to have a capillary content of 5 grams of reduced hemoglobin per 100 ml of blood. The correlation is shown of arterial oxygen saturation and tension with reduced hemoglobin content in capillary blood for bloods of hemoglobin contents of 15 and 10 grams per 100 ml of blood. *A* represents a normal blood flow and assumes that a capillary will contain approximately one third arterial and two thirds venous blood. An arteriovenous reduced hemoglobin difference of 3.75 grams per 100 ml of blood is assumed. *B* represents the high flow state (flow is doubled) and assumes that capillary blood contains equal parts arterial and venous blood. The arteriovenous reduced hemoglobin difference is assumed to be 1.90 grams per 100 ml of blood. *C* represents the low flow state (flow is reduced by one third) and assumes that the capillary contains about nine parts venous and one part arterial blood. The arteriovenous reduced hemoglobin difference is assumed to be 5.60 grams per 100 ml of blood. (From Bendixen, H. H., et al.: Respiratory Care. St. Louis, C. V. Mosby Company, 1965.)

of reduced hemoglobin. On the one hand, a patient with a low flow such as C will have cyanosis even when oxygenation is normal. On the other hand, a patient with a high flow such as B will develop cyanosis only when the hemoglobin saturation or P_{O_2} is very low (P_{O_2} about 38 mm Hg with a normal 15 gm hemoglobin). If hemoglobin is 10 gm, cyanosis does not manifest in high flow states until P_{O_2} is about 28 mm Hg. The most reliable means of evaluating oxygenation are blood gas and pH measurement.

CLINICAL CAUSES OF HYPOXEMIA

When patients are hypoxemic, it is necessary to determine the underlying cause. The defects of oxygen transport which can result in hypoxemia and some of the adverse influences of surgery upon oxygenation have previously been discussed. The major cause of hypoxemia is atelectasis.

Atelectasis

Clinical manifestations.   Atelectasis means collapse of a portion of the lung; it is the most common pulmonary complication occurring in cardiac surgical patients.

Cardiac surgical patients are predisposed to atelectasis by the location of the incision, by direct effects upon the lung from bypass systems, and by the frequent underlying congestive changes that are associated with severe heart disease. Atelectasis is manifestly more important in cardiac patients because the effects of atelectasis upon oxygenation are greater when cardiac output is reduced. The *downside lung syndrome* is a good example of this complication. During lateral thoracotomy (particularly for mitral stenosis operations), the dependence of the lung on the side opposite the operation commonly promotes edema, inadequate ventilation, and atelectasis. The predictable frequency with which this complication occurs alerts the nursing staff to the problem.

Usually, however, postoperative atelectasis is less obvious and may be quite diffuse and patchy. It often occurs without obvious physical findings or x-ray film abnormalities. When the atelectasis is more extensive and better localized, the clinical diagnosis is made by observing diaphoresis and shallow ventilations and by finding tubular (bronchial) breathing tones; the P_{O_2} usually is somewhat low, and there is always a significant alveolar-arterial gradient (A-a gradient). Localized collapse of a portion of the lung can often be seen by chest x-ray examination.

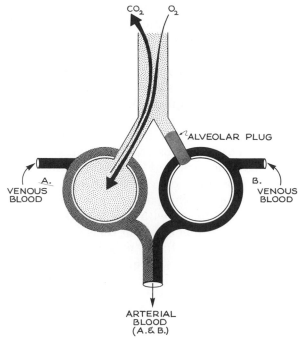

Figure 6–27. Schematic illustration of intrapulmonary shunting of blood in a nonfunctioning respiratory exchange unit. (After Comroe, J. H., Jr., et al.: Physiology of Respiration. Chicago, Year Book Medical Publishers, Inc., 1965.)

Physiologic effects. Impaired oxygenation occurs because there are multiple shunt units as illustrated in Figure 6–27. Some alveoli are normally ventilated and perfused and enjoy normal oxygen exchange. Other alveoli, however, are perfused but not ventilated, and blood leaves the alveolar capillary without having taken up any oxygen. This unoxygenated blood returns to the systemic (arterial) circulation and physiologically simulates a right-to-left cardiac shunt. Collapse of alveoli and larger airways will also cause airway obstruction and will lead to decreased lung compliance.

Predicting who will get atelectasis. Atelectasis must be prevented when possible and promptly treated when it occurs. One of the keys to prevention of pulmonary complications and the promotion of good oxygenation is to anticipate that atelectasis will occur. Patients most likely to have pulmonary complications can be predicted by history, physical, and pulmonary function tests. An example of a patient who is very likely to develop atelectasis postoperatively would be someone with a past history of pulmonary infections, who is a persistent heavy smoker, and who has emphysema and a chronic cough productive of purulent sputum. Obesity, old age, and a low pain threshold would make it even worse.

Prevention and treatment of atelectasis.   Prevention and treatment of atelectasis can be concentrated into three main areas: (1) obtaining the patient's cooperation, (2) maintaining a clear airway, and (3) keeping the lung expanded in apposition to the chest wall.

OBTAINING PATIENT COOPERATION.   The patient's cooperation is secured preoperatively by discussion of the forthcoming operation, including an explanation of equipment and a reassurance concerning the strength of the incisional closure. He should be encouraged to stop smoking, preferably two or three weeks prior to surgery. Ask the patient to cough and deep breathe. Many patients simply do not know how to cough adequately. Physiotherapy may be of value in training patients to breathe, cough effectively, clear secretions, or perform postural drainage. The patient should be allowed to use a respirator to familiarize himself with how it works, and overcome any fears of its use or claustrophobia from the face mask. The patient's ability to cooperate postoperatively may be enhanced by judicious use of analgesics, nerve blocks, nonrestrictive dressings, and early chest movement and by manual support of the patient's chest when coughing or deep breathing.

MAINTAIN A CLEAR AIRWAY.   Maintenance of a clear airway is greatly facilitated in the postoperative phase if the preoperative preparation has been adequate. During the operation, proper position of the patient, adequate ventilation of the lungs, and aspiration of secretions are important maneuvers to minimize postoperative pulmonary complications.

After the operation, clearing of secretions may be facilitated by postural drainage, antibiotic therapy, and the use of a respirator with bronchodilators. In addition, measures to thin secretions by systemic hydration and humidification of the inspired gas can be important. The use of expectorants such as intravenous sodium iodide, vaporized detergents such as Mucomist, or proteolytic enzymes may be helpful in selected patients. The patient's position is changed regularly. Deep breathing, coughing, ambulation, and blowing up a balloon or glove will increase intraluminal pressure within the airway, prevent atelectasis, and re-expand alveoli. When, despite all these measures, the patient is unable to clear secretions, nasotracheal or endotracheal suction, bronchoscopy, or tracheostomy may be utilized.

OBLITERATE PLEURAL SPACE.   Apposition of the visceral and parietal layers of the pleura is necessary to obtain adequate lung expansion or to achieve an effective cough. At the time of operation every effort is made to eliminate or minimize leakage of air from the lung. Chest tubes are used if the pleural space has been entered; residual air and fluid are removed. Temporary clamping of chest tubes prior to vigorous coughing or suctioning enhances the effectiveness of the cough.

Accumulation of blood or loculation of fluid around the lung prevents adequate lung expansion, coughing, or clearing of secretions. Periodic position changes, "milking" of the chest tubes, and proper function of the chest tube suction apparatus are important to prevent this accumulation.

Other Causes of Hypoxemia in Surgical Patients

Seldom is there a single isolated cause of hypoxemia in surgical patients; multiple interrelated factors are involved. Among these contributing factors are the following:
1. Bronchial and Parenchymal Diseases
   Airway obstruction:
   a. Upper airway obstruction (foreign body, tumor, and so on)
   b. Asthma
   c. Chronic bronchitis
   d. Emphysema
   Decrease in the volume of functioning lung tissue:
   a. Pulmonary edema
   b. Atelectasis
   c. Consolidation
2. Obliterative Pulmonary Vascular Disease
   Idiopathic and thrombotic pulmonary hypertension
3. Limitation of Lung Expansion
   a. Pleural effusion
   b. Pneumothorax
   c. Fibrothorax
   d. Pulmonary fibrosis
   e. Pleural fibrosis
4. Limitation of Thoracic Wall Expansion
   Pain:
   Thoracic or upper abdominal surgery; sternal, costal, and spinal injuries
   Bony deformities:
   Sternal, costal, and spinal
5. Limitation of Diaphragmatic Excursion
   a. Obesity
   b. Ascites
   c. Surgery
   d. Eventration
6. Neuromuscular Problems
   a. Muscular blocking agent, such as curare, succinylcholine
   b. Brain, spinal cord, or peripheral nerve injuries
7. Respiratory Center Depression or Damage
   a. Anesthetics

b. Narcotics
c. Barbiturates
d. Increased intracranial pressure

CHRONIC LUNG DISEASE

Chronic lung disease is not infrequently associated with cardiac disease, because in both there is a similar age incidence, an association with smoking or obesity, and a possibility that primary disease of one system can cause secondary disease of the other. Chronic bronchitis and emphysema are the most frequent forms of obstructive pulmonary disease. The differential clinical diagnosis of one or the other is often arbitrary and may be based primarily upon the amount of secretions the patient brings up.

Chronic bronchitis is a pulmonary disease of particular importance, because these patients have thick tenacious secretions which can cause major areas of atelectasis, can predispose to pneumonia, and can result in pulmonary failure. There is a strong causal relationship to smoking. Bacterial growth in the secretions is usual, but it is not thought to be the usual initiating cause of chronic bronchitis. When chronic bronchitis is advanced, bronchiectasis (dilatation of the airways which collapse during expiration) can occur. Chronic bronchitis is not uncommonly associated with emphysema.

Emphysema, with or without bronchitis, is associated with loss of elastic and cartilagenous support of the airways, so that obstruction of the airways occurs, especially during expiration. Positive airway pressure is often required to empty the lungs and patients often "purse" their lips to facilitate expiration. Mucous plugs are not necessarily present. In emphysema, unlike chronic bronchitis, there is often associated vascular obliteration and eventually right ventricular hypertrophy results; when heart failure occurs under these circumstances, it is called *cor pulmonale*. Recently, emphysema patients have been categorized clinically as either "blue bloaters" or "pink puffers."

The pink puffers are patients who have relatively little bronchitis but have lost all components of many respiratory exchange units at once (i.e., components of both ventilation and perfusion). They are not cyanotic (pink), but have a marked increase in the work of breathing (puffer). Chest x-ray examination of these patients usually shows relatively overinflated lungs with flattened diaphragms, increased anterior-posterior diameter of the chest, and diminished bronchovascular markings. The blue bloaters (bloater is an English colloquialism meaning "to spit") are patients who have associated chronic bronchitis and emphysema. The clinical picture explains the terminology because they are cyanotic (blue) and have a productive cough (bloaters). Physiologically, they are cyanotic because plugs of mucous in the airways prevent ventilation of alveoli that are still perfused. X-ray findings in the cyanotic group are increased vascular markings and may resemble the appearance of the "dirty chest" associated with chronic bronchitis. Overinflation of the lungs with flattening of the diaphragm is a less prominent feature in these patients than in patients with pure emphysema.

Pulmonary Therapy or Care

Our greatly expanded present state of knowledge has evolved from coronary care or intensive care unit experience and the associated mechanical and technological advancements. These developments have not eliminated the need for good patient care, but rather have intensified the requirement. We are learning to use equipment and are seeing disease and problems that we heretofore had not seen because the patient usually expired before they developed. Good nursing and pulmonary care can minimize the complications and mortality in this group of critically ill patients.

PREVENTION OF PULMONARY COMPLICATIONS

Prevention is the ultimate in therapy. The daily routines of good nursing care are by far more effective in contributing to large numbers of patient survivals than are some of our more dramatic recuperative efforts used after the complication has occurred.

MECHANICAL DEVICES, ROUTINES, AND METHODS USED IN PULMONARY CARE

Mechanical Devices

Ventilators. TYPES OF VENTILATORS. Although there are numerous manufacturers of ventilators and certain models have several special features, the basic design of ventilators is of two major types: pressure-regulated and volume-regulated. Manufacturers of respirators have recently changed designs frequently in order to include newly recognized desirable features, such as periodic hyperinflation, expiratory resistance, and oxygen concentration adjustment, as well as to eliminate some of the deficiencies of older models. In

evaluating the performance of a ventilator, the following characteristics should be considered:

Criteria Rated*

A. General
   1. Noise
   2. Durability
   3. Ease of operation
   4. Convenience
   5. Cost
B. Respirator controls
   1. Time-cycled accuracy
   2. Ease of adjustment rate
   3. Variable ratio of inspiration-expiration
   4. Range of respiratory rates
C. Tidal volume exchange
   1. Tidal volume, no resistance
   2. Tidal volume, with resistance
   3. Measured tidal volume
   4. One-way valve efficiency
   5. Expiratory resistance
   6. Peak pressure
   7. Intermittent large inflations
D. Oxygen, humidity
   1. Accuracy range O_2 concentration
   2. Danger, excessive O_2
   3. Smog
   4. Controlled humidity

As an example of some of these features, Figure 6–28 shows the
dial settings of the Bennett MA-1 ventilator.

Pressure-regulated Ventilators. Pressure-regulated ventilators
are designed to continue to inflate the lungs until a preset pressure
has been achieved. At that point, gas flow is terminated, inspiration
stops, and the expiratory phase begins. The tidal volumes achieved
by the preset pressure are determined by resistance from the endotracheal tube, elastic and airway resistance of the patient's lungs,
pleura, chest wall or dressings, and the inspiratory flow rate. Since
the pulmonary compliance and airway resistance can change very
abruptly, the expired minute volume, tidal volume, and alveolar
ventilation may be unpredictable. Commonly, incisional chest pain
will cause the patient to "clench down" or resist the inflation of his
lungs by the ventilator, the so-called *clenched chest syndrome.* It is
necessary to check adjustments frequently. Low tidal volumes over

---

*(After Peters, R. M., and Hutchin, P.: Adequacy of available respirators to their
tasks. Ann. Thorac. Surg. 3:414, 1967.)

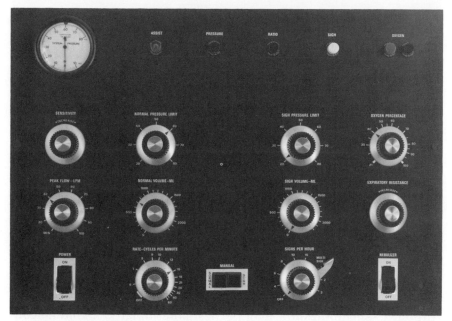

Figure 6–28. Photograph of the front panel of the Bennett MA-1 ventilator. Note the settings for patient sensitivity and rate of maximum inspiratory flow (*left*); pressure limit, volume limit, and cycles per minute for "normal" breaths (*left center*); pressure limit, volume limit, and cycles per hour for "sighs" (*right center*); and oxygen percentage and resistance to expiratory flow (*right*). Above are the pressure dial and indicator lights for patient assist, excessive pressure, abnormal inspiratory-expiratory ratio, sighs, and oxygen percentage.

a period of time can aggravate or cause atelectasis in themselves. It is generally agreed that pressure-regulated ventilators are safest, but familiarity with their deficiencies is mandatory.

Volume-regulated Ventilators. Volume-regulated ventilators usually have an inflow reservoir that can be adjusted to any desired gas flow, frequency, stroke volume, or gas mixture. The predetermined volumes of gas for each tidal volume are delivered (more or less) regardless of resistance until some preset safety release is activated. This is most frequently accomplished by a pressure relief system that interrupts the inspiratory phase when the preset maximum pressure is obtained. The advantage of the volume respirators is that a (more or less) constant alveolar ventilation is accomplished. The hazard is that excessive pressure can be generated within the airway and may cause a rupture of alveoli, resulting in a pneumothorax.

THE LEVEL OF VENTILATOR SUPPORT. The terminology describing ventilatory support is based upon its extent or completeness in replacing the patient's own efforts. *Assisted ventilation* usually denotes that the patient, working with the respirator, initiates and terminates inspiration. The gas flow rate or depth of inspiration can be modified to some extent by adjustment of the ventilator. Most assisted ventilation is done with pressure-regulated respirators. Therapy can be administered either intermittently or continuously. *Intermittent assisted ventilation* is most commonly used with a face mask in patients who are not intubated. The purpose is to periodically improve ventilation, administer aerosolized medications, or humidify and thin secretions. The work of breathing is temporarily reduced during the time of therapy, which can be most of the time or widely spaced and brief intervals. *Continuous assisted ventilation* is most often used in patients who have indwelling endotracheal tubes, but who are awake and able to cooperate. *Controlled ventilation* means that the patient's rate and depth of respiration are determined by the ventilator alone and the patient's inspiratory effort and control are eliminated. Either pressure-cycled ventilators or volume-cycled ventilators can be used. Successfully controlled ventilation is more difficult to achieve with pressure-controlled models and may initially require synchronization of the ventilator with the patient's respiration. Although synchronization may be desirable initially, a volume-controlled ventilator can, if necessary, deliver the preset volume more or less regardless of patient resistance.

INDICATIONS FOR VENTILATORY SUPPORT. The prime purpose for using a mechanical ventilator is to provide adequate alveolar ventilation and oxygenation. If the patient cannot do this on his own, he requires ventilatory support. In formulating a decision about the use of ventilatory support, the factors of excessive oxygen demand, increased work of breathing, causes of hypoxia, and defects of the oxygen transport system are considered. Use of the ventilator may be either prophylactic or therapeutic. For example, patients who are quite vulnerable to pulmonary complications, such as cardiac surgery patients, are treated in one sense prophylactically and in another sense therapeutically. Use of a ventilator permits use of enriched oxygen mixtures, aids in preventing atelectasis, minimizes pulmonary edema, and allows the use of aerosolized medications. The oxygen consumption and demand for cardiac output is decreased because the work of breathing is reduced. Oxygen consumption is further reduced by permitting sedation or muscle relaxation and decreasing combativeness without risk of respiratory depression.

There are also inherent hazards to mechanical ventilation which may be related to the mechanical failures of the ventilator, such as over- or underventilation or asphyxiation, if therapy to a dependent patient is interrupted for any reason. Pulmonary complications can be caused by the ventilator or the accessory equipment that is used. Endotracheal tubes cause tracheal injuries; humidifiers or vaporizers cause infection; enriched oxygen mixtures cause lung toxicity, or prolonged ventilatory support causes lung water retention.

ADJUSTMENT OF THE VENTILATOR. When establishing use of a ventilator in a critically ill patient, it is important that it be as near fail-safe as possible. Everything must be prepared and working before the equipment is connected to the patient. Adequate air or oxygen supply (turned on), airway control (endotracheal tube with a functioning cuff), and suction equipment are some of the essentials.

For purposes of discussion, we shall consider a patient (either serious cardiac or postcardiac surgical) who requires cuffed endotracheal intubation and discuss establishing the use of the ventilator, management during use, and methods to wean the patient from respirator support.

Ventilation Rate. Adjustment of the ventilator must be adequate to meet the patient's present needs, but is also subject to frequent reassessment and revision if the desired effect is not obtained or his situation changes. During the initiation phase of ventilation

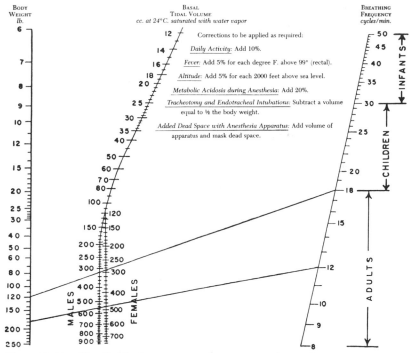

Figure 6–29. The Radford nomogram. A nomogram from which standard (basal) ventilation can be obtained from the breathing frequency, body weight, and sex. This nomogram applies only, as stressed by Radford, to patients with normal lungs. (From Radford, E. P., Jr., et al.: New Eng. J. Med. *251*:877, 1954. Reprinted with permission of the New England Journal of Medicine.)

support, judiciously regulated hyperventilation may be used to obtain "control" of the patient's respiration. After this phase, excessive ventilation is avoided because a respiratory alkalosis can be induced by decreasing P_{CO_2} below 30 mm Hg and this may have adverse effects upon cerebral blood flow, metabolic stability, and cardiac rhythmicity. The best indication of the adequacy of alveolar ventilation is the arterial P_{CO_2}. The amount of alveolar ventilation needed for a person of a certain size is determined by both tidal volume and respiratory rate. The Radford nomogram (Fig. 6–29) gives the basal ventilation requirements and corrections for activity, fever, altitude, and anesthesia.

Normal Patterns of Ventilation. We used to think that a healthy pattern of respiration was a regular, constant-volume rhythmic occurrence. In fact, normal breathing is usually quite irregular. Normally, we take periodic deep breaths or hyperinflate our lungs in the form of sighs, yawns, coughing, or sneezing. Critically ill patients often require narcotics or sedatives and, like postsurgical patients with residual anesthesia, these reflex hyperinflations are then depressed or eliminated. Patients whose respiration is controlled also cannot sigh or deep breathe unless the ventilatory therapy is regulated to provide them.

Adjusting Ventilation and Functional Reserve Capacity. When ventilators are set to deliver prolonged, constant low tidal volumes, atelectasis will surely occur. By such a technique we will, in fact, be promoting pulmonary failure (exactly opposite from our objective). Alveoli collapse when the baseline lung volume or functional residual capacity (FRC) is reached and when this resting position is maintained until the next inspiration. If normal periodic re-expansion of the cumulative alveolar collapse is not done, then the functional reserve capacity progressively decreases (Fig. 6–30). A brief review

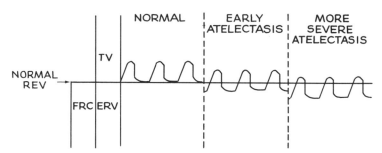

Figure 6–30. Effect of progressive alveolar collapse on resting expiratory volume (REV). Note that as atelectasis becomes more severe, the tidal volume progressively encroaches upon the expiratory reserve volume (part of the functional reserve capacity, see Figure 6–4). Similarly, the level of the resting expiratory volume is displaced downward.

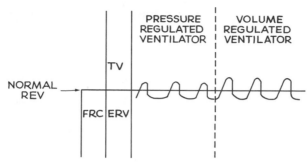

Figure 6–31. Effect of pressure-regulated and volume-regulated ventilators upon the tidal volume (TV). In this example, the lung compliance and the resting expiratory volume are already reduced below normal; the effect of the two types of ventilators can be seen.

of Figure 6–4 will remind us that the lung volume at the time of reaching resting expiratory level (when pressure in the airways is equal to atmospheric pressure) is the volume of the lung called the functional reserve capacity. Collapse of alveoli (atelectasis) not only decreases FRC but also decreases compliance. The lungs are stiffer and more resistant to expansion. When a patient is treated with a pressure-regulated ventilator, peak inspiratory pressure is unchanged, and since the lungs are stiffer, tidal volume and alveolar ventilation decrease, perpetuating the deteriorating cycle. In the same situation, volume-regulated respirators would continue to give the same tidal volume, but it would be noted that increasingly higher peak inspiratory pressure would be required (Fig. 6–31). When higher peak inspiratory pressures are required, it is more likely that an alveolus will rupture and pneumothorax will develop. When peak inspiratory pressure exceeds 35 mm Hg, the possibility of pneumothorax increases.

Methods of Ventilator Adjustment Used to Prevent Atelectasis. Atelectasis produced by ventilator therapy is preventable to a large extent. Four main approaches are used: (1) continuous positive pressure breathing (CPPB), also called positive expiratory plateau pressure (PEPP) or positive end-expiratory pressure (PEEP); (2) periodic hyperinflation or artificial "sighing"; (3) continuous sighing using large tidal volumes; and (4) retarded expiration. As mentioned, alveolar collapse causes a decrease of the functional residual capacity (FRC) and of the number of alveoli open to ventilation. Most ventilatory assistance regimens attempt to prevent the tendency for the FRC to decrease either by periodically re-expanding alveoli (sighing) or by maintaining a state of relative hyperinflation by preventing a return of airway pressure to atmospheric pressure (Fig. 6–32).

Continuous Positive Pressure Breathing (CPPB). Continuous

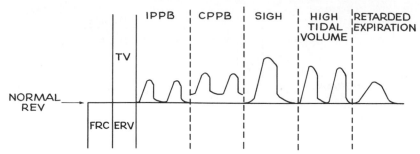

Figure 6–32. Breathing patterns in different types of respiratory support. See text for discussion.

positive pressure breathing is a modification of intermittent positive pressure breathing (IPPB). It has been shown that if modest positive pressure (6 to 10 mm Hg) is maintained during the expiratory phase, atelectasis is less likely to occur (Fig. 6–33). Because of the danger of pneumothorax, and because cardiac output may be reduced with higher pressure, the continuous positive intrathoracic pressure can cause decreased return of venous blood to the heart. CPPB with high pressures should be used cautiously in cardiac patients. CPPB is often used with fairly large tidal volumes of 8 to 14 ml per kg body weight and without sighing; respiratory rate is determined by the arterial P_{CO_2}. The ratio of inspiration to expiration is usually set at

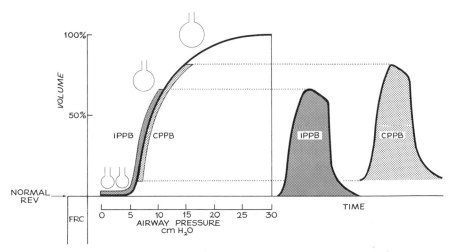

Figure 6–33. Effect of IPPB and CPPB on the resting expiratory volume. Note that as the inflation volumes become larger, the pressure required to produce this volume also increases. CPPB does not allow the lung volume to return to the resting level (as IPPB does), thereby maintaining slight hyperinflation and reducing atelectasis.

about 1:2 or 1:3. Peak airway pressures of 25 cm H₂O or less are usually adequate, unless compliance is reduced.

Sighing. Periodic hyperinflation or sighing is being used as the principal method of preventing atelectasis and it should be done frequently. When IPPB of relatively low tidal volumes is used, seven to 10 sighs per hour are required because the alveoli will begin to recollapse during the interval phase between sighs (Fig. 6–34). When sighing is used to prevent atelectasis and the lungs are adequately compliant, the volume of the sigh can be safely set to two, or sometimes three, times the tidal volume without significant risk of alveolar rupture and pneumothorax. The volume of a sigh is relatively unpredictable with pressure-regulated respirators; sighing is sometimes better accomplished manually using a resuscitation bag device. When volume-regulated respirators are used, the peak inspiration pressure does not necessarily limit the volume of sighing, so the hazard of pneumothorax may be increased.

Continuous High Tidal Volume. The principle of high tidal volume therapy or continuous sighing is the use of substantially larger-than-normal tidal volumes. With this technique, overventilation and respiratory alkalosis are prevented by decreasing the rate of respiration. For example, a tidal volume of 1200 ml may be given six or eight times per minute. When a large tidal volume is required at a rate rapid enough to cause hyperventilation, respiratory alkalosis can

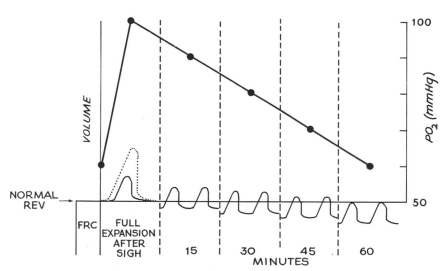

Figure 6–34. Effect of sighing upon the resting expiratory volume and the arterial P$_{O_2}$. Note the progressive decrease in the inspiratory volume, the reduction of the arterial P$_{O_2}$ and the downward displacement of the level of the resting expiratory volume with the passage of time after the full expansion of a sigh. Sighing must be repeated frequently.

be prevented by increasing the respiratory dead space. This is accomplished by adding lengths of tubing between the patient and the exhalation valve or by introducing a rebreathing mechanism to the system.

Temporary hyperventilation with high tidal volumes to obtain control of respiration is often done, particularly in patients whose spontaneous respiratory drive is intense. Patients with fever, metabolic acidosis, pneumonia, or central nervous system disturbances may require treatment in this manner; however, use of excessively high tidal volumes may itself adversely affect the lungs. There is evidence that sustained hyperventilation depletes surfactant.

Retarded Expiration. Retardation of the expiratory phase may be necessary in patients with collapsing airways, many of whom do not require CPPB. Retardation of expiration by the respirator has the same effect as an emphysematous patient pursing his lips. There is an increased resistance to expiration, preventing airway collapse; the expiratory phase is prolonged, allowing more complete emptying of the lungs.

HAZARDS AND SPECIAL PROBLEMS OF CONTROLLED VENTILATION. Assisted ventilation may be inappropriate when the patient is unable to cooperate. He may trigger the rate either inadequately or excessively. Spontaneous respiration, if not synchronous with the ventilator, may interfere with ventilation. In this situation, the patient will be better ventilated if he is permitted to breathe on his own without ventilatory assistance. Fighting a respirator can cause the work of breathing and oxygen expenditure for breathing to be markedly increased; oxygen availability is reduced. When an intubated patient defies control or is combative or shivering, it is possible and may even be desirable to obtain control of respiration by use of sedation and muscle relaxation. Sedation can be obtained with incremental dosages (1 to 4 mg) of intravenous morphine or 10 to 20 mg of Valium, or neuromuscular blockade may be achieved with agents such as d-tubocurare (6 to 12 mg) or succinyl choline (20 to 30 mg) given intravenously. Oftentimes, these measures will be necessary only temporarily, and once control is established they can be discontinued. Shivering is often benefitted by the administration of chlorpromazine, but the drug must be administered cautiously because of its tendency to decrease blood pressure and lower cardiac output.

Sedation and administration of muscle relaxants is usually used sparingly. When a patient is fighting a respirator or is seemingly "unable to cooperate," the first thought must be that he may be inadequately oxygenated and hypoxemic. Sedation and relaxation would be used only after it was certain that the gas supply and mixture, mechanical function of the respirator, and arterial oxygenation were satisfactory.

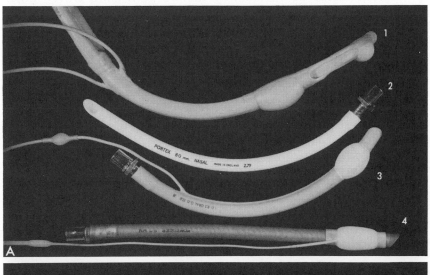
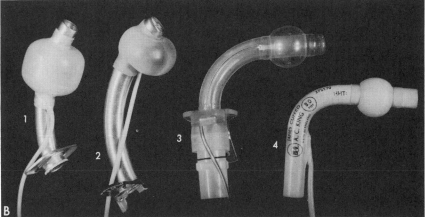

Figure 6–35. Photograph of ventilator tubes. *A*, Endotracheal tubes (from top to bottom): (1) The Robert-Shaw double-lumen tube to isolate the flow to each lung. Note the individual inflatable cuffs for the trachea and the left bronchus; (2) The Portex nasotracheal tube, without attached cuff; (3) An orotracheal tube with attached inflatable cuff (very commonly used); and (4) The LA (Latex-Armored) tube. Note the spiral winding to prevent kinking. *B*, Tracheostomy tubes (from left to right): (1) The Hollinger tracheostomy tube with separately attached "Sof-Cuf" cuff. Note the relatively shallow curve of the tube and the evenly inflated (low-pressure) cuff; (2) The Jackson tracheostomy tube with separately attached cuff. Note the relatively sharp angle of the tube and the eccentrically inflated (high-pressure) cuff; (3) The Portex plastic tracheostomy tube with attached cuff which inflates evenly at relatively high pressure; and (4) The James tracheostomy tube with attached cuff which inflates evenly; this tube is occasionally used in short-necked patients.

Control of the airway itself is also mandatory when a patient is receiving controlled ventilation. Even brief obstruction, disconnection, dislodgment, or mechanical failure can soon prove lethal. Trained personnel, capable of correcting the situation, should be in constant attendance. Whenever bottled gas is used, spare tanks, and manual ventilatory devices, such as Ambu bags or the equivalent, must be available for some unforeseen mechanical failure and be used until the problem is rectified.

Endotracheal tubes. VARIETIES OF ENDOTRACHEAL TUBES. A wide variety of tubes is available for nasotracheal or orotracheal placement. Each has special uses, advantages, and disadvantages. All are available with inflatable cuffs near the tip of the tube (Fig. 6–35A).

Tracheostomy cannulas may be made of disposable plastic, stainless steel, or sterling silver (Fig. 6–35B). They may be short (end tracheostomy) or long (such as the Hollinger tube) and may have angles of 60 or 90 degrees. The 60 degree shorter version is generally preferred for most patients. The components of a metal tracheal cannula are the outer cannula, inner cannula, and stylet. Metal cannulas come in various sizes graded in millimeters; an average adult size is 6 to 8 mm. The inner cannula is designed to be removed and cleaned. The entire cannula apparatus should be changed frequently, daily if necessary. Tracheostomies are becoming less routine and have been reserved for situations in which prolonged respiratory care is anticipated, or in which they are substituted for nasotracheal or orotracheal tubes after 48 to 72 hours.

Cuffed orotracheal tubes are often preferred for initial therapy in most patients. Orotracheal tubes have the advantage of not causing hemorrhage from the nasal passages, as occasionally happens with nasotracheal tubes. This bleeding can be bothersome and persistent, both during and after the operation, particularly when anticoagulation for total cardiopulmonary bypass has been required. Orotracheal tubes are also larger, permitting more adequate suction; however, too large a tube can cause injury to the larynx. Patients will accept prolonged use of orotracheal tubes as well as nasotracheal tubes if they are instructed in the objectives of therapy preoperatively or prior to insertion. If endotracheal intubation is required, an orotracheal tube is always preferred to a tracheostomy, and is usually tolerated very well. It has only rarely been necessary to change to a nasotracheal tube, or to perform a tracheostomy because of orotracheal tube intolerance. Either nasotracheal or orotracheal tubes can be left in place, without complication, for many days; usually three to four days is maximum. This is not to say that complications may not occur before this. Tracheal stenosis following orotracheal intubation has been seen after only 17 hours' duration. Unlike tracheostomy cannulae, orotracheal and nasotracheal tubes do not have inner cannulae that can be removed for cleaning, and it is impractical to make daily changes of the entire tube.

Uncontrolled leaks of air around any of these tubes make ventilation therapy ineffective and inaccurate; alveolar ventilation may be inadequate. Volume respirators are especially difficult to use under these circumstances and are therefore almost always used with cuffed tubes. The balloon or cuff of the endotracheal tube should be tested before use. When in place, they should be inflated to just the minimum pressure that will prevent air leakage. Periodic deflation of the cuff may minimize the hazard of tracheal injury. When this is done, it should be preceded by careful suctioning of the hypopharynx so that accumulated secretions above the balloon do not gain access to the lungs. As there is considerable variation in cuff design, one should be chosen that requires minimal inflation pressure, inflates evenly and uniformly over a broad area, and is composed of material which is neither irritating to tissue or subject to leakage.

HAZARDS OF ENDOTRACHEAL INTUBATION. There are many hazards from indwelling endotracheal tubes, some of them so serious and distressingly frequent that additional comment is required. The major complications of indwelling endotracheal tubes are (a) tracheal injuries, which include tracheal stenosis, tracheoesophageal fistula, and erosion through the trachea into the innominate artery; (b) respiratory infection; (c) hypoxia, cardiac arrhythmias, and death.

Tracheal Injury. Tracheal injuries occur because of local tissue trauma related to the indwelling cannulas. They occur whether or not a tracheostomy is performed. Figure 6–36 illustrates the varieties of injuries that occur.

Excessive inflation pressure of the cuff is the commonest cause of tracheal stenosis, but it also occurs frequently at the site of the tracheostomy stoma. Excessive movement of the endotracheal tube because of improper fixation to the mouth, nose, or neck, or "dragging" on the indwelling tube because of inadequate support of the cannula and its connecting tubing are other important causes of injury.

The tip of a malpositioned tracheostomy cannula can erode the anterior wall of the trachea, and subsequently cause massive bleeding from the innominate artery. Erosion through the posterior wall can cause a fistula between the trachea and the esophagus. These complications may be caused by an incorrect site of the tracheostomy, improper cannula length, or by angulation or improper fixation of the cannula. The proper site and placement of a tracheostomy is illustrated in Figure 6–37.

Occasionally, the cuff of the tube will not deflate and continuous and excessive pressure is applied to the tracheal wall. Adding more air to reinflate the cuff only causes more hyperinflation. This compli-

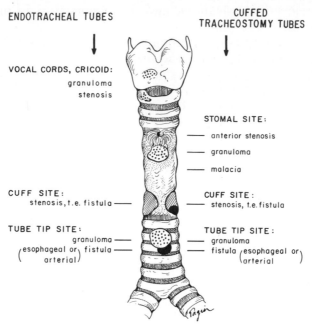

ENDOTRACHEAL TUBES

CUFFED
TRACHEOSTOMY TUBES

VOCAL CORDS, CRICOID:
granuloma
stenosis

STOMAL SITE:
—— anterior stenosis
—— granuloma
—— malacia

CUFF SITE:
stenosis, t.e. fistula ——

CUFF SITE:
—— stenosis, t.e. fistula

TUBE TIP SITE:
granuloma ——
(esophageal or) fistula ——
(arterial   )

TUBE TIP SITE:
—— granuloma
—— fistula (esophageal or)
(arterial   )

Figure 6–36.   Tracheal injuries produced by cuffed endotracheal and tracheostomy tubes. (From Grillo, H. C.: Surgery of the trachea. Curr. Probl. Surg July 1970.)

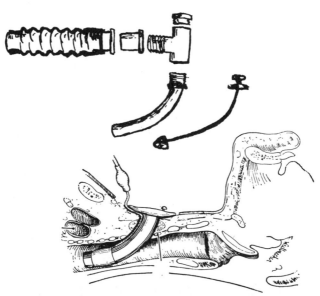

Figure 6–37.   Proper position of head, tracheal cannula, and ventilatory equipment. (From Safar, P.: Recognition and management of airway obstruction. J.A.M.A.
208:1010, 1969.)

cation usually occurs after a clamp has been placed across the tiny tubing used to inflate the cuff. The clamp causes the two walls to "stick together" and prevents cuff deflation. The remedy to this situation is to use a three-way stopcock or other device to keep air in the cuff rather than to clamp the tubing. If the block cannot be relieved by massaging the tiny tubing, it will have to be cut "downstream" from where it was clamped.

Tracheal injury can further be caused by the suction catheters placed through the endotracheal tube. The catheter tip can physically irritate or erode the tracheal or bronchial mucosa.

Respiratory Infection. Respiratory infection may range in severity from minor tracheostomy stomal infections to massive confluent pneumonitis. Normally, the glottis protects the airway from bacteria and the trachea and other airways are usually sterile. However, when an endotracheal tube is placed, this barrier to bacterial invasion is removed. Bacterial exposure can also be increased because of the equipment used in respiratory care. There is a propensity for gram-negative organisms to grow in tubing, vaporizers, and other nooks and crannies of ventilator equipment. Often these organisms are resistant to the antibiotic the patient is receiving. When these organisms have colonized the ventilatory equipment, they perpetuate the infectious problem by continuously reinfecting the patient. Epidemics of pulmonary infections have been traced to respiratory equipment. Because of this hazard, it may be necessary to change all equipment daily, including the vaporizer. Tracheostomy cannulas are changed daily, but nasotracheal and orotracheal tubes usually cannot be. The most common organisms are *Staphylococcus aureus, Pseudomonas pyocyanea,* bacillus *Proteus, Escherichia coli,* and several organisms usually not pathogens, such as *Serratia marcescens.*

Infection of the respiratory tract can be minimized by (a) careful, aseptic intratracheal and intrabronchial suctioning; (b) prevention of atelectasis and prompt re-expansion of collapsed lung segments; (c) aseptic and atraumatic tracheostomy care; (d) prevention of cross-infection by using isolation precautions; and (e) daily sterilization of humidifiers, tubes, and valves.

Hypoxemia, Cardiac Arrhythmias, and Death. Hypoxemic complications from endotracheal intubation may occur from dislodgment, plugging, or malposition of the endotracheal tube in ventilator-dependent patients. Prolonged, excessive endotracheal suction is also a very common cause of hypoxemia in these patients, as will be discussed later.

When the patient gags, coughs violently, or thrashes about in bed, nasotracheal and orotracheal tubes are easily dislodged if not carefully secured to the face. After the application of tincture of benzoin, adhesive tape is wrapped around the tube and then extended

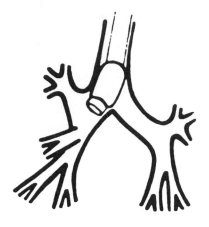

Figure 6–38. Intubation of the right mainstem bronchus, preventing ventilation of left lung. (From Bain, J. A., and Spoerel, W. E.: Canad. Anaesth. Soc. J. *11*:598, 1964.)

on the face on both sides, securely fixing the tube in place. If the patient is particularly active (especially in children), it may be necessary to immobilize the head by placing sandbags on either side. Should the tube be positioned poorly, either at the time of insertion or from subsequent patient motion, there may be inadequate ventilation of all lung segments. For example, the tube may slip inward and pass into the right mainstem bronchus, completely occluding the entire left lung (Fig. 6–38). Plugging of the tube usually does not occur if humidification is adequate. It is most likely to occur when a patient is not breathing humidified gas from a ventilator, but after he has been weaned from the ventilator and is breathing ambient air that is relatively dry. There are several humidification devices available to prevent this complication.

Endotracheal suctioning. NORMAL CLEARING OF SECRETIONS. Sometimes we overestimate the therapeutic value of the devices that we use. This is probably true concerning the extent of our use of ventilatory equipment. Although some of the mechanical properties of aeration are provided by a ventilator, these benefits are sometimes exchanged for other problems. Indwelling endotracheal tubes not only increase the amount of secretions, but also reduce the ability to cough explosively and clear them. Clearing of secretions may also be less efficient in postoperative patients because of incisional pain and sedation. The management of secretions is, therefore, of paramount importance to ensure airway patency, maintain ventilation, and prevent infection. The amount of secretions can sometimes be minimized by preventive measures, which were discussed in the section on atelectasis. Assistance to the patient in clearing secretions should include chest support when coughing, positioning, and judicious use of analgesics. Despite adequate hydration, humidification, and patient cooperation, there will be occasions when it is not mechanically possible for the patient to clear thick, voluminous secretions. In this situation, tracheal suctioning can effectively stimulate coughing and mechanically remove secretions. During this procedure, violent coughing may be stimulated. In postoperative patients, the chest tubes are temporarily clamped to limit the dissipation of the effort and force of the cough; otherwise, a significant dampening of peak negative and positive pressures occurs and energy is expended to draw water up the tubing from the underwater seal during inspiration and to expel the air in the pleural space during expiration. Tracheal suction is used when secretions are audibly present, not just as a routine "to see if there are secretions present."

TECHNIQUE OF NASOTRACHEAL SUCTIONING. The entire procedure should be accomplished using sterile gloves, catheters, and irrigation solution. It is best to discard this equipment after each use. The proper route for the suction catheter is to go past the posterior oropharynx, around the epiglottis, then through the vocal cords. The

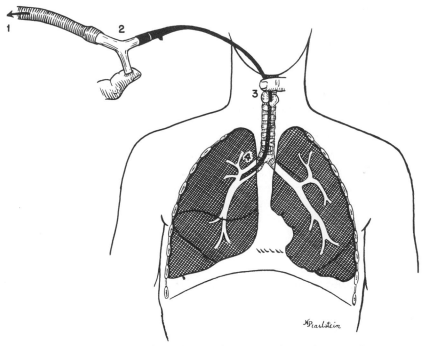

Figure 6–39. Suctioning through a tracheostomy tube. A drawing illustrating the suction setup: suction source (*1*), connecting tubing with Y glass tube occluded (*2*) by the operator's thumb is closed, and the selective bronchial suction catheter is already inserted through the fenestration (*3*) and its tip is in position for suctioning (*4*). (From Rockey, E. E., and Thompson, S. A.: Selective bronchial suction catheters and their clinical application. Amer. J. Surg. 96:552, 1958.)

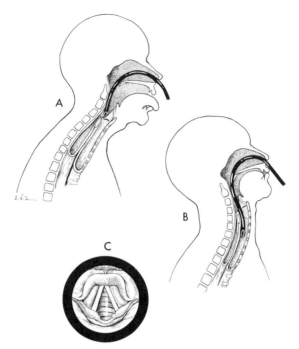

Figure 6-40. Technique of nasotracheal suctioning. *A,* Optimal position of head in order to direct catheter tip anteriorly into the trachea. The neck is flexed and the head is extended. The tongue is protruded (and held there by a gauze 4 × 4). *B,* After the catheter has been advanced into the trachea, the tongue is released and the patient's head may be more comfortably positioned. *C,* View of the vocal cords from above. The cords are most widely separated during inspiration.

cords, which are located anteriorly in the midline, may be partially closed, but will open with inspiration. The trachea bifurcates into the right and left mainstem bronchi (Fig. 6–39), normally the right mainstem bronchus has a 15 degree angle to the vertical, whereas the left bronchus is more acutely angled, 25 to 35 degrees. Using a catheter with a slightly curved tip, it is possible to intubate either the left or right side by rotation of the catheter tip and by angulation of the head and neck to one side.

The technique of nasotracheal suction is as follows: the patient should be sitting with his back supported from behind. His head position should be looking straight forward with the neck flexed and the head extended. The patient's mouth should be widely open. If an assistant is available, he should be positioned behind the patient and can hold the protruded tongue with a 4 × 4 gauze (Fig. 6–40). For adults, a No. 14 or No. 16 Fr. red Robinson catheter with a curved tip, that has one hole located at the end, is used. The catheter is connected to a wall suction or other suction device with a glass or plastic

Y connector. The patient is asked to breathe through the mouth. The Robinson catheter is passed through the more widely patent nostril into the hypopharynx after orienting the curved tip to the Y connector, so that the direction of the tip is known. The depth of the insertion required to reach the vocal cords can be determined by measurement before passage. Proximity of the tip of the catheter to the vocal cords can be determined if one listens to the patient's respiration next to the open side of the Y connector (with suction off). The tip is slowly advanced. It is important that the head, tongue, and catheter tip position all be properly aligned, then the patient is asked to take a deep breath and the catheter is rapidly advanced about 2 inches unless resistance is met; the catheter should not be connected to suction. If the catheter is in the trachea, the patient may be acutely restless and he should be reassured. He will not be able to talk because the vocal cords cannot approximate. The catheter position can be maintained by holding the catheter near the patient's nose to prevent withdrawal. Tracheal suction is accomplished by intermittent occlusion at the Y connector orifice with the thumb, listening for air movement around the catheter tip. With sufficient rest periods, advance down both the right and left mainstem bronchi. Suction is applied only at the time of withdrawal and only after any wedging of the catheter tip has been corrected by withdrawing the catheter 1 or 2 cm. Release the suction if aspiration sounds stop (the catheter may be occluded by mucus), or if the tip seems stuck and won't withdraw freely. During rest periods, the suction must be turned off, but the catheter need not be removed. Irrigate each side with 5 cc sterile water or saline, if indicated, and repeat the suctioning procedure. Patients are distressed by this procedure and deserve every consideration, and they often benefit from frequent reassurance.

COMPLICATIONS OF NASOTRACHEAL OR ENDOTRACHEAL SUCTIONING. *Hypoxia.* Negative pressure from the suction may cause

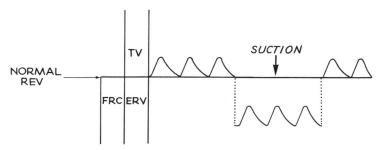

Figure 6–41. Effect of tracheal suction on the resting expiratory volume. During suctioning, the level of the resting expiratory volume is displaced acutely downward; hypoxemia can easily result.

such a negative pressure in the lungs that the air in the patient's major airways is aspirated (Fig. 6–41). Such a circumstance can easily cause hypoxemia, particularly if the suction is prolonged. In order to avoid this complication, it is often advisable to "preoxygenate" the patients prior to or during suctioning.

Lobar Collapse. If the airway is too small, relative to the size of the endotracheal tube (a narrow airway or an oversized tube), air cannot enter into a segment of lung, thus producing lobar collapse. This complication may be avoided by using a proper-sized tube and by not wedging the catheter out in the bronchus.

Ulceration of Respiratory Epithelium. The suction catheter should be smooth, soft, not too large, and handled gently in order to prevent trauma to the mucosal lining.

Sudden Death. Continuous suctioning for periods exceeding 15 to 30 seconds should be avoided. In critically ill, poorly oxygenated patients, 15 seconds with apnea is maximum, and then only after they have been hyperoxygenated.

The possible causes of sudden death with tracheal suction include the following: (a) anoxia from prolonged suctioning which frequently causes severe cardiac arrhythmias; (b) respiratory tract reflexes which can initiate both bronchospasm and bradycardia, and (c) dilatation of the superior vena cava and pulmonary artery; after the apnea stops, venous return is started once again and the heart may become distended with the blood from the dilated vessels. These effects may be cumulative and additive and may cause sudden death in the marginal, critically ill cardiac patient.

Humidity and vaporizers. Whatever method of oxygen therapy is used, it is important to remember that oxygen is a completely dry gas and, if not humidified, it will take up considerable amounts of water when it contacts the moist respiratory mucosa. Injury to the mucosa and thickening of the secretions result.

The formation and transport of mucus is very important to the normal function of respiratory mucosa and an important cause of impairment of this function is lack of adequate humidification of the inspired gas. The inspired gas should reach the trachea fully saturated with water vapor at body temperature. Various types of humidifiers, nebulizers, and vaporizers are available. Ultrasonic nebulizers are probably the most efficient.

Humidifying devices can complicate the effectiveness of ventilatory therapy. Condensation may form in the tubes leading from the nebulizer to the patient and project a bolus of water through the tubes into the tracheobronchial tree with the inspiratory phase. When a pressure-limited respirator is used, condensed water may partially block the inspiratory tube, causing a sharp decrease in effective ventilation. Continuous ventilation with fully humidified gas may result in a positive water balance and must be carefully considered in the oliguric patient. The tracheobronchial tree can absorb 400 ml of water in 24 hours when continuous ventilation is used.

Chest tubes and bottles. The general principles of the management of chest tubes and underwater seal and negative pressure apparatuses are well covered in several texts. The important principles of management would apply to patients receiving ventilator support. In artificially ventilated patients, pneumothorax is one of the most frequent problems seen, especially in patients with severe pulmonary disease. The patients most likely to develop pneumothorax are those who require high inflation pressures, usually more than 35 mm Hg.

When an alveolus or terminal bronchus ruptures, air enters the pleural space during inspiration, but often cannot return during expiration. The lung is externally compressed by the gas in the pleural space, which increases in volume with each cycle of the ventilator. The suddenness of this development can be dramatic, because the volume respirator that delivers a fixed tidal volume will continue to pump air into the trachea and if the ruptured airway offers little resistance, tension pneumothorax will develop rapidly. A tension pneumothorax causes the mediastinum to shift over to the opposite side and this, in turn, compresses the other lung (the "good" lung).

It is surprising how often the diagnosis of pneumothorax is missed. Although breath sounds may be decreased on the side of the pneumothorax and the trachea shifted to the other side, these findings often are not obvious and are sometimes inadequate to make the diagnosis. When a patient who has required ventilatory control with high pressures unexpectedly deteriorates, becomes hypotensive, appears blue and flushed, shows engorged neck veins, and demonstrates an abruptly increased A-a gradient, he should be considered to have a tension pneumothorax until proven otherwise. Treatment is aimed at deflating the affected side by inserting a needle to relieve the tension, and then placing a chest tube connected to suction as more definitive treatment. After treatment, ventilation may require adjustment commensurate with the percentage of the tidal volume that is lost to the underwater seal apparatus.

Oxygen Therapy

The general importance of oxygen is obvious, but only recently have we appreciated the need to define criteria for the adequacy of oxygenation based upon an analysis of tissue oxygen requirements relative to the patient's ability to supply it. The balance of oxygen supply and demand has moved from the laboratory to an impor-

TABLE 6–7*

Cause of Hypoxemia	Therapy
1. Inadequate oxygenation of normal lung	
a. Deficiency of O_2 in atmosphere	Restore P_{O_2} of inspired gas to 159 mm Hg
b. Airway obstruction; neuromuscular disorders	Adequate ventilation with air
2. Inadequate oxygenation of abnormal lung	
a. Hypoventilation	Adequate ventilation with air
b. Uneven alveolar ventilation per pulmonary capillary blood flow	Hyperventilation with air; inhalation of O_2
c. Impaired diffusion	Hyperventilation with air; inhalation of O_2
3. Venous-to-arterial shunts	Close shunt; O_2 inhalation corrects anoxemia only partially
4. Inadequate circulatory transport of O_2	
a. Anemia; abnormal Hb	Increase amount of active Hb
b. General circulatory deficiency	Increase systemic blood flow
c. Localized circulatory deficiency	Increase local blood flow
5. Inadequate tissue oxygenation	
a. Tissue edema	Inhalation of O_2 (?)
b. Abnormal tissue demand	Inhalation of O_2 (?)
c. Poisoning of cellular enzymes	Inhalation of O_2 of no value

*(From THE LUNG: CLINICAL PHYSIOLOGY AND PULMONARY FUNCTION TESTS, 2nd edition by Julius H. Comroe, Jr., et al. Copyright © 1962, Year Book Medical Publishers, Inc. Used by permission.)

tant role in the care of critically ill patients. This broadened perspective in medical care is largely the result of the growing clinical application of methods for measuring (1) blood gases and pH; (2) ventilation—tidal volume and flow, and (3) cardiac stroke volume and flow. Blood gases and pH are now readily available in most hospitals.

Rationale for use of enriched oxygen mixtures. Oxygenation must be considered separately from ventilation and should be adjusted to the patient's requirements.

There are some general indications for oxygen therapy. It must be appreciated that adjustment of ventilation is determined by different considerations than the decision to give an enriched oxygen mixture, and both of these differ from the therapy for inadequate oxygen-carrying capacity. Table 6–7 outlines some of the causes of hypoxemia and the role oxygen therapy might have in those situations.

Methods of oxygen delivery. When it is decided to use enriched oxygen mixtures, one of the first questions to ask is what concentration to use. The correct concentration may not be known initially and will have to be determined by titration to the patient's needs. The methods of administration of oxygen are summarized in Table 6–8.

Nasal catheters or prongs are the most commonly used way of giving enriched oxygen mixtures and are the least expensive. They must be used with humidified gas, and will achieve relatively modest oxygen concentrations. Oxygen flow rates can be varied to a maximum of 6 or 8 L per min. They are not really uncomfortable, but patients do not like tubes in their noses. The tip of a nasal catheter must be carefully advanced to just below the soft palate to avoid stimulation of swallowing reflexes which might cause gastric distension. Prolonged use is irritating to the nasal mucosa.

Face hoods or tents are best used when an enriched oxygen concentration is not mandatory, but humidification is desired. Tightly fitting face masks usually have nonrebreathing valves and reservoir bags. They provide the highest oxygen concentrations of these listed methods; with a reservoir bag 90 per cent concentration can often be attained. They are simple to use and many patients find them quite comfortable. Some patients tolerate them poorly because they dislike the tight fit around the face.

Oxygen tents are now seldom used because they are cumbersome and make the patient relatively inaccessible to nursing care. They require high flow rates (12 to 14 L per min) and achieve a maximal oxygen concentration of only about 50 per cent. Other disadvantages are that the oxygen tension falls rapidly when the tent is open and then requires time to build back up; some patients become claustrophobic in the tent.

Patients with endotracheal tubes may be treated with a T-piece in which flows can be adjusted to 12 L per min and the maximum oxygen concentration achieved is about 50 per cent. The only really certain way of delivering 100 per cent oxygen is with a closed system and a ventilator delivery unit. It should be realized that oxygen is injurious to lungs and the concentration used should be based entirely upon the measured need of the patient.

Monitoring oxygen requirements. The concentration of oxygen required is based upon the arterial P_{O_2}. Normally, an arterial P_{O_2} of 80 to 100 mm Hg is adequate and provides some margin of safety in regard to hemoglobin saturation. Under some circumstances, the $P_{a_{O_2}}$ may need to be increased to compensate for reduced hemoglobin content or inadequate cardiac output; whenever possible, the anemia should be corrected and cardiac output improved.

In some situations, in which severe chronic pulmonary shunting exists, a patient may tolerate a P_{O_2} as low as 40 mm Hg either inter-

TABLE 6–8.   *Methods of Oxygen Administration**

METHOD	MAX PER CENT OXYGEN	FLOW (L/min)	COMMENTS
A. *Nasal catheter*	30–40%	6–8	Comfortable. Higher flows provide up to 40% oxygen, but can cause respiratory depression and drying of mucosa.
B. *Nasal prongs*	30–40%	6–8	Comfortable. Higher flows provide up to 40% oxygen, but can cause respiratory depression and drying of mucosa.
C. *T-piece*	40–60%	4–12	Provides enriched oxygen mixtures and humidification. Used most often in weaning patients from ventilator assistance before endotracheal tube is removed.

*After Weiss, E. B. et al.: Acute Respiratory Failure in Chronic Obstructive Pulmonary Disease. Part II: Treatment. Chicago, Year Book Medical Publishers, Inc., 1969.

(Table continued on opposite page.)

TABLE 6–8.   *Methods of Oxygen Administration* (Continued)

D. *Face tent*	30–55%	4–8	Well tolerated. Good for supplying extra humidity.
E. *Venturi masks*	25–35%	4–8	Mask well tolerated. Accurate concentrations delivered.
F. *Mask without bag*	35–45% 45–55% 55–65%	6–8 10 10–12	Poorly tolerated. Significant CO_2 rebreathing possible at low flows. Highest percentage requires tight mask fit.

(Table continued on following page.)

TABLE 6–8.   *Methods of Oxygen Administration* (Continued)

G. *Mask with bag*	40–55%	6	Poorly tolerated.
	50–60%	8	Significant CO_2
	90 + %	8–12	rebreathing possible at low flows. Highest percentage requires tight mask fit and a large bag.

H. *Pressure-regulated ventilator*	40–100%	Direct from supply	Oxygen per cent unpredictable

I. *Volume-regulated ventilator*	20–100%	Direct from fupply	Bennett MA1, Ohio 560 can be set to any desired per cent.

mittently or temporarily. Usually in patients with severe pulmonary complications, such as "pump lung," "shock lung," or pulmonary embolus, it is impossible to achieve normal oxygenation of arterial blood and one must, of necessity, settle for a 60 to 80 mm Hg $P_{a_{O_2}}$.

Pressure-regulated ventilators are frequently very inaccurate when set to "40 per cent air mix" and may actually be delivering the equivalent of 90 per cent oxygen to the patient. It is necessary in all supported ventilation to regularly confirm the $P_{I_{O_2}}$ of the mixture being delivered. Most of the newer volume respirators, such as the Bennett MA-1 or Ohio 560, have accurate regulating devices to vary the oxygen concentration. In older equipment, modification of the oxygen content may be accomplished by using air or oxygen in either the vaporizer or ventilator lines and adjusting flow to achieve the desired concentration. Enriched oxygen-air mixtures of any desired P_{O_2} can also be purchased.

Complications of oxygen treatment. The complications of oxygen therapy are (1) respiratory depression due to removal of the hypoxic stimulus to respiration, (2) circulatory depression due to reduction of sympathetic compensatory response to hypoxia, (3) atelectasis, (4) tracheobronchitis, and (5) pulmonary injury or toxicity, which is now a well recognized hazard. It appears that 100 per cent oxygen may be tolerated eight to 12 hours in most normal patients, and air-oxygen mixtures with a P_{O_2} less than 300 mm Hg are usually safe for several days. However, oxygen partial pressures exceeding 300 mm Hg are hazardous, must be avoided, and can occasionally be lethal. Of course, 100 per cent oxygen is sometimes required and is used when necessary to prevent hypoxemia.

Weaning from Enriched Oxygen Mixtures and from the Respiratory Support Apparatus

Weaning is accomplished gradually. Patients who require continuous-controlled ventilation and intubation must be decannulated only after a sequential "de-escalation" of respiratory support has been achieved. Parallel decreases in the amount of enriched oxygen concentration and the peak respiratory pressure requirements are usually the first signs that support can be diminished. Sometimes tidal volume, vital capacity, or inspiratory or expiratory force are measured. The patient will demonstrate that he can trigger or initiate respiration on his own and will then need only continuous-assisted ventilation and later intermittent-assisted ventilation. Intervals off the ventilator, supported by a T-piece with enriched oxygen mixtures, are tolerated better, for longer periods, and with lower $P_{I_{O_2}}$

requirements to maintain adequate $P_{a_{O_2}}$. The adequacy of oxygenation ($P_{a_{O_2}}$) and ventilation ($P_{a_{CO_2}}$) must be established. When extubation is accomplished, the patient may be given supportive oxygen therapy by use of a mask with a rebreathing bag, then perhaps he will tolerate less support, such as nasal prongs. The patient must not be permitted to become hypoxemic or acidotic; however, somewhat less than ideal oxygenation may be accepted temporarily in order to establish self-sufficiency.

Commonly Used Medications in Respiratory Care

Bronchodilators. Aminophylline is used intravenously or by rectal suppository. The adrenergic drugs such as epinephrine and isoproterenol are the most potent.

Analeptics or central nervous system stimulants. These have not yet been established to be of proven benefit in stimulating respiration. There is a secondary central stimulation of respiration from aminophylline.

Sedatives. These are often used in respiratory care to permit the patient to "disengage himself" from the environment. Most CCUs or ICUs are not restful! Valium may be preferable to barbiturates, which sometimes depress cardiac function. Sedation is also used to suppress resistance to ventilatory control and to decrease the work of breathing.

Analgesics. Morphine and Demerol are used for similar purposes as are the sedatives. They are also used for pain relief if this is a problem. Aspirin is used to reduce temperature as well as to provide analgesia.

Diuretics. One of the complications of prolonged continuous-assisted or controlled ventilation is deterioration of pulmonary function, which may be related to excessive fluid retention. Usually there is weight gain and the chest x-ray film may have the appearance of pulmonary edema. Administration of diuretics can be dramatic in its effect of improving oxygenation. Mercurials, Diamox, ethacrynic acid, and Lasix are used. With these agents, electrolyte abnormalities, especially hypokalemia, must be anticipated and avoided.

Medications for secretions. Mucomyst is sometimes used in the vaporizers to decrease vapor particle size. Sodium iodide may be given intravenously to thin secretions. Purulent secretions may be thinned and mobilized by using a variety of enzyme preparations. Some medications, such as anticholinergics and antihistamines, thicken secretions and are hazardous in certain situations.

Bibliography

Bendixen, H. H., Egbert, L. D., Hedley-Whyte, J., Laver, H., and Pontoppidan, H.: Respiratory Care. St. Louis, C. V. Mosby Company, 1965.

Comroe, J. H., Jr., Forster, R. E., II, Dubois, A. B., Briscoe, W. A., and Carlsen, E.: The Lung, Clinical Physiology and Pulmonary Function Tests. 2nd ed. Chicago, Year Book Medical Publishers, Inc., 1962.

Comroe, J. H., Jr.: Physiology of Respiration. Chicago, Year Book Medical Publishers, Inc., 1965.

Kinney, J. M.: Oxygen Availability and Oxygen Consumption, Lecture Outline. American College of Surgeons, October 10–14, 1966.

Secor, J.: Patient Care in Respiratory Problems. Philadelphia, W. B. Saunders Company, 1969.

CHAPTER 7

Cardiac Drugs

By Richard G. Sanderson, M.D. *and*
Mervin J. Goldman, M.D.

Each physician has his own favorites in the therapeutic arma-
mentarium of cardiac drugs in use today. A full description of all the
different preparations is beyond the scope of this chapter, which
shall be limited to the drugs most frequently used in the care of
cardiac patients. The discussion will be confined to the cardiac and
pertinent extracardiac actions of the drugs, their indications and
contraindications, dosages and route of administration, and signs of
drug toxicity. Details of the investigational and more theoretical
aspects and the biochemistry of the drugs will be omitted. When
practical, comparative graphs of related drugs will be illustrated.

The discussion of cardiovascular drugs will be divided into the
following sections: cardiotonic agents, drugs which effect the autonomic nervous system, antiarrhythmic drugs, diuretics, anticoagulant
drugs, abnormalities of water and electrolyte metabolism, and antihypertensive drugs.

Cardiotonic Agents

Most patients with serious congenital or acquired heart disease
eventually reach a stage in which an effective cardiac output is no

longer maintained. This results in the clinical manifestations of heart failure. Cardiotonic agents increase the force of cardiac contractions (inotropic action), thereby increasing cardiac output.

CARDIAC GLYCOSIDES (DIGITALIS PREPARATIONS)

These glycosides are found in a large number of plants, classically foxglove, and are the most commonly used drugs in the treatment of heart failure and the atrial tachy-arrhythmias. The drugs have cardiac and extracardiac effects.

Cardiac Effects

A major effect is the increase in myocardial contractility (inotropic action) with resulting increase in cardiac output and reversal of heart failure. The increased cardiac output increases glomerular filtration in the kidney, resulting in diuresis and reduction in the expanded circulatory blood volume.

Digitalis slows conduction through the AV node, which results from a direct action of the drug on the AV node and the indirect vagal action of digitalis (dromotropic action). The effect is a slowing of the ventricular rate in atrial fibrillation and atrial flutter. A slower ventricular rate (e.g., change from 200 to 100) permits an increase in diastolic filling of the ventricles with a resulting increase in systolic ejection volume, thereby increasing cardiac output. Digitalis is also effective in terminating an atrial tachycardia with a 1:1 atrioventricular conduction largely by its vagal action.

A relatively weak action of digitalis is a slowing of the rate of discharge from the sinus node (chronotropic action). It is relatively ineffective in directly slowing the rate in sinus tachycardia, a finding which led earlier investigators to believe that digitalis was ineffective in the presence of sinus rhythm. This is obviously not true in view of the inotropic action of the drug.

There is some evidence to indicate that digitalis has a direct action on the kidney tubules, resulting in sodium and water excretion. If true, this is a minor action.

Extracardiac Effects

Digitalis produces constriction of veins, especially in the hepatic circulation. This reduces venous return to the heart. In the heart failure patient with an expanded blood volume, this effect reduces the inflow load on the dilated heart, resulting in more effective contraction and increased output. In the normal heart, however, with a normal blood volume, this decreased venous return reduces output. This latter effect is balanced by the inotropic action of the drug, so that the net effect is no appreciable change in cardiac output.

Digitalis produces temporary arteriolar constriction. This effect is of little clinical significance.

Toxicity, Side Effects, and Dangers

Digitalis effect can be observed in the clinical response of the patient and by electrocardiographic changes, such as slight prolongation of the PR interval, ST segment depression, decreased magnitude of the T wave, and decreased QT interval. These ECG changes due to digitalis are not signs of toxicity nor can they be used to evaluate effective dosage.

Digitalis toxicity is a frequent and serious complication of the use of this drug and, when unrecognized, can be fatal. The extracardiac toxic effects of digitalis preparations include anorexia, nausea and vomiting, diarrhea, yellow or green vision, and acute mental changes. These are more commonly seen with digitalis leaf and digitoxin than with digoxin. The cardiac toxicity is manifested by the following arrhythmias:

Ventricular arrhythmias (in order of increasing severity)
  Premature ventricular contractions, unifocal
  Ventricular bigeminy
  Multifocal premature ventricular contractions
  Ventricular tachycardia (may be bi-directional)
  Ventricular fibrillation
Atrial arrhythmias
  Paroxysmal atrial tachycardia (PAT), more commonly with
    AV block (e.g., 2:1), but may occur with 1:1 conduction
  Premature atrial contractions
  Atrial flutter or atrial fibrillation (rare)
Disturbances of AV conduction
  First, second, or third degree AV block
  AV junctional rhythms, including AV dissociation

A major predisposing factor to digitalis toxicity is hypokalemia, as commonly results from diuretic therapy. Most diuretics (see later) cause an appreciable loss of potassium through the kidneys, decreasing the serum potassium concentration. Since digitalis (especially digoxin) is largely excreted through the kidney, patients with severe renal disease become toxic unless small doses of the drug are used. Alkalosis, either metabolic or respiratory (e.g., hyperventilation from improper use of respirators), also lowers the serum potassium. Similar hypokalemic states result from gastrointestinal losses (vomiting, gastrointestinal suction, chronic diarrhea), salt-losing renal disease, and certain endocrine diseases (Cushing's syndrome and hyper-aldosteronism). A normal serum potassium level (3.5 to 5.5 mEq per liter) does not exclude the possibility of a deficiency in total body potassium. Since less than 2 per cent of the total body potassium is in the serum, there can be appreciable intracellular potassium loss which may not be reflected in the serum level.

Hypokalemia sensitizes the myocardium to the toxic effects of digitalis, since both similarly affect cell membrane potential. Other clinical states which render the patient more sensitive to digitalis include hypothyroidism, chronic lung disease, and advanced age (over 70 years). Caution must be observed in the digitalis-treated, uremic, and hyperkalemic patient who is undergoing renal dialysis. Correction of the hyperkalemia by this procedure permits digitalis toxicity to become manifest. On the other hand, patients with hyper-thyroidism, persistent hyperkalemia, or spontaneous atrial flutter commonly require and tolerate relatively high doses of digitalis.

There is no linear correlation between digitalis toxicity and therapeutic effect. If the digitalis toxicity can be corrected (potassium replacement in hypokalemic states) or treated effectively with drugs, further digitalis can then be given with resulting effectiveness and without recurrence of the toxic arrhythmia.

Indications

Digitalis is used in the presence of heart failure secondary to congenital, acquired valvular, arteriosclerotic, hypertensive, and most primary myocardial diseases. It is also indicated in the treatment of paroxysmal supraventricular tachycardias, atrial fibrillation and atrial flutter. It is not necessarily contraindicated in spontaneous ventricular tachycardia associated with heart failure.

Contraindications to the administration of digitalis are digitalis toxicity, the presence of hypertrophic subaortic stenosis (the inotropic action of digitalis increases the left ventricular outflow obstruction), and bradycardia or incomplete heart block (particularly in the early postoperative period after heart surgery). It is usually withheld one or two days before cardiac surgery to reduce the possibility of a digitalis-induced arrhythmia in the postoperative period owing to the multiplicity of metabolic changes secondary to anesthesia and surgery. It is withheld for two to three days before elective cardio-version because of the effects of countershock on cell membrane po-tential which sensitize the myocardium to the effects of digitalis.

Preparations, Administration, and Dosage

The choice of the digitalis preparation and method of administration will depend on the desired speed of action, on the duration of action, and largely on the physician's personal experience and preference.

Digoxin and digitoxin are purified preparations of digitalis leaf. In contrast to the leaf, the former preparations are accurately assayed and are reliably well absorbed from the gastrointestinal tract.

Digoxin is more rapidly effective than digitoxin or digitalis leaf. The duration of action of digoxin is shorter than the other drugs. Thus, there is usually a shorter duration of digitalis toxicity resulting from digoxin. On the other hand, there will be a greater loss of effectiveness if digoxin is not taken for two or three days, in contrast to digitoxin or digitalis leaf.

Intravenous administration offers the greatest speed of onset of action. In decreasing order of onset of action are ouabain, Cedilanid, digoxin, and digitoxin. Intramuscular preparations result in a slower onset of action than oral administration and are rarely indicated.

The preparation, onset of action, maximum effect, duration of effect, and average doses are listed in the following Table 7–1.

TABLE 7–1.   Comparison of Various Cardiac Glycosides

Preparation	Onset of Action	Maximum Effect	Duration of Effect	Average Digitalizing Dose	Average Daily Maintenance Dose
Digitalis folia* (oral)	2–6 hr	8–24 hr	14–21 days	1.0–2.0 gm over 3–4 days	.1 gm
Digitoxin (oral)	2–4 hr	6–8 hr	14–21 days	1.2–1.6 mgm over 24–48 hr	.1 mgm
(IV)	30 min– 2 hr	6–8 hr	14–21 days	1.2–1.6 mgm over 24–48 hr	.1 mgm
Cedilanid-D (Deslanoside) (IV)	3 min	20 min	3–5 days	1.2–2.0 mgm	—
Digoxin (oral)	1–3 hr	6 hr	3–6 days	1.5–3.0 mgm over 48 hr	.25 mgm
(IV)	5–10 min	1–3 hr	3–6 days	1.0–2.0 mgm over 24 hr	.25 mgm
(IM)	½–2 hr	1–3 hr	3–6 days	1.0–2.0 mgm over 24 hr	.25 mgm
Ouabain (G-Strophanthin) (IV)	5 min	30 min– 1 hr	12 hr– 2 days	0.1–0.5 mgm	—

*No intravenous digitalis preparation should be administered without full knowledge and appreciation of prior digitalis administration.

ISOPROTERENOL (ISUPREL)

This is a potent sympathetic amine which acts by stimulating beta-receptor sites (see later). Its actions on the heart and peripheral vascular system explain its clinical values, especially in the patient with a reduced cardiac output and an expanded blood volume.

Cardiac Actions

Isoproterenol is a potent inotropic drug similar to digitalis and can be used concurrently with digitalis. It increases the force of myocardial contraction, thereby increasing stroke volume and cardiac output.

Effects on automaticity. The drug increases the rate of discharge at pacemaker sites (chronotropic action). It therefore increases the sinus rhythm and is of value in the patient with sinus bradycardia which requires treatment, as in the setting of acute myocardial infarction with a low cardiac output. It also increases the rate of secondary pacemakers and thereby can increase the rate in AV junctional rhythm and idioventricular rhythm.

Effects on AV conduction. The drug may increase conductivity through the AV node and thereby revert a second or third degree AV block into a lesser degree block.

Peripheral Vascular Actions

The drug dilates the peripheral vascular tree, thereby lowering peripheral vascular resistance. This increases blood flow to vital organs, such as the kidney and the brain. The reduction in peripheral resistance reduces the venous return to the heart and, in the patient with an expanded blood volume, this effect will permit the compromised myocardium to more efficiently contract and eject blood. Although this effect on vascular resistance can lower blood pressure, it is often counterbalanced by a rise in cardiac output owing to the inotropic action of the drug and the reduced venous overload, resulting in an increase in blood pressure.

Dangers

By its action on increasing automaticity in pacemaker sites, potential pacemakers which are not in operation can be stimulated (as in the Purkinje system), resulting in ectopic discharge (e.g., ventricular ectopic beats), ventricular tachycardia, and ventricular fibrillation. Therefore, patients receiving this drug must be carefully monitored and the drug discontinued or the dose reduced when such arrhythmias appear. Similarly, excessive sinus tachycardia must be avoided, since in the patient with a diseased myocardium, aortic stenosis, or mitral stenosis, a critical rate will be reached above which cardiac output will fall.

As stated before, the fall in peripheral vascular resistance can produce hypotension unless this is counterbalanced by a reduction in venous return, as evidenced by a reduction of an elevated central venous pressure, and an increase in cardiac output. Therefore, the drug should not be used in a patient with a low central venous pressure (CVP). The central venous pressure and blood pressure must be monitored during administration of the drug.

As with digitalis, the inotropic action of the drug increases left ventricular outflow obstruction in patients with hypertrophic subaortic stenosis and is therefore contraindicated.

Indications

Isoproterenol is used in (1) the patient who is in failure and who is hypotensive (typically the acute myocardial infarction or cardiac surgery patient) and (2) the medical treatment of sinus bradycardia, of slow AV junctional rhythms, and of advanced degree of heart block. Admittedly, in many of the previous situations, electrical pacing will be more reliable and more effective with less hazard.

Administration and Dosage

Isoproterenol is most effective when given intravenously using a pediatric microdripper. Usually 2 to 5 mg (maximal dose may be 15) are diluted to 1000 ml 5 per cent dextrose in water (D/W), and the drip is adjusted to administer 1 to 5 μgm per minute. The concentration may be increased and the minute dose kept constant in order to reduce the fluid intake. As stated before, the patient must be constantly monitored by ECG, blood pressure, CVP, urine output, and clinical features (skin temperature, mental status, and so on).

Isoproterenol linguets (5 and 10 mg) are available and may be of some value in the treatment of chronic advanced AV block; however, because of the short duration of action of the drug and its unreliability it should not be used when electric pacing is indicated.

Drugs Which Affect the Autonomic Nervous System

Transmission along a nerve fiber occurs by the spread of the electrical activation wave; however, transmission between the nerve ending and the target organ which is innervated is by a chemical mediator which is liberated at the nerve ending. Norepinephrine is the chemical mediator liberated at sympathetic nerve endings. Acetylcholine is the mediator at all (sympathetic and parasympathetic) ganglionic synapses, at parasympathetic nerve endings, and at the nerve-voluntary muscle junctions. Epinephrine and a small amount of norepinephrine are secreted by the adrenal medulla.

PARASYMPATHETIC-LIKE DRUGS

Choline Esters

Methacholine (Mecholyl) and Bethanechol (Urecholine) are choline esters which mimic the action of the physiologic mediator, acetylcholine, but are of longer duration. The major indication for methacholine is in the treatment of paroxysmal atrial tachycardia (vagal action). The usual dose is 1 to 2 mg intravenously. It is not commonly used for this condition because of the availability of more effective and less troublesome drugs. Its other physiologic actions include contraction of nonvascular smooth muscle in the gastro-intestinal tract, urinary bladder, and bronchioles and thereby can be used in the treatment of a paralytic ileus and an atonic bladder. It also decreases pupil size and increases the flow of saliva, sweat, and respiratory tract secretions.

Cholinesterase Inhibitors

These drugs inhibit cholinesterase (the enzyme that hydrolyzes acetylcholine), allowing acetylcholine accumulation at its normal sites of action. These drugs are similar to the choline amines and the major cardiac indication is the treatment of paroxysmal atrial tachycardia. The commonly available drugs are neostigmine (Prostigmine) and edrophonium (Tensilon). These drugs are also of value in terminating the action of curare-alkaloids used in anesthesia.

PARASYMPATHOLYTIC DRUGS

These drugs block the action of acetylcholine at receptor sites but do not prevent the release of acetylcholine. The action is therefore competitive with acetylcholine. The major indication in the cardiac patient is to increase the heart rate in sinus bradycardia and to improve AV conduction in acute AV heart block. Atropine is the primary drug and is administered intravenously or orally in doses of 0.5 to 1.0 mg. It can cause postural hypotension, in addition to other undesirable physiologic effects—dry mouth, dilated pupils, impairment of bowel and bladder function, and mental changes.

SYMPATHOMIMETIC DRUGS

Catecholamines are chemicals (naturally secreted or drugs) which mimic the effects of sympathetic nerve stimulation and act directly on effector tissues (heart, glands, smooth muscle). The effect of these drugs fall into two categories, which are explained on two different receptor sites in the effector tissues. These are arbitrarily called alpha and beta sites.

Drugs Which Activate Alpha Receptor Sites

These actions result in vasoconstriction, contraction of smooth muscle organs, and pupillary dilatation. There is no direct cardiac action, but owing to the resulting vasoconstriction and rise in blood pressure there may be reflex slowing of the heart rate. In spite of the resulting rise in blood pressure, cardiac output may not rise or may actually fall in the presence of a diseased myocardium. The peripheral vasoconstriction can reduce blood flow to many organs (kidney, liver, brain, and other organs) and thereby impair the functions of these organs. Methoxamine (Vasoxyl) is a pure alpha-stimulating drug.

Drugs Which Activate Beta-receptor Sites

These actions result in vasodilatation, relaxation of nonvascular smooth muscles (e.g., in gastrointestinal tract, bronchi, and so on), and increase in the strength of myocardial contraction. Isoproterenol is a pure beta-adrenergic stimulating drug, and has been discussed earlier.

Drugs Which are Both Alpha- and Beta-adrenergic Stimulators

Aside from methoxamine and isoproterenol, most of the other commonly used drugs have both actions.

TABLE 7–2. *Adrenergic-stimulating Agents*

PREPARATION	ADREN-ERGIC EFFECT	EFFECT ON BLOOD PRESSURE	EFFECT ON HEART RATE	INO-TROPIC EFFECT	DOSAGE FOR INTRAVENOUS DRIP SOLUTIONS
Norepinephrine (Levophed, Levarterenol)	Alpha and beta	++++	0 –	+	1–4 amps/1000 ml (4–16 mgm)
Epinephrine (Adrenalin)	Alpha and beta	++	++	++	7 cc 1:1000 solution/1000 ml (multiply as necessary for fluid restriction)
Isoproterenol (Isuprel)	Pure beta	0 +	+++	++++	3–16 mgm/1000 ml
Metaraminol (Aramine)	Alpha and beta	+++	0 +	+	100 mgm/1000 ml

Norepinephrine (Levophed, Levarteranol). This drug is mainly an alpha stimulator, thereby producing vasoconstriction. It has weak beta action which does result in a minor degree of inotropic effect on the myocardium.

Metaraminol (Aramine). The action of this drug is identical to norepinephrine. It causes release of normal stores of norepinephrine. Therefore, when the latter stores are exhausted, the drug will become ineffective.

Epinephrine. This drug has equal alpha and beta actions. It constricts blood vessels in the skin (producing blanching) and splanchnic areas, but dilates arterioles elsewhere. The net effect is vasodilatation and lowering of peripheral vascular resistance. By its beta action on the myocardium, inotropic and chronotropic effects are obtained.

Mephenteramine (Wyamine) and phenylephrine (Neosynephrine). These drugs are intermediary in their action between norepinephrine and epinephrine.

Indications

The most common clinical indication for these sympathomimetic drugs is the shock state. In the cardiac patient, these agents are used to support the failing myocardium (beta action resulting in inotropic effect), to increase heart rate in sinus bradycardia or AV block (beta action), and to elevate blood pressure (direct alpha action or indirect beta action by improving cardiac output). The drugs with major alpha action can be used in the treatment of paroxysmal atrial tachycardia in patients without serious cardiovascular disease. The mechanism by which this is effective is the production of hypertension which, in turn, reflexly produces strong vagal stimulation, thereby slowing the heart rate.

Dangers

These include (1) Cardiac arrhythmias resulting from increased automaticity (beta stimulation); (2) ischemic injury to vital organs (heart, liver, kidneys, and so on), resulting from vasoconstriction (alpha action); (3) extravasation into subcutaneous tissues, causing tissue slough (phentolamine [Regitine] should be infiltrated into the tissues to counteract their effect); and (4) prolonged infusions resulting in a resistant state which requires ever increasing amounts of the agent to maintain blood pressure (tachyphylaxis). This is especially true of norepinephrine.

SYMPATHOPLEGIC DRUGS

These drugs block the action of the sympathomimetic catecholamines or reduce sympathetic outflow.

Alpha-adrenergic Blocking Agents

These block the action of circulating catecholamines, especially at the end-organ effector site.

Phentolamine (Regitine) is a short-acting antagonist to catecholamines. It is of major value in the diagnosis and treatment of pheochromocytoma (an adrenal medullary tumor which secretes norepinephrine or epinephrine, or both). As a diagnostic test, 10 mg is administered intravenously and blood pressures are determined every 30 seconds for the next five minutes. A fall in blood pressure in excess of 35/25 mm Hg is consistent with a diagnosis of pheochromocytoma. Phentolamine is also used to prevent local necrosis following the accidental infiltration into subcutaneous tissues of levarteranol, isoproterenol, and potassium chloride. The drug is infiltrated locally.

Phenoxybenzamine (Dibenzylene) is a long-acting alpha-adrenergic blocking agent. It produces vasodilatation and thereby increases blood flow to vital organs. Its use in the shock state is still investigational. The intravenous dose is 1 mg per kg body weight. The drug is also used in peripheral vascular disease (orally 10 mg three times a day), but its value is questionable.

Beta-adrenergic Blocking Drugs

Propranolol (Inderal) is the only commercially available drug in this category. By blocking adrenergic action at beta receptor sites, this drug (1) depresses pacemaker activity, thus slowing the rate of discharge in the sinus node and suppressing ectopic pacemaker discharge; (2) depresses AV conduction, thereby slowing the ventricular rate in atrial flutter or fibrillation; (3) depresses myocardial contractility (anisotropic), thereby reducing cardiac output; and (4) produces bronchoconstriction.

Clinical indications

(a) To slow undesirable sinus tachycardia.

(b) To slow the ventricular rate in atrial flutter or atrial fibrillation. The drug is commonly used in conjunction with digitalis for this purpose.

(c) To suppress ventricular arrhythmias, especially those due to digitalis toxicity (see later).

(d) To revert 1:1 atrial tachycardia to sinus rhythm when other drugs are ineffective.

(e) To treat idiopathic hypertrophic subaortic stenosis when a significant left ventricular outflow obstruction is documented. This is accomplished by the depression of cardiac contractility, which reduces the muscular outflow obstruction.

(f) To treat hypertensive states which are associated with high cardiac outputs. The reduction of cardiac output can thereby reduce blood pressure even though peripheral vascular resistance is unchanged. The recognition of such patients is difficult and this modality of therapy is investigational.

(g) To treat dissecting aneurysm of the aorta (by reducing the strength of ventricular contraction, which in turn lessens the pressure wave in the dissecting channel).

(h) To treat angina pectoris: although some current reports are optimistic, this is an experimental and investigational approach at the present time.

Contraindications

(a) Bronchospasm (as in bronchial asthma, bronchitis, and so forth), since the drug produces bronchoconstriction.

(b) Congestive heart failure. By depressing cardiac contractility, the drug can produce or worsen heart failure. This effect is readily appreciated at surgery when deterioration of myocardial contractility is readily visible following administration of the drug.

(c) Presence of advanced degrees of heart block. By increasing AV block, a more serious degree of heart block will result.

Doses

INTRAVENOUS. One tenth mg per kg body weight is administered slowly with continuous electrocardiographic and blood pressure monitoring. Usually 1 mg is given intravenously every two to three minutes until either a desirable or toxic effect is achieved. The total dose should not exceed 7 to 10 mg. If indicated, the dose may be repeated in two to four hours.

ORAL. Ten to 40 mg three to four times daily under close clinical observation.

Ganglion Blocking Drugs

These block the transmission of impulses across sympathetic and parasympathetic ganglia. Their primary indication is in the treatment of hypertension (see later).

Postganglionic Blocking Drugs

These drugs prevent the liberation of norepinephrine at sympathetic nerve endings. They act distal to the ganglion and hence have no effect on parasympathetic action. They are used in the treatment of hypertension (see later).

Antiarrhythmic Agents

The commonly used antiarrhythmic drugs are quinidine, procainamide (Pronestyl), lidocaine (Xylocaine), diphenylhydantoin (Dilantin), and propranolol (Inderal).

QUINIDINE

This drug has many cardiac and extracardiac actions. Its cardiac actions include (1) suppression of pacemaker activity by alteration of cell membrane potential. It suppresses secondary pacemakers in the ventricles and atria, thereby abolishing ectopic rhythms. It can also suppress primary pacemaker function in the sinoatrial node, or important secondary atrioventricular junctional pacemakers. (2) It decreases conductivity in Purkinje's fibers, thereby eliminating ectopic rhythms which are related to disturbances in conductivity (re-entry), (3) increases conductivity in the AV node in therapeutic dose ranges and suppresses conductivity in the AV node in toxic doses, and (4) depresses myocardial contractility. The extracardiac effects include (1) peripheral vasodilatation with a resultant fall in blood pressure; (2) anorexia, nausea, vomiting, or diarrhea; (3) mental disturbances, such as lethargy and clouding of the sensorium; (4) toxic effects on the bone marrow with thrombocytopenia (uncommon), anemia, and agranulocytosis (rare); (5) toxic skin eruptions; (6) fever; and (7) rare idiosyncratic reactions with shock, coma, and convulsions.

Administration, Dosage, and Side Effects

Quinidine is usually given orally in doses of 200 to 400 mg every two to six hours. The drug is well absorbed from the gastrointestinal tract. Onset of action occurs in 15 minutes; maximum effect is attained in two to four hours. Only 25 per cent remains in the blood after 12 hours. Similar doses may be given intramuscularly. Intravenous administration is rarely indicated.

The cardiotoxic effects of quinidine are monitored electrocardiographically and are evidenced by prolongation of the QT interval (upper limit of normal is 0.44 sec), widening of QRS complex to 50 per cent or more above baseline measurement, prolongation of the PR interval, and appearance of ventricular arrhythmias. The latter seems paradoxical, since a major indication is the treatment of ventricular arrhythmias. This is explainable by its effects on conductivity in the Purkinje system and automaticity (pacemaker suppression), both of which can suppress ectopic discharge in therapeutic dose ranges and produce ectopic discharge in toxic dose ranges. A guide to dosage can be obtained from quinidine blood levels. A value of 4 to 7 mg per liter is within the usual therapeutic range with lesser chances of toxicity (but toxicity still can be manifest at these levels); values of 8 mg per liter and higher greatly increase the risk of toxicity. The other side effects and toxicity have been discussed earlier.

Indications

Quinidine is used most commonly to revert atrial fibrillation or flutter to sinus rhythm (or maintain sinus rhythm after cardioversion). In these circumstances, digitalis must be given initially to control the ventricular rate. Quinidine is also used to control ventricular ectopic discharge (ventricular premature beats or ventricular tachycardia) and paroxysmal atrial tachycardia.

PROCAINAMIDE (PRONESTYL)

The cardiac effects and toxicity are similar to those of quinidine. It is useful in the control of ventricular arrhythmias (premature ventricular contractions and ventricular tachycardia) but is relatively ineffective in the treatment of the atrial arrhythmias (this is in contrast to quinidine, which is effective in the atrial arrhythmias). Like quinidine, it impairs myocardial contraction (thereby lowering cardiac output) and lowers systemic blood pressure. Procainamide is rapidly absorbed from the gastrointestinal tract. Peak levels are reached in one to two hours and decline to minimal levels in four to six hours. The oral dose ranges from 250 to 1000 mg three to four times daily. Intramuscular administration produces maximal blood levels in one half to 1 hour. The intramuscular dose is 100 to 200 mg every four to six hours. Intravenous administration requires constant electrocardiographic and blood pressure monitoring. The dose should not exceed 50 mg per min and the maximal dose at any one time usually should not exceed 1000 mg.

LIDOCAINE (XYLOCAINE)

The cardiac effects are similar to quinidine in the treatment of the ventricular arrhythmias. It is much less effective than quinidine in the treatment of atrial arrhythmias. It is preferable to quinidine and procaineamide in the acute management of ventricular arrhythmias (i.e., in acute myocardial infarction and the cardiac surgical patient), because it has lesser adverse effects, e.g., less depression of cardiac contractility and less hypotension. The antiarrhythmic effect is apparent within seconds of intravenous administration and persists for 10 to 20 minutes. It is commonly given in 50 mg intravenous doses (2.5 ml of 2 per cent lidocaine) and repeated as necessary. For persisting ectopic ventricular activity, an intravenous drip of 1 to 4 mg per min (200 to 800 mg in 500 ml 5 per cent D/W) is utilized. With doses of 5 mg or more per minute the drug can produce depression of respiration, convulsive seizures, and suppression of normal conduction pathways, with resultant ventricular arrhythmias.

DIPHENYLHYDANTOIN (DILANTIN)

This drug is effective in the control of ventricular arrhythmias, especially those produced by digitalis. Like all the antiarrhythmic drugs, it does have a depressant action on myocardial contractility. It does not depress AV conduction and hence is the drug of choice in the treatment of ventricular ectopic discharge due to digitalis toxicity when associated with AV block. The dose is 100 to 250 mgm given intravenously over five to 10 minutes. The dose may be repeated every one to two hours, but the total daily dose should not exceed 800 to 1000 mg per 24 hours.

PROPRANOLOL (INDERAL) (SEE EARLIER)

This drug has a dual action in the therapy of the arrhythmias. By it beta-adrenergic blocking action it suppresses automaticity, thereby slowing the heart rate in sinus tachycardia and abolishing ectopic discharge, especially of ventricular origin. It depresses AV conduction with resultant slowing of the ventricular rate in atrial fibrillation and atrial flutter. In addition it has a quinidine-like action which further increases its efficacy as an antiarrhythmic agent.

Diuretics

Congestive heart failure and often other edematous states (cirrhosis of the liver, nephrosis, and so on) are characterized by sodium retention, with resulting retention of water and expansion of the blood volume and extracellular fluid volume. The diuretic agents act to promote sodium and water excretion and thereby reduce this circulatory overload.

MERCURIAL DIURETICS

These drugs act primarily on the proximal convoluted tubule of the kidney and reduce the normal (85 per cent) reabsorption of sodium at that site. As a result, less water is passively absorbed. A greater load of sodium (and water) will be presented to the distal renal tubule which will exchange hydrogen and potassium ions (with chloride ion) for the sodium reabsorbed in the distal tubule. The net result will be an increased urinary loss of sodium, water, chloride, and some potassium. Prolonged use of these drugs with resultant potassium and chloride loss can produce a hypochloremic and hypokalemic alkalosis. For maximal effectiveness of the mercurial diuretics, the serum chloride concentration must be adequate; therefore, when indicated, supplementation with potassium chloride is helpful.

The two common mercurial drugs are meralluride sodium with theophylline (Mercuhydrin) and mercaptomerin sodium (Thiomerin). One to 2 ml are given intramuscularly or intravenously. The intramuscular injections are at times painful. The injection must never be given into edematous sites (such as the buttock which may be edematous in patients with congestive heart failure), since absorption and hence therapeutic effect will be poor. Diuresis begins in one to two hours, is maximal by eight hours, and continues for 24 hours. For the patient's comfort it is best given in the early morning hours, so major diuresis will occur during the usual waking hours of the patient. The dangers of mercurial diuretics include electrolyte and acid-base disturbances due to excess potassium and chloride loss and additional water (with electrolyte) loss, resulting in hypotension and possible thrombotic episodes. Potassium loss is a common reason for the appearance of digitalis toxicity in patients taking digitalis.

THIAZIDE DIURETICS

These drugs, in addition to a major action on the proximal renal tubule (like the mercurial diuretics), also act on the distal renal tubule to reduce ion exchange, with resultant sodium (and water) loss in the urine. The major advantage of these drugs is their effectiveness when given orally. They are also effective in the treatment of hypertension, which is a common cause of heart failure. These favorable effects of the drug are counterbalanced by many undesirable actions which include (1) electrolyte, acid-base, and volume disturbances and digitalis toxicity, similar to the mercurial diuretics, (2) diminished excretion of uric acid with resultant increase in serum uric acid levels and clinical manifestations of acute gouty arthritis, (3) impairment of carbohydrate tolerance with resultant hyperglycemia in the unsuspected diabetic or known diabetic patient, and (4) occasional skin eruptions and hematologic disturbances (agranulocytosis, thrombocytopenia, and anemia) which occur as sensitivity reactions. Most

TABLE 7–3.   *Comparison of the More Common Oral Diuretic Agents*

PREPARATION	DAILY DOSAGE (ORAL)	DURATION OF ACTION
1. Chlorothiazide (Diuril)	500 mgm–1 gm	6–12 hours
2. Hydrochlorothiazide (Hydrodiuril, Esidrix)	25–200 mgm	12–18 hours
3. Trichlormethiazide (Naqua)	2–4 mgm	+ 24 hours
4. Chlorthalidone (Hygroton)	50–200 mgm usually every other day	48–72 hours
5. Triamterene (Dyrenium)	100–200 mgm 1–3 days to reach maximal effect	24–48 hours
6. Spironolactone (Aldactone A)	50–150 mgm 3–5 days to reach maximal effect	2–3 days
7. Ethacrynic Acid (Edecrin)	50–150 mgm (25–50 mg IV)	3–12 hours (15 min–1 hr IV)
8. Furosemide (Lasix)	40–80 mgm	2–24 hours

patients receiving the drug require 50 to 100 mEq of potassium supplementation daily. Orange juice and apricots contain potassium, but generally, potassium chloride elixir is still necessary. Commercial preparations of a thiazide with potassium chloride in enteric-coated tablets have been available. These have been incriminated in the production of upper gastrointestinal ulceration owing to the local caustic action of potassium chloride on the intestinal mucosa. The various types of thiazide diuretics commonly used are listed in Table 7–3.

OTHER DIURETIC AGENTS

Triamterene (Dyrenium)

This drug is similar in action and side effects to the thiazides with one major difference. It reduces potassium excretion and may result in potassium retention. Therefore, routine potassium supplementation is contraindicated. Its action is potentiated by combination with a thiazide diuretic.

Spironolactone (Aldactone A)

This drug competitively antagonizes the effect of aldosterone, the normally produced adrenal mineralocorticoid hormone. Aldosterone acts on the distal renal tubule to promote sodium absorption and potassium excretion. By blocking this action, spironolactone produces sodium (and water) excretion with potassium retention. Therefore, potassium supplementation is contraindicated in the presence of a normal serum potassium. Serial blood potassium measurements are necessary to avoid hyperkalemia, even when supplementary potassium therapy is not given. Used alone, spironolactone is not a potent agent, but is most effective when combined with a mercurial or thiazide diuretic. For maximal effect the drug must be continued for at least three days.

Ethacrynic Acid (Edecrin) and Furosemide (Lasix)

These drugs are extremely potent diuretics with relatively rapid onset of action, thereby being effective agents in the treatment of pulmonary edema. They cause greater sodium and potassium loss than produced by maximum doses of thiazide diuretics. Because of their potency, frequent determinations of serum electrolytes are necessary and potassium and chloride supplementations are usually mandatory. Elevation of serum uric acid and glucose may also result.

Agents Which Alter Coagulation

Open heart surgery is performed in a completely anticoagulated system; otherwise, the extra corporeal circuit would clot and cease to function. The use of anticoagulants in the postoperative course of patients who have undergone valve replacement is commonplace in order to lessen the incidence of clot formation on the prosthetic valves. Anticoagulants are also used in the treatment of thrombophlebitis, pulmonary embolism, and other thromboembolic states. Its use remains controversial in the treatment of coronary artery disease.

Heparin sodium

This drug is used for anticoagulation during open heart surgery and in the treatment of various thromboembolic conditions. Its effect, as measured by a more than twofold prolongation of the coagulation time, occurs in less than one minute and persists for two to four hours when administered intravenously. When given subcutaneously, the onset of effect occurs in one hour and lasts for eight to 12 hours, dependent upon the dose given. Subcutaneous administration may result in pain and hematoma formation.

Actions

The mechanisms by which heparin is known to prolong the clotting time are (a) neutralization of formed thrombin; thrombin is necessary to convert fibrinogen to fibrin (with resulting clot); hence, suppression of thrombin inhibits the clot formation; (b) inhibition of the actions of plasma thromboplastin antecedent (PTA or factor XI) and plasma thromboplastin component (PTC or factor IX), thereby preventing the conversion of prothrombin to thrombin (this latter effect explains the prolonged prothrombin time obtained during heparin therapy); and (c) prevention of the thrombin-induced aggregation of platelets, which is often the initiating event in thrombus formation.

Preparations

Heparin is commonly measured in U.S.P. units; 100 units of heparin is equal to 0.83 mg, or 120 units equals 1 mg. Heparin is commercially available in vials containing 1000, 5000, 10,000, 20,000, and 40,000 units per ml. Great care must be used in giving the correct concentration. Confining hospital supplies to only two concentrations (1000 units per ml for intravenous use and 40,000 units per ml for subcutaneous administration) will eliminate much of the confusion in administration.

Dosage

In the open heart operating room, anticoagulation of the entire circuit (patient plus extracorporeal system) is accomplished by a dose of 300 to 400 units per kg body weight, supplemented by 100 units per kg every hour while the patient is on cardiopulmonary by-pass. On the ward, heparin may be given intravenously, subcutaneously, or in combination. One method is the administration of 5000 to 10,000 units intravenously every four to six hours, or by continuous intravenous infusion. The initial dose may be given intravenously in order to obtain immediate effect, followed by a subcutaneous injection of 7500 to 15,000 units within two hours, and then every six hours. No matter what schedule is used, the effectiveness should be checked by clotting times (Lee-White), aiming for levels of two to three times the control. Meticulous care must be used when administering subcutaneous heparin in order to get the desired prolongation of the anticoagulation effect. If not carefully done, absorption will be more rapid and duration of action will be reduced (approximating intravenous use), thereby defeating the purpose of such use. Subcutaneous injection is made deep into fatty sites (iliac fat pad, abdominal wall). A 25 gauge needle on a tuberculin syringe containing the least volume (most concentrated preparation) is used. The skin is not rubbed vigorously before or after injection and aspiration is not done before the injection.

PROTAMINE SULFATE

Protamine neutralizes heparin by a colloidal effect. The positively charged protamine neutralizes the negatively charged heparin, thus inactivating it. It is administered to the patient at the completion of cardiopulmonary by-pass to reverse the anticoagulation effect of heparin.

A 1 per cent solution is given intravenously, 1 mg per mg of heparin. Its effect lasts about four hours. It should be administered slowly (over five to 10 minutes) in order to prevent hypotension. Excessive doses of protamine paradoxically act as an anticoagulant.

WARFARIN SODIUM (COUMADIN)

Warfarin is one of the common group of coumarin derivates (another being bishydroxy-Coumadin [Dicumarol]) which act by inhibition of prothrombin synthesis. The drug interferes with the utilization of vitamin K, produced by the gastrointestinal tract bacteria, which is essential for the formation of prothrombin. Although the term prothrombin inhibition is commonly used, the drug not only inhibits the formation of prothrombin (factor II) but also proconvertin (factor VII), plasma thromboplastin component (PTC or factor IX), and the Stuart-Prower factor (X). Since this action involves the synthesis of the clotting factors (in the liver), warfarin, in contrast to heparin, will have no *in vitro* action.

The onset of action of warfarin is about 12 hours, therapeutic levels can be reached in 24 hours, dependent upon the dose used, and the peak effect occurs in 36 hours; the duration of action is usually two to five days.

A common dosage schedule (not in cardiac surgery patients) is the administration of 30 to 50 mg (orally) over a 24 to 48 hour period, if the basal prothrombin time is normal. If the prothrombin time is reduced before administration of warfarin, this dose must be reduced. If the prothrombin time is already at a level of 30 per cent or less, the drug cannot be used. Daily maintenance doses of 2.5 to 10 mg follow the initial primary doses, the exact amount dependent upon the daily prothrombin time, aiming for a value of 15 to 25 per cent activity, or a prothrombin time of twice the control value (in seconds).

Coumadin therapy is generally started on patients who have undergone valvular replacement one to two days after removal of the chest drainage tubes. Effective doses are generally 20 mg on the first day, 10 mg on the second day, and 2.5 mg. to 7.5 mg per day thereafter, dependent upon the prothrombin time. Abnormalities of hepatic function, which itself lowers the prothrombin time, will dictate the use of lower doses. As cardiac performance improves with resultant improvement in hepatic function (by lessening of hepatic congestion), the daily dose may have to be raised to five to 10 mg per day.

Many drugs interfere with the action of warfarin with a resultant alteration of the prothrombin time. The commonly used drugs which elevate the prothrombin time and therefore result in a higher dose requirement of warfarin include the barbiturates, chloral hydrate, diphenylhydantoin, and the oral contraceptives. Drugs which further suppress the prothrombin time, thereby requiring smaller doses of warfarin and at times precipitating bleeding, include aspirin, phenylbutazone, and clofibrate. Therefore, the physician and the nurse must be aware of these drug interactions in order to maintain therapeutically effective, and not dangerous, utilization of warfarin.

PHYTONANDIONE – VITAMIN K_1 (AQUAMEPHYTON)

This agent reverses the prothrombin deficiency induced by warfarin. The effects of vitamin K_1 appear in 15 minutes and a therapeutic level is reached in three to six hours following intramuscular or intravenous administration. In emergent bleeding situations secondary to warfarin therapy, fresh blood is indicated immediately to provide a source of prothrombin. In patients with prosthetic heart valves, vitamin K_1 should not be used unless a real emergency exists. The occurrence of thrombi on the valve with resultant peripheral embolization is closely correlated with rapid changes in prothrombin activity.

Water and Electrolyte Metabolism

SODIUM AND WATER

Cardiac patients in congestive right heart failure have excess total body sodium and water. The total body water in the edematous cardiac patient is reflected in an expanded blood volume (mainly plasma) in excess of the normal 72 ± 3 ml per kg body weight. Patients with only left heart failure often have a normal blood volume. The serum concentration of sodium is not a true reflection of total body sodium. The factors which determine serum sodium concentration are total body sodium, total body potassium, and total body water. This can be expressed as:

Na_s (serum sodium concentration) $=$

$$\frac{Na_e \text{ (total body Na)} + K_e \text{ (total body K)}^*}{TBW \text{ (total body water)}}$$

With rare exceptions every edematous cardiac patient has an elevated total body sodium content. However, the serum sodium concentration is commonly low (130 mEq/L or less). This is due to

---

*e equals exchangeable Na and K as measured by isotope techniques.

an increase of total body water in excess of sodium or a reduced total body potassium, or both. Severe hyponatremia (below 120 mEq/L) occurs in the cardiac patient usually as a result of excessive diuretic therapy. The treatment of this is obviously not sodium replacement, but rigid water restriction (750 ml per day or less) and supplemental potassium as indicated. The normal physiologic responses to surgery cause additional sodium and water retention, the latter the result of antidiuretic hormone secretion. Thus, careful attention must be paid to the amount of fluid and sodium given in the immediate postoperative period to avoid further expansion of the blood volume with aggravation of heart failure.

POTASSIUM

Approximately 98 per cent of the total body potassium is intracellular. Therefore, the serum potassium concentration is not an accurate measurement of total body potassium. The serum potassium concentration is normally maintained between 3.5 to 5.5 mEq/L and any deviation from these values can produce serious metabolic abnormalities, especially on the heart.

Hypokalemia

This is defined by a serum potassium concentration below 3.5 mEq/L. In the cardiac patient it is often the result of diuretic therapy (urinary loss). Other contributing factors are gastrointestinal losses (vomiting, gastric suction, diarrhea), poor dietary intake of potassium, and excess urinary losses due to associated renal disease (salt-losing nephritis) and excess mineralocorticoid activity (hyperaldosteronism, Cushing's disease, and corticoid therapy). The use of osmotic diuretics (e.g., mannitol) during cardiac surgery increases potassium losses in the urine. Respiratory alkalosis due to mechanical hyperventilation in the patient with respiratory support further accentuates the hypokalemia. Therefore, the serum potassium concentration and the daily losses (urine, gastric suction, and stool, if excessive) must be measured and adequate supplementary therapy given. In the presence of renal insufficiency and a serum potassium concentration exceeding normal values, no potassium should be administered.

Hypokalemia produces important cardiac abnormalities. It increases automaticity which results in ectopic discharge (atrial, AV nodal and ventricular arrhythmias). This effect is accentuated in the patient who is receiving digitalis. It slows conduction from the sinus node to the ventricles, which is reflected in a prolongation of the

PR interval. Ventricular repolarization is altered and prolonged and is evidenced in the electrocardiogram by ST depression, lowered or inverted T waves, and very prominent U waves (see Fig. 4–46 and Fig. 4–48*D*).

Hyperkalemia

This is defined as a serum potassium concentration in excess of 5.5 mEq/L. Although the serum level is elevated, the total body potassium is often reduced, indicating a shift of intracellular potassium to the extracellular spaces. It most commonly results from retention of potassium in patients with renal disease. Other types of metabolic acidosis (diabetic) and severe tissue necrosis contribute to hyperkalemia. Injudicious use of potassium-retaining diuretics (e.g., Aldactone) is unfortunately not an uncommon cause. The major and potentially life-threatening toxicity of hyperkalemia is the effect on the heart. Ventricular repolarization is altered, producing very tall and slender T waves in the electrocardiogram (usually at levels over 6 mEq/L). Conduction through the Purkinje fibers and myocardium is markedly slowed, which is manifested by a widening of the QRS complexes (over 0.12 sec) and a loss of the P waves (usually at potassium levels over 7.5 mEq/L) (see Fig. 4–47 and Fig. 4–48*B* and *C*). With further elevation of the serum potassium, ventricular tachycardia and fibrillation ensue. Emergency treatment includes the use of intravenous calcium (1 gm calcium gluconate) or hypertonic glucose (50 to 100 ml of 50 per cent glucose) with regular insulin (10 to 20 units) intravenously. This drives the potassium into the cells and promptly lowers the serum potassium concentration. To hasten excretion of potassium, sodium polysterone sulfonate (Kayexalate) is effective by exchanging sodium for potassium (3 mEq sodium exchanges with 1 mEq potassium). It is given orally in a dose of 10 to 15 gm every three to six hours with a cathartic. It can also be given rectally, 20 to 40 gm in 200 ml of 25 per cent sorbitol every six hours. In patients with severe renal insufficiency, peritoneal or hemodialysis may be necessary to control the hyperkalemia and the uremic state.

CALCIUM

Abnormalities in serum calcium concentration are rarely seen in the cardiac patient unless there is an independent disease which produces such abnormalities. Patients who have large replacements of bank blood containing citrate can have a marked drop of the serum calcium concentration because of the binding of calcium with citrate. Supplementary calcium is indicated (intravenously) to keep the serum calcium within the normal range (9 to 11 mg per cent or 4.5 to 5 mEq/L). Intravenous calcium is indicated in the emergency treatment of hyperkalemia (see before). Calcium is the important ion which acts on the actin and myosin filaments in the heart muscle to produce cardiac contractility. Although there is no positive evidence to prove its efficacy, calcium may be used in the operating room in an attempt to improve cardiac contractility when all other measures fail. It must be used cautiously, since an increase in serum calcium concentration (above 12 mg per cent) can produce ventricular ectopic rhythms, especially in the patients who have received digitalis. The commonly used preparations are 10 per cent calcium gluconate or 10 per cent calcium chloride, administered intravenously in doses of 10 ml.

Antihypertensive Drug Therapy

GENERAL PRINCIPLES

In the treatment of nonemergent hypertensive states, the aim is a gradual reduction of the blood pressure to normal or near-normal levels without the production of side effects. Acute hypotension from therapy can result in a serious reduction in blood flow to the brain, heart, and kidneys and thereby result in cerebral thrombosis, coronary insufficiency (angina or infarction), and deterioration in renal function.

The ganglionic and postganglionic blocking drugs (see section on drugs which affect the autonomic nervous system for mode of action) produce postural hypotension. This is also true for hydralazine and methyldopa, but to a lesser degree. Therefore, patients receiving these drugs must have their blood pressure recorded in the standing position and these values used as a guide in dosage. In addition, the patient must be informed about the symptoms of postural hypotension, i.e., dizziness and syncope. The patient should be instructed to stand erect and motionless for one to two minutes before taking the next dose of the drug and, if the above symptoms occur, that dose should be omitted.

DRUGS

The following drugs are listed in order of increasing potency.

Reserpine

The usual oral dose is 0.25 mg per day. The maximum effect will not be evident for 10 to 14 days. Nasal stuffiness and drowsiness are common side effects of this dose range. Higher doses are not recommended for long-term therapy because of resultant mental depression (to suicide), peptic ulceration, and sodium retention. Reserpine is of value in the mildly hypertensive patient, but is of greater value when given in combination with other antihypertensive drugs.

Thiazides

These (see earlier for dosage and side effects) are commonly effective in the management of mild-to-moderate hypertension, especially when used in combination with reserpine. When used in combination with more potent antihypertensive drugs, the thiazides will potentiate the action of the second drug and often permit a reduction of its dose.

Hydralazine (Apresoline)

The initial oral dose is 10 mg two to four times daily, progressively increasing every three to five days as indicated to a maximum dose of 200 mg per day. Headache and tachycardia can result because of an increase in cardiac output. Renal blood flow is not decreased and therefore hydralazine is of value in treatment of the hypertensive patient with renal insufficiency. Hydralazine can produce a clinical syndrome resembling disseminated lupus erythematosis, which is usually reversible following discontinuation of the drug.

Methyldopa (Aldomet)

The initial oral dose is 250 mg two to three times daily, increasing at intervals of two to three days to a maximum of 2 gm per day. Methyldopa, like hydralazine, does not reduce renal blood flow. Fever and hemolytic anemia (Coombs' positive) are rare complications.

Ganglion Blocking Drugs

Pentolinium tartrate (Ansolysen), chlorisondamine chloride (Ecolid), and mecamylamine (Inversine) are drugs which produce sympathetic and parasympathetic blockade (see before). Mecamylamine is preferable because of more reliable intestinal absorption. The initial dose is 1 to 2.5 mg two to three times daily and may be increased to 10 mg three times a day. In addition to its hypotensive action, which is mainly postural, it produces constipation, urinary retention, blurred vision, dry mouth, and failure of ejaculation.

Postganglionic Blocking Drug

Guanethidine (Ismelin) is the commonly used drug in this category (see before). Since it does not produce parasympathetic blockade, constipation, urinary retention, blurred vision, and dry mouth do not occur. Diarrhea and loss of ejaculation are troublesome side effects. Since the drug has a long duration of action, a single daily dose is effective. The initial oral dose is 10 mg, increasing as needed at weekly intervals to a maximum of 100 mg per day.

COMMON ANTIHYPERTENSIVE DRUG COMBINATIONS

Since combinations of antihypertensive drugs are frequently more effective and often permit smaller doses of either drug, the following combinations are recommended. Empirical dosages cannot be given. One should begin with minimal doses and adjust these in accordance with the clinical response of the patient.

Mild-Moderate Hypertension

Reserpine + Thiazide
Reserpine + Thiazide + Methyldopa (or Hydralazine)
Thiazide + Methyldopa (or Hydralazine)

Severe-Malignant Hypertension

Thiazide + Guanethidine
Methyldopa (or Hydralazine) + Guanethidine

Acute Hypertensive Emergencies

Acute hypertensive encephalopathy, acute pulmonary edema in association with marked hypertension, dissecting aortic aneurysm in association with hypertension, and the severe hypertension which may follow surgical repair of coarctation of the aorta are medical emergencies which require immediate parenteral therapy.

Effective drugs

RESERPINE. One to 2.5 mg IM every four to eight hours. The antihypertensive effect will not appear for at least one hour and therefore this is not the drug of choice in acute life-threatening situations.

HYDRALAZINE. Five to 20 mg IM every two to four hours.

METHYLDOPA. Five hundred to 750 mg in 500 ml 5 per cent D/W given as an intravenous drip.

TRIMETHAPHAN (ARFONAD). This is a ganglion blocking drug. The dose is 5 mg in 500 ml 5 per cent D/W given as an intravenous drip. It is effective within minutes. Constant blood pressure monitoring (preferably by indwelling arterial catheter) and repeated adjustments of the rate of infusion are mandatory. Since the drug has a marked postural hypotensive action, this must be appreciated if the patient's position is changed from reclining to more upright.

Bibliography

The references chosen are largely current comprehensive reviews of the subject rather than original articles. This list will permit the individual to obtain a review in depth. Each article, in turn, contains an extensive bibliography.

DIGITALIS

Bristow, J. D., and Griswold, H. E.: The use of digitalis in cardiovascular surgery. Progr. Cardiovasc. Dis. 7:387, 1965.

Ellis, J. G., and Dimond, E. G.: Newer concepts of digitalis. Amer. J. Cardiol. *17*:759, 1966.

Mason, D. T., Spann, J. F., Jr., and Zelis, R.: New developments in the understanding of the actions of the digitalis glycosides. Prog. Cardiovasc. Dis. *11*:443, 1969.

McIntosh, H. D., and Morris, J. J., Jr.: Use of digitalis in heart failure. Progr. Cardiovasc. Dis. 7:360, 1965.

Sodeman, W. A.: Diagnosis and treatment of digitalis toxicity. New Eng. J. Med. *273*:35 and 93, 1965.

Wilson, W. S.: Metabolism of digitalis. Progr. Cardiovasc. Dis. *11*:479, 1969.

ISOPROTERENOL

Elliott, W. C., and Gorlin, R.: Isoproterenol in treatment of heart disease. J.A.M.A. *197*:315, 1966.

Friedberg, C. K.: Diseases of the Heart. Philadelphia, W. B. Saunders Company, 1966.

Kardos, G. G.: Isoproterenol in treatment of shock. New Eng. J. Med. *274*:868, 1966.

Nissen, N. I., and Thomsen, A. C.: Oral treatment of AV block with isoprenaline (Isoproterenol). Brit. Heart J. 27:926, 1965.

AUTONOMIC NERVOUS SYSTEM DRUGS

Mecholyl

Friedberg, C. K.: Diseases of the Heart. Philadelphia, W. B. Saunders Company, 1966. p. 521.

Neostigmine
Friedberg, C. K.: Diseases of the Heart. Philadelphia, W. B. Saunders Company, 1966.
p. 521.
Edrophonium
Moss, A. J., and Aledort, L. M.: Use of edrophonium in supraventricular tachycardias.
Amer. J. Cardiol. *17*:58, 1966.
Atropine
Friedberg, C. K.: Disease of the Heart. Philadelphia, W. B. Saunders Company, 1966.
p. 600–601.

ALPHA RECEPTOR STIMULATORS

Chidsey, C. A.: Norepinephrine stores and contractile force. Circulation *33*:43, 1966.
Friedberg, C. K.: Diseases of the Heart. Philadelphia, W. B. Saunders Company, 1966.
p. 458–460.
Smulyan, H.: Hemodynamic aspects of pressor agents. J.A.M.A. *190*:188, 1964.

SYMPATHOPLEGIC DRUGS

Amery, A.: Critical review of diagnostic tests for pheochromocytoma. Amer. Heart J.
73:129, 1967.
Bay, G.: Hemodynamic effects of propranalol. Brit. Med. J. *1*:141, 1967.
Eckenhoff, J. E., and Cooperman, C. H.: The clinical application of phenoxybenzamine.
Surg. Gynec. Obstet. *121*:483, 1965.
Keelan, P. J.: Propranolol in angina pectoris. Brit. Med. J. *1*:897, 1965.

ANTIARRHYTHMIC AGENTS

Bigger, J. T., Jr., and Heissenbuttel, R. H.: The use of procaine amide and lidocaine in
the treatment of cardiac arrhythmias. Progr. Cardiovasc. Dis. *11*:515, 1969.
Covino, B. G., and D'Amato, H. E.: Current status of antiarrhythmic drug therapy. J.
Electrocardiol. *1*:141, 1968.
Damato, A. N.: Diphenylhydantoin: Pharmacological and clinical use. Progr. Cardio-
vasc. Dis. *12*:1, 1969.
Dreifus, L. S.: Arrhythmias in the post operative period. Amer. J. Cardiol. *12*:431,
1963.
Gibson, D., and Sowton, E.: The use of beta-adrenergic receptor blocking drugs in
dysrhythmias. Prog. Cardiovasc. Dis. *12*:16, 1969.
Goldman, M. J.: Management of chronic atrial fibrillation. Progr. Cardiovasc. Dis.
2:465, 1960.
Hoffman, B. F., and Cranefield, P. F.: The physiologic basis of cardiac arrhythmias.
Amer. J. Med. *37*:670, 1964.
Singer, D., and Ten Eick, E.: Pharmacology of cardiac arrhythmias. Progr. Cardiovasc.
Dis. *11*:488, 1969.

DIURETICS

Cannon, P. J., and Kilcoyne, M. M.: Ethacrynic acid and furosemide: Pharmacology
and clinical use. Progr. Cardiovasc. Dis. *12*:52, 1969.
DeGraff, A. C., and Lyon, A. G.: Diuretic therapy. Amer. Heart J. *67*:840, 1964.
Early, L. E.: Thiazide diuretics. Ann. Rev. Med. *15*:149, 1964.
Friedberg, C. K.: Diseases of the Heart. Philadelphia, W. B. Saunders Company, 1966.
p. 389–414.
Gantt, C. L.: Aldosterone antagonists. New York J. Med. *61*:756, 1961.
Swartz, C.: Evaluation of diuretic agents. Circulation *28*:1042, 1963.

ANTICOAGULATION THERAPY

Barrett, D. W., and Jordan, C. S.: Anticoagulant drugs in the treatment of pulmonary
embolism. Lancet *1*:1309, 1960.

Cooperative study: Heparin vs. warfarin in acute myocardial infarction. J.A.M.A. *189*:555, 1964.
Hughes, M. L., Jr.: Long term heparin and anticoagulant therapy in patients with severe angina pectoris. Amer. Heart J. *65*:615, 1963.
Mersky, C., and Drapkin, A.: Anticoagulant therapy, critical review. Blood *25*:567, 1965.
Symposium on heparin: Amer. J. Cardiol. *14*:1–68, 1964.
Thomas, D. P.: Treatment of pulmonary embolic disease. New Eng. J. Med. *273*:885, 1965.
VA cooperative study: Long term anticoagulant therapy after myocardial infarction. J.A.M.A. *193*:929, 1965.
Wessler, S., and Gaston, L. W.: Pharmacologic and clinical aspects of heparin therapy. Anesthesiology *27*:475, 1966.

WATER AND ELECTROLYTES

Blumentals, A. S.: Symposium on acid base balance. Arch. Int. Med. *116*:647, 1965.
Brozek, J.: Body Composition. Ann. N. Y. Acad. Sci. *110*:1, 1963.
Carson, S. A.: Acid-base management for open heart surgery. Circulation *29*:456, 1964.
Chamberlain, M. J.: Emergency treatment of hyperkalemia. Lancet *1*:464, 1964.
Edelman, I. S., and Leibman, J.: Anatomy of body water and electrolytes. Amer. J. Med. *27*:256, 1959.
Edelman, I. S., and Maffly, R. H.: The rate of sodium, potassium and water in heart failure. Progr. Cardiovasc. Disc. *4*:88, 1961.
Epstein, F. H.: Cerebral hyponatremia. New Eng. J. Med. *265*:513, 1961.
Forland, M., and Pullman, T. N.: Electrolyte complications of drug therapy. Med. Clin. N. Amer. *47*:113, 1963.
Kassiser, J. P.: The critical role of chloride in the correction of hypokalemic alkalosis. Amer. J. Med. *38*:172, 1965.
Luckey, E. H., and Ruben, A. L.: The correction of hyponatremia in congestive heart failure. Circulation *21*:229, 1960.
Norman, J. N., and Clark, R. G.: Metabolic acidosis in general surgery. Lancet *1*:348, 1964.
Santos, R. F., and Leaf, A.: Physiologic mechanisms in potassium deficiency. New Eng. J. Med. *264*:335, 1961.
Schwartz, W. B., and Waters, W. L.: Lactate vs. bicarbonate. Amer. J. Med. *32*:831, 1962.
Surawicz, B.: Electrolytes and electrocardiogram. Amer. J. Cardiol. *12*:656, 1963.
Symposium on modern concepts of fluids and electrolytes. Amer. J. Surg. *103*:283, 1962.
Virtue, R. W.: Fluid shifts during surgical period. Amer. Surg. *163*:523, 1966.

ANTIHYPERTENSIVE DRUG THERAPY

Dollery, C. T.: Methyldopa in the treatment of hypertension. Progr. Cardiovasc. Dis. *8*:278, 1965.
Freis, E. D.: Guanethidine. Progr. Cardiovasc. Dis. *8*:183, 1965.
Gaffney, T. E.: The clinical pharmacology of antihypertensive drugs. Progr. Cardiovasc. Dis. *12*:52, 1969.
Hollander, W., and Wilkins, R. W.: The pharmacology and clinical use of rauwolfia, hydralazine, thiazides, and aldosterone antagonists in arterial hypertension. Progr. Cardiovasc. Dis. *8*:291, 1965.
Sokolow, M., and Perloff, D.: The choice of drugs and the management of essential hypertension. Progr. Cardiovasc. Dis. *8*:253, 1965.
VA cooperative study on antihypertensive agents. Arch. Int. Med. *106*:81, 1960; *110*: 222, 1962; *110*:230, 1962.

CHAPTER 8

Specialized Equipment

By RICHARD G. SANDERSON, M.D.

The specialized equipment developed for use in the care of cardiac patients has provided a tremendous saving in time and energy for the nurse, greatly improved patient survival, and, at the same time, evoked considerable apprehension. The complexity of the equipment has caused the inexperienced nurse to shy away, thereby limiting its usefulness. Basic concepts and uses of the various types of specialized equipment will be stressed in this chapter.

Monitoring Equipment

Electronic monitoring of physiologic parameters is used to supplement clinical observation of the patient and to facilitate the collection of important physiologic data which can then be analyzed further. The three phases of this monitoring process are data collection, data processing, and data display. Although this specialized equipment is extremely useful in caring for cardiac patients, the information obtained in the monitoring process must always be correlated with the patient's condition. Treatment should be based on clinical observation, as well as upon the results obtained from the monitoring system. "Treat the patient, not the machine."

346

DATA COLLECTION EQUIPMENT

A wide variety of physiologic parameters may be monitored in the care of an acute coronary patient or in the postoperative period following cardiac surgery. Each parameter involves converting the energy produced by the patient (electrical, pressure, or thermal) into a form which can be amplified and then appropriately displayed.

Electrocardiogram

The electrical activity of the heart can be picked up by *leads* which are placed on three extremities (with a fourth one as *ground*) or on the chest wall. The lead wires are usually three or five in number and are connected to an oscilloscopic monitor either directly or through a lead selector switch. For a patient who is moderately active in bed or in whom gross observation of rate and rhythm are to be made, the three-lead chest system is sufficient. Usually two of the leads are placed over the base and apex of the heart and the ground lead (often color-coded black) is placed elsewhere on the chest.

In patients who are relatively quiet in bed, whose chests are partially covered with dressings, whose heart and lungs are examined at frequent intervals, or in whom standardized ECG tracings are desired, the five-lead ECG monitoring system is preferred. Often, this five-lead system is color-coded so that the right arm is white, the right leg is green, the left arm is black, the left leg is red, and the chest lead is brown. The following list outlines the leads used to obtain the routine ECG traces:

Lead 1	LA	RA
Lead 2	LL	RA
Lead 3	LL	LA
avR	RA	LL and LA
avL	LA	LL and RA
avF	LL	LA and RA
V	C	LL and LA and RA

The contact points on the patient may be by metal plates, conductive bandaids, biopotential skin electrodes, or by needles (Fig. 8–1).

The metal plates are attached to the patient either by adhesive tape or by a rubber strap which encircles the extremity or the chest. Electrode paste or small, saline-dampened sponges provide the contact between the patient and the plate, and should be renewed once or twice daily if the transmitted tracing is to be accurate. Connections of the lead wires to the plates should be oriented in such a direction

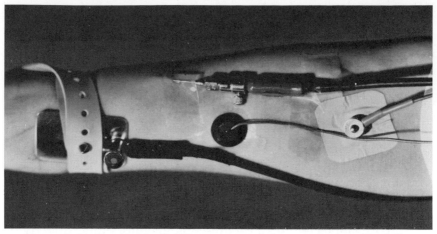

Figure 8–1. Photograph of different types of electrocardiogram "leads." From left to right the leads are plates, needles, biopotential skin electrodes, and conductive bandaids.

that there is a minimum of torsion on the plates. Plates are easy to apply, but cause many artifacts, particularly when the patient moves. The lead cables are usually quite heavy and uncomfortable if the patient lies upon them.

The "conductive" bandaids and biopotential skin electrodes provide lasting contact because the electrode paste is held within a closed space surrounded by adhesive and, therefore, need not be renewed frequently. The connecting wires are usually thin and unobtrusive. The least amount of artifact is produced by these leads and the motion of the patient affects the electrocardiographic tracing but slightly.

With ECG plates, conductive bandaids, or biopotential skin electrodes, the skin should be adequately cleansed before applying a small amount of electrode paste beneath the electrode; maximum contact is thus assured.

Needles are placed into the subcutaneous tissues of the extremities and therefore provide lasting contact. However, they cause some slight discomfort, may cause superficial infection if left in place over many days, and must be adapted to the ends of the connecting leads.

Any of the electrical equipment attached to the patient should be connected with the oscilloscope or ECG machine by the same grounded outlet. If 60 cycle interference waves persist on the tracing, the power plug should be reversed (if possible) or a ground wire should be connected from the oscilloscope or ECG machine to an unpainted metal ground (water faucet, radiator, and so forth). Figure 8–2 demonstrates the artifacts commonly seen on the electrocardiographic tracings.

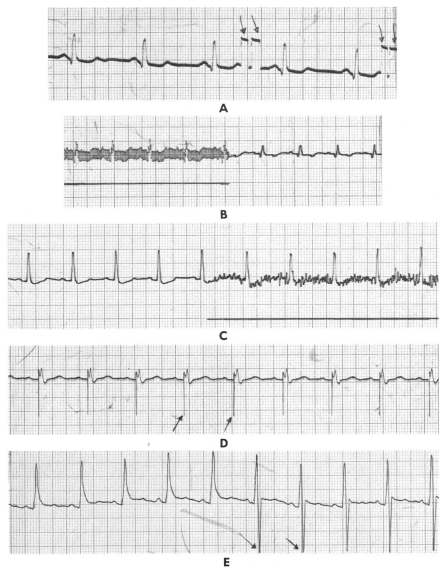

Figure 8-2. Artifacts seen in ECG tracings. *A,* Artifact of the 1 millivolt calibration signal of the ECG machine. *B,* 60 cycle electrical artifact (usually due to poor grounding). *C,* Artifact from patient movement. The QRS complexes can still be seen even though the baseline is very irregular. *D,* Artifact of fixed-rate pacemaker. Each QRS complex is preceded by a brisk downward deflection (the pacing artifact). *E,* Artifact produced by the synchronizer output of the defibrillator. Note that the synchronizer artifact occurs on the R wave and not on the T wave (see Figure 8-6).

Electroencephalogram

Needle or "stick-on" leads are usually used to transmit the electrical activity of the brain. Similar grounding precautions are exercised as explained for the ECG equipment.

Pressure Transducer

The pressure within a cardiac chamber, an artery, or a vein is usually obtained by placing a cannula into the appropriate area, interposing a length of connecting tubing, and then connecting it to a transducer (a strain gauge). Often, the arterial pressure line is attached to the transducer by an intervening manifold which facilitates flushing the pressure line and removing air or blood from the transducer. A typical manifold is diagrammed in Appendix A.

The pressure transducer is a delicate (and expensive) instrument which should be handled with great care. Within the transducer is a sensitive diaphragm which, when displaced by pressure changes, transmits a wave form through the electrical circuitry to a display system (Fig. 8–3). High pressure should not be applied directly to the diaphragm (as by flushing against it), as it is easily damaged. Appendix B provides instructions for the assembly of the pressure transducer. Certain artifacts should be kept constantly in mind when monitoring pressure wave forms (Fig. 8–4).

The most common and most important artifact is seen when the wave form "dampens out" (Fig. 8–4A and B). This dampening is usually caused by a blood clot or air bubble which partially obstructs the system. As a similarly dampened wave form can be produced by a rapidly failing heart, the patient's clinical condition should be correlated closely with this tracing. A knowing glance at the patient or a check of the blood pressure with the sphygmomanometer will usually resolve the confusion. Flushing gently through the monitoring system will usually restore the wave form to its original configuration.

Most systems for monitoring pressures have a length of hard-core nylon tubing that connects the cannula (arterial, venous, or cardiac chamber) to the transducer. When this tubing is moved quickly, as commonly occurs when one is working near the patient, a distinctive high frequency artifact is produced (Fig. 8–4C). As this connecting tubing has very little distensibility, the transmitted arterial wave forms tend to have very sharp "spikes," which peak 10 to 15 mm Hg above the systolic pressure as determined by the sphygmomanometer. Miniaturized transducers, which connect directly to the arterial cannula, eliminate this artifact, inscribing an arterial wave form with a more physiologic, rounded apex; peak systolic pressure is then very

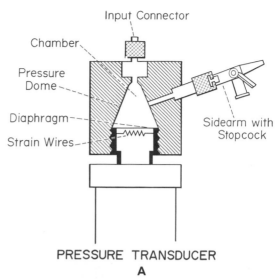

PRESSURE TRANSDUCER

A

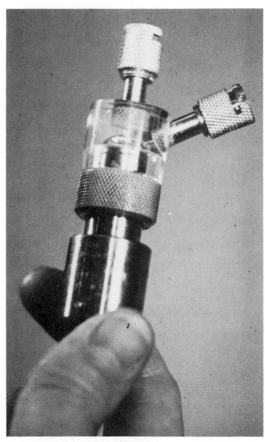

Figure 8–3. Pressure transducer (strain gauge). *A*, Schematic drawing. *B*, Actual photograph. The strain gauge diaphragm can be seen at the base of the plastic pressure dome. The connection on the top is for the connecting tubing from the cannula and the sidearm is for flushing the air out of the dome.

B

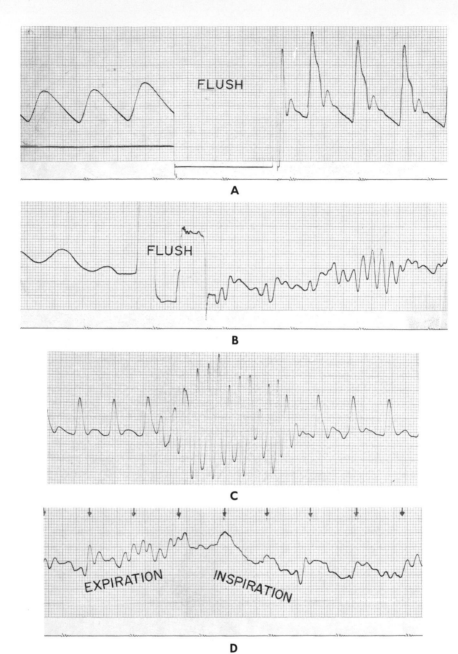

Figure 8-4. Artifacts in pressure wave forms. *A,* Dampening of the arterial wave form. Note the rounded, smooth wave form on the left. Following flushing of the arterial line, the typical undampened, peaked wave form with its dicrotic notch is seen. *B,* Dampening of the venous pressure wave form. Note the rounded undulating wave form on the left, the flushing of the line and the undampened phasic form on the right. *C,* Artifact of movement of the connecting tubing. The sequence of arterial wave forms is interrupted by the sharp "spikes" produced when the connecting tubing is moved. *D,* Variations of central venous pressure (CVP) with the phases of respiration. With inspiration, the intrathoracic pressure falls (as does the CVP pressure); with expiration these pressures rise. The phasic wave form of the right atrium is repeated at regular intervals (*see arrows on tracing*), as is seen in sinus rhythm.

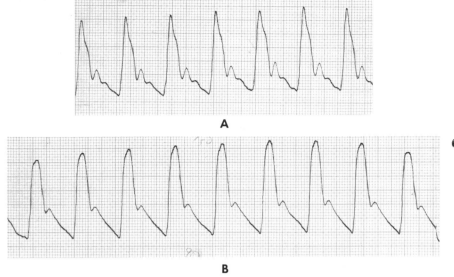

Figure 8–5. Transmission of wave forms. *A*, A sharply peaked wave form is inscribed when a hard-core tubing transmits the wave form from the monitoring cannula to the strain gauge. The dicrotic notch is also abnormally peaked. *B*, When the arterial pressure wave is received directly by the strain gauge (without interposed tubing), the wave form has a smooth rounded apex and dicrotic notch.

similar to that recorded by the arm cuff. Figure 8–5 compares these two types of wave form transmissions.

The wave form of the central venous pressure has regular impulses that correspond to the cardiac beats. There is also normally a 3 to 5 mm Hg variation of the peaks of these waves with respiration (Fig. 8–4*D*). When the monitoring system is partially obstructed (by clot or air), the tracing loses both the cardiac waves and respiratory variations (Fig. 8–4*B*). If the venous cannula is in the inferior vena cava, pressing on the patient's abdomen (increasing intra-abdominal pressure) will no longer cause a sharp rise in the venous pressure. Again, gentle flushing will usually remedy the situation. If the pressure line cannot be cleared, clinical observation alone will become the monitoring guideline.

Plethysmograph

The arterial pulse wave may be observed indirectly by recording its arrival at a peripheral site. In a photoelectric plethysmograph, light is transmitted through the tissues by a small, incandescent bulb. Light intensity changes produced by the pulsatile blood flow are picked up by the adjacent photoelectric cell. Similar voltage changes can be detected by a sensitive column of mercury in the "strain-gauge plethysmograph." The voltage signal is then amplified, fed through an amplifier, and presented on the oscilloscope as a pulse wave.

Temperature

Thermal sensitive probes may be placed in the esophagus, in the rectum, or on the skin. The patient's temperature may then be electronically transmitted to a display system.

Miscellaneous

Other physiologic parameters which can be monitored by more complex equipment include blood volume, cardiac output, and blood gases (P_{O_2}, P_{CO_2}, pH, and so on).

Many of these physiologic parameters may be monitored simultaneously in a single patient. Each piece of the data acquisition equipment has its own connecting wires or tubing. In order to facilitate and simplify the transmission of the data, a "clearing station" or "input junction box" may be provided near the patient. From the different monitored parameters, the multiple wires lead into the bedside junction box and then are transmitted by a single composite cable to the display equipment.

DATA PROCESSING EQUIPMENT

After the acquired data has been converted into electrical energy, it must be processed further before it can be displayed.

Preamplifiers

The input signal (i.e., the wave forms of the different physiologic parameters) must be appropriately amplified before transmission to the oscilloscope or other recording device. ECG preamplifiers are usually calibrated so that a 1 mv calibration signal will cause a 10 mm deflection of the tracing (Fig. 8–2A). Carrier (pressure) preamplifiers are calibrated so that a standardized signal will produce an appropriate deflection of the tracing (e.g., a 5 mm Hg calibration signal for venous pressures or a 100 mm Hg calibration signal for arterial pressures). Diagrams of ECG and carrier preamplifiers and instructions for balancing and calibrating them are found in Appendix C.

Converting Equipment

Sometimes this data is processed further by converting a wave form or series of wave forms into a numerical read-out. For example, the number of QRS complexes of the electrocardiogram per minute is converted to a meter read-out of heart rate. In a more complex fashion, the arterial pressure wave form may be analyzed electronically and converted into numerical values for systolic, diastolic, and mean pressures (digital read-out).

Centralizing Equipment

In a large intensive care unit, so much data is obtained from each bedside monitoring set that a large staff of professional personnel would be required to handle it effectively. Instead, the data is relayed from the bedside to a central monitoring station, where the data from each bed may be simultaneously displayed and observed by a single person.

At this central station, the work of observing the data from the individual beds and detecting physiologic abnormalities may also be performed electronically. The equipment at the central monitoring station can be connected to a programmer which scans the data from each bedside at a predetermined interval and displays it appropriately. By connecting the programmed scanner to an electronic typewriter, the vital signs from each unit may be typed out, thereby relieving the nurse of the onerous task of "charting."

The range of acceptable values of the physiologic parameters of each individual bed may be pre-established in such a way that if a patient's values exceed this range, an "alarm condition" will exist and appropriate electronic or audio notification can be made. The central station scanner can be further programmed so that if such a condition occurs, the abnormal data can be continuously monitored and recorded during the alarm period.

Storage Equipment

Physiologic data obtained from the patient can also be stored for future analysis. After the information has been collected and processed, it may then be transferred onto punched cards, punched tape, or magnetic tapes. At a later date, these tapes or cards may be reprocessed through appropriate equipment and the data analyzed at leisure.

Memory loops are reels of magnetic tape which constantly record a physiologic parameter for a set period of time. When this time limit is exceeded, the tape is automatically erased and the parameter continues to be recorded. In the event of an alarm condition, the loop can be replayed in order to document the events preceding the alarm period.

DATA DISPLAY EQUIPMENT

In order to make the information achieved from the data collecting systems available for interpretation, it must be displayed in an appropriate form. Parameters which fall within a narrow range and which change slowly need only simple display equipment, while rapidly changing parameters with complex wave forms require oscilloscopic display. Some parameters should be recorded at varying intervals and included in the clinical chart; additional recording equipment is then necessary.

Meter Read-out

Central venous pressure (CVP), mean left atrial pressure (LAP), heart rate, and temperature are physiologic parameters which change relatively slowly. Although saline manometers may be used for the CVP or mean LAP, the continuous meter display is more convenient and less time-consuming for the nursing staff. A heart rate meter which can be activated either by the peripheral arterial wave form or by the QRS complex of the electrocardiogram saves valuable time in determining the patient's cardiac rate. (Newer equipment has T wave discriminators which electronically eliminate the T wave artifacts of rate counting.) A display of the patient's temperature from an indwelling rectal or esophageal probe can relieve the nurse of the burden of intermittently taking the patient's temperature.

Oscilloscopic Display

The cathode ray tube of an oscilloscope projects the variations of electrical energy of a transmitted wave form onto a phosphorescent screen where it can be viewed. The electrocardiogram, electroencephalogram, and plethysmograph can then be interpreted by the configuration and amplitude of the wave forms. The oscilloscope may display a single physiologic parameter or multiple parameters, depending upon its size and the number of input channels available.

Systolic, diastolic, and mean arterial pressures may be displayed on a meter read-out, but the wave form itself is more valuable when viewed on the oscilloscope. When a calibrated grid is super-imposed onto the oscilloscope tracing, the systolic and diastolic pressure of each wave form can be viewed instantly. By switching the preamplifier control to "AVG" (average), the mean arterial pressure can also be determined. Although intermittent checks of the blood pressure by a sphygmomanometer may reassure the nurse, the electronic measuring of arterial pressures is a tremendous saving in time and effort by the nursing personnel.

An audio signal may be used with the ECG monitor so that each QRS may be detected as a "beep" and the nurse need not watch the ECG oscilloscope constantly. Because of the "persistence" of a tracing on the oscilloscope, the wave form can be seen until the tracing dims from view (usually for 4 to 6 beats). If an extra-systole (or a run of extra-systoles) is heard via the audio system, the nurse can quickly turn to the oscilloscope and observe the abnormality.

Digital Read-out

The thinking process of perceiving an arterial pressure involves the visual observation of the arterial wave form on the oscilloscope, correlating it with the calibrated oscilloscope grid, and then finally realizing the numerical figures in one's brain. The digital read-out equipment eliminates the first two steps of this process by analyzing the wave form electronically and converting it to numerical figures directly. With this equipment, the numerical values of systolic and diastolic arterial pressures, venous or left atrial pressures, and heart rate may be seen at one quick glance.

Recording Equipment

Commonly, a permanent record of the wave forms obtained from the collecting equipment is desired. For example, cardiac arrhythmias are recorded on paper so that they may be analyzed at leisure and later incorporated into the patient's chart. Most bedside monitoring units have a strip chart recorder for documentation of these ECG abnormalities. In some units, the recorder is automatically activated by a preset timing sequence or activated when an alarm condition occurs. In more complex units (usually used in research situations), a multichannel recording system (two to 14 channels) records simultaneously a wide variety of physiologic parameters.

In summary, physiologic monitoring requires sensitive and expensive equipment. The data is collected from the patient, converted into electrical energy, standardized and processed, and then transmitted to display equipment appropriate for the individual parameter being monitored. Diagrammatic schema for an individual bedside monitoring unit and for an entire programmed and computerized system are presented in Appendix D.

Defibrillators

Electrical conversion of cardiac arrhythmias has become common practice in the care of cardiac patients. Ventricular fibrillation, ventricular tachycardia, atrial flutter, and atrial fibrillation are the arrhythmias most commonly treated by this modality. The prompt and proper application of a defibrillating electrical current can often be lifesaving.

When a heart is defibrillated, an electrical shock is sent through the entire mass of cardiac muscle, depolarizing all the individual fibers. During the forced refractory period which follows, no impulses can be initiated and the muscle cells are at a standstill. If the patient's oxygenation and metabolic status are adequate, the heart will usually resume rhythmic coordinated contractions following defibrillation.

CONTACT

Correct placement of the electrodes is necessary if the electrical current is to pass through the heart. In the open chest, one paddle is applied to the left ventricle and the other to the right atrium (see Fig. 9–15). In the intact chest, the electrodes are placed over the apex and the base of the heart (see Fig. 9–14). Electrode paste or moistened saline sponges are used to ensure good contact. *When the electrical discharge is made, no one should be in direct contact with the patient or his bed.* The operator is protected from the electrical current by the insulated electrode handles.

ENERGY LEVEL

The energy level necessary to convert an arrhythmia depends not only upon the type of rhythm disturbance but also upon the efficiency of the contact points and the thickness of the tissues separating the heart from the electrodes. Either alternating current (AC) or direct current (DC) shocks may be utilized; DC is now used more commonly. In the open chest, a defibrillating shock of 120 to 180 volts AC for 0.1 to 0.2 seconds or 10 to 40 watt-seconds (joules) DC is used. With an intact chest wall, ventricular defibrillation may be accomplished by an AC shock of 440 volts for 0.25 seconds; 880 volts is occasionally required. DC shocks as low as 100 watt-seconds occasionally may be effective, but 200 to 400 watt-seconds are more often necessary for defibrillation. Cardioversion for atrial flutter generally requires only 100 watt-seconds, while 300 watt-seconds are usually necessary for atrial fibrillation.

DISCHARGE

Depending upon the type of defibrillator, discharge of the electrical current is made at the electrode handle, at the machine (by an assistant), or by a foot pedal connected to the defibrillator. During cardioversion of rhythms other than ventricular fibrillation, the timing of the discharge is important. Ventricular fibrillation may be induced during certain portions of the cardiac cycle. Zones of vulnerability (the areas of the cardiac cycle when the applied current can produce atrial or ventricular fibrillation) are seen in Figure 8–6. Therefore, an electronic synchronizing device is used to time the

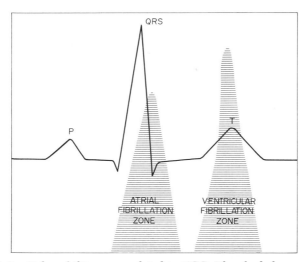

Figure 8–6. Vulnerability zones related to ECG. The shaded areas indicate the times when an induced electrical current can produce atrial or ventricular fibrillation. The peak of the T wave is the most critical time for producing ventricular fibrillation (a situation similar to the R-on-T phenomenon discussed in Chapter 4).

electrical discharge to the apex of the R wave of the electrocardiogram, preventing discharge in the vulnerable zone. The synchronizing artifact is seen in Figure 8–2E.

Pacemakers

In the normal heart, the hierarchy of pacemaking activity is initiated by the sinoatrial node, transmitted across the atrium to the atrioventricular node, where, after a short delay, the impulse is transmitted down the bundle of His, through the bundle branches, out into the Purkinje fiber system, and into the ventricular musculature (Figure 8–7). Any obstruction in this electrical conduction system results in heart block and produces abnormal cardiac rhythms (e.g., nodal rhythm, idioventricular rhythm, cardiac standstill). Serious hemodynamic consequences attend heart rates of 30 to 40 beats per minute (particularly in older persons), and many patients will faint or even have a cardiac arrest at such slow rates.

Pacemakers are electrical devices designed to stimulate the electrical activity of the heart. From a pulse generator circuit (powered by batteries or by electricity), the pacemaking impulse is carried through the electrodes to the heart. From the point of contact at the tip of the electrode, the impulse spreads to the contractile areas of the heart, causing it to beat.

Pacemakers are most commonly utilized in treating severe bradycardia, but may also be used to suppress ventricular arrhythmias and to augment a failing cardiac output by increasing cardiac rate. In

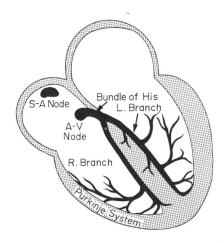

Figure 8–7. Cardiac conduction tissue. Note the component parts of the conduction system. See Figure 4–2 for a more detailed drawing.

some patients, electrical pacemaking assistance is required for only short intervals, while in others there is long-term dependence upon the artificial pacemaking stimuli.

TEMPORARY PACEMAKERS (EXTERNAL PACEMAKERS)

The pulse generator is kept outside the body and the power is provided either by batteries or by a regular electrical current (Fig. 8–8).

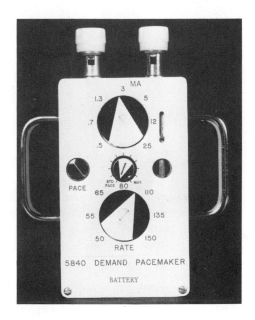

Figure 8-8. External battery-powered pacemaker, demand type. The connectors for the electrodes are on top of the unit. The two large dials are for adjustment of milliamperage (*above*) and rate (*below*). The sensitivity of the demand mode is adjusted by the small dial (*center*). The pacemaker is activated by releasing the button on the right; the timing of the pacing stimulus is seen by the deflections of the dial (*center left*).

Transvenous

A unipolar or bipolar catheter electrode (Fig. 8–9) is passed retrograde under fluoroscopic control from a peripheral vein (median basilic, femoral, or jugular) back into the heart. Here pacing can be then accomplished at the following sites.

Atrial. The atrial site is near the junction of the superior vena cava and the right atrium, in close proximity to the sinoatrial node.

Ventricular or nodal. The catheter is intentionally impinged in trabeculations of the right ventricle. If the catheter is caught in the apex of the heart, a right ventricular focus will be apparent; if caught in the outflow tract of the right ventricle, a junctional configuration will be evoked.

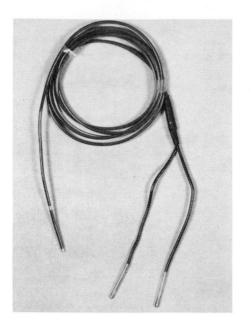

Figure 8-9. Bipolar transvenous pacing catheter electrode. The two long metal tips (*right lower corner*) are for connecting the electrode to an external pacemaker. The metal inserts on the other end of the catheter electrode are the active contact points for the pacemaking signal.

Implanted

Operative. At the close of cardiac operations, pacemaking electrodes are sometimes affixed to the surface of the heart with fine epicardial sutures and are brought out through the incision (Fig. 8–10). Atrial pacing is accomplished if the electrodes are affixed near

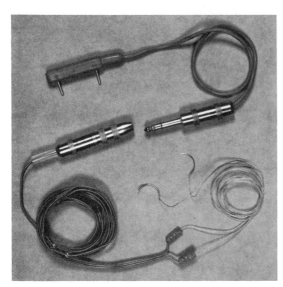

Figure 8-10. Epicardial pacing wires. In the right lower corner are the epicardial pacing wires and the "swaged-on" needles used to affix them to the heart. In this illustration the pacing wires are crimped to an electrical wire whose end is a "female" phonojack. Connection of this system to the external power source is facilitated by the "male" phonojack (*upper right*).

the sinoatrial node, and ventricular pacing will ensue if they are placed on an available avascular area of the right or left ventricles. In the postoperative period these electrodes can be connected to an external pulse generator (external pacemaker) if pacing is required. When the electrodes have served their usefulness, gentle traction will break the fine restraining epicardial sutures, allowing the electrodes to be removed.

Percutaneous. Under emergency circumstances, a pacing electrode can be introduced into the left ventricle by percutaneous needle puncture, and then connected to the pulse generator.

The electrodes leading away from the heart are usually shielded with a nonconductive plastic to a point near to the connecting end. These bared wires may be connected to the terminals of the external pacemaker either directly or through an extra length of wire, the ends of which have been fashioned into a "phono-jack" or "alligator clip" arrangement (Fig. 8–11). In order to effectively "take over" pacemaking function, the rate must generally exceed the patient's intrinsic rate by 5 to 10 beats per minute. Often a very low amperage (2 to 5 milliamperes) is required for transvenous or implanted epicardial electrodes; however, with scarring around the implanted electrodes or depressed myocardial contractility, amperage as high as 15 to 20 milliamperes may be necessary.

To institute external pacemaking, the following steps should be carried out under constant electrocardiographic monitoring: (1) turn rate control to a rate of 5 to 10 beats faster than patient's own rate;

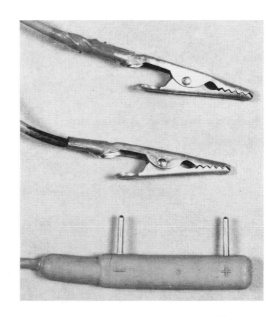

Figure 8–11. Alligator clip connection. An intermediary wire, with alligator clips on one end (to grasp the ends of the pacing electrodes) and a connector bar on the other end (to fit into the terminals of the external pacemaker), is used to connect the components of this system.

(2) turn amperage control as low as possible; (3) turn pacemaker on (most pacemakers have small neon flashers or oscillating meters to indicate when the pacer is functioning); (4) slowly turn up amperage control (the pacemaking artifact on the ECG should appear small at first and become larger as the amperage is increased); (5) continue turning amperage control until a QRS complex follows immediately after each pacing artifact; and (6) after pacemaker has "taken over," make sure all connecting wires cannot come apart. *New batteries should always be available.*

External

Occasionally external electrodes are applied to the chest wall, and the pacemaking impulse, which of necessity must be of much higher amperage, is transmitted to the heart.

PERMANENT PACEMAKERS (IMPLANTED PACEMAKERS)

The pulse generator of these pacemakers is composed of tiny mercury-zinc batteries, appropriate electronic circuitry, and connections for the electrodes. All these components are encased in a nonreactive plastic covering. The entire unit, measuring approximately $2 \times 2 \times 1$ inches, is implanted into a subcutaneous pocket in the abdomen, axilla, or infraclavicular fossa (Fig. 8–12). Just as in the temporary pacemaker, the electrodes can be passed in through a peripheral vein; alternately, they may be implanted in the heart muscle itself through a thoracotomy.

No implanted pacemaker is truly permanent. Battery life is only 15 to 36 months, and replacement of the power unit (usually not the electrodes) is usually required after 18 to 24 months. Diagnosis of a failing pacemaker is made when the pacing impulse fails to consistently evoke a ventricular contraction, when the rate changes, or when the synchronous pacemaker functions as a fixed-rate pacemaker (see later).

Fixed Rate

The heart rate and amperage of these pacemakers are preset at the factory (generally 68 to 72 beats per minute and 3 milliamperes) and cannot be adjusted. They are usually adequate for elderly, relatively inactive, patients. Some of the manufacturers of fixed-rate pacemakers have developed external rate control devices that (through an induction coil placed on the skin overlying the battery pack) increase the cardiac rate in the immediate postoperative period.

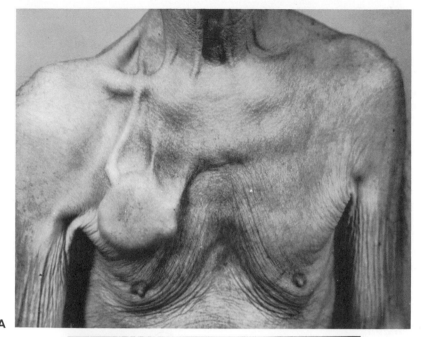

A

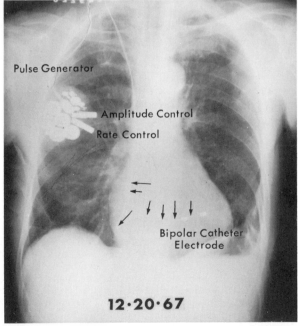

Pulse Generator

Amplitude Control

Rate Control

Bipolar Catheter
Electrode

12·20·67

B

Figure 8–12. A, Photograph of a patient with an implanted transvenous permanent pacemaker. The pulse generator lying on the pectoral muscles and the catheter electrode leading up to the jugular vein can easily be seen in this thin patient. B, X-ray of the same patient. Note the radioopaque electronic components and batteries in the pulse generator, and the course of the bipolar catheter electrode as it passes through the venous system to the apex of the right ventricle.

Variable Rate and Amplitude

Attached to the side of these pacing units are two protruding receptacles for the control of rate and amplitude (see Fig. 8–12B). When one of these parameters requires adjustment, a Keith skin needle is inserted percutaneously into the receptacle and turned until the appropriate rate (or amperage) is achieved.

Dual Rate

This pacer was designed for people who intermittently need a faster heart rate. Conversion from the slower rate to the faster rate is accomplished by placing beiefly a magnetic *pencil* on the skin overlying the pulse generator. When the rapid rate is no longer needed, the pencil is replaced again, now in the reverse direction over the battery pack and the circuitry returns the rate to the slower level.

Demand

The internal circuitry of this pacemaker allows it to fire a pacemaking impulse only if the patient's rate falls below a certain predetermined level. If a bradycardia develops, the pacemaker will automatically "take over." When the sensing circuit of the demand pacemaker "senses" a QRS complex from the patient himself, it will inhibit the next pacemaking impulse. Then, if another QRS complex does not appear (within the predetermined time interval), the pacer will initiate the pacing impulse.

Figure 8–13.   ECG patterns of different types of pacemakers. *A,* Fixed rate (asynchronous) pacemaker. Note the 1:1 ventricular response to the pacing artifact. There is no ventricular response to the patient's P waves (third degree heart block). *B,* Failing fixed rate pacemaker. Note that the pacing artifact is of low amplitude and is not followed by a ventricular response. Atrial rate is 110/min; ventricular rate is 30/min; pacing rate is 58/min. *C,* Synchronous pacemaker. Note that the pacing artifact appears 0.16 seconds after each P wave and that there is a 1:1 ventricular response to each pacing artifact. If second degree heart block were not present and the QRS was initiated before 0.16 seconds, the pacing artifact would be inhibited. *D,* Failing synchronous pacemaker. Note that the pacing artifact does not follow the P waves and only occasionally evokes a ventricular response. *E,* Demand pacemaker. Note that the first six QRS complexes are evoked by the pacemaker. The patient's own QRS complex (7) occurs before the next pacing stimulus and thereby inhibits it (by the demand mode of the pacemaker.) The pacemaker then resumes its function in QRS complex 8. *F,* Failing demand pacemaker. This unit is working only intermittently: although the patient's

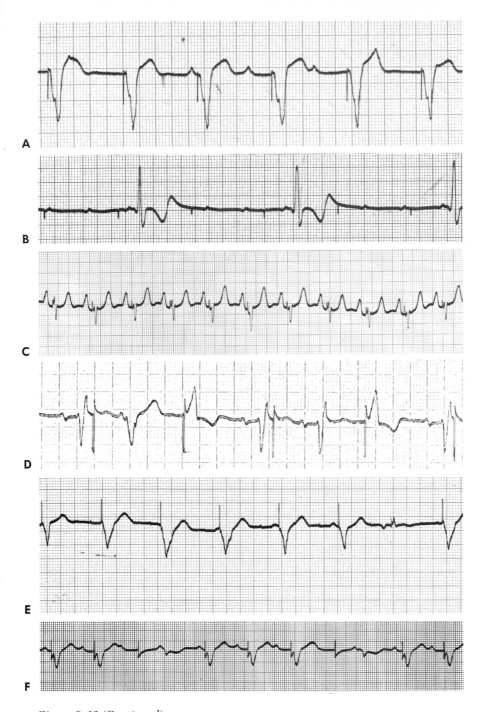

Figure 8–13 *(Continued).*
own QRS complexes inhibit the pacing artifact in complexes 3 and 7 (sensing unit functioning correctly), failure to capture is evidenced by the absence of a QRS complex after the pacing artifact between complexes 2 and 3 and 6 and 7. Appropriate capture occurs in complexes 1, 2, 4, 5, 6, 8, and 9.

Synchronous

This type of pacemaker is used in patients who have intermittent heart block. As long as the patient's cardiac rate is determined by his own atrial activity (and correct transmission of that electrical impulse), the pacer does not function. However, if the interval between atrial activation and the ventricular response exceeds a certain interval (0.16 seconds), the pacemaker impulse will be evoked and ventricular contraction will follow immediately.

The cardiac nurse should learn to identify the artifact of the pacing impulse on the electrocardiogram as well as the patterns of pacemaker malfunction. Figure 8–13 will demonstrate some of these ECG patterns.

Pleural Drainage Systems

Normal respiration depends upon the integrity of the chest wall to maintain proper pressure relationships. The pressure within the pleural cavity starts at about −5 mm Hg. During inspiration, the rib cage expands, the diaphragm descends, and the negative intrapleural pressure is increased to −7 to −15 mm Hg, depending upon the depth of inspiration. Relaxation of the muscles of respiration and elastic

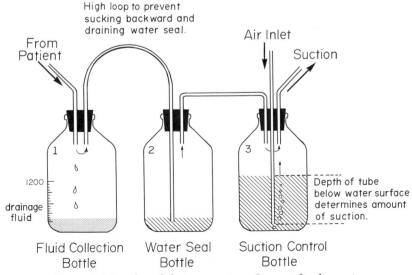

Figure 8–14. Pleural drainage system. See text for discussion.

recoil of the lung during expiration cause a return of the intrapleural pressure to the original level.

When the continuity of the pleural surface is interrupted (by thoracotomy incision, open pneumothorax, and so on), ambient atmospheric pressure is found in the pleural cavity as well as in the tracheobronchial tree. Unless positive pressure is applied to the lungs from within, the lung will collapse.

The purpose of pleural drainage systems is to evacuate the air from the pleural space and to re-establish the normal negative pressure relationships. Further, the drainage system removes excess intrapleural fluid, allowing full expansion of the lungs. If there is air escaping from a damaged surface of the lung, a vacuum system is usually necessary to keep up with this air leak.

The three-bottle suction system (Fig. 8–14) is used routinely in the postoperative care of patients who have undergone heart or lung operations and in patients who have suffered a pneumothorax. It is composed of the following parts:

THE FLUID COLLECTION BOTTLE, LABELED NO. 1

Fluid from the operative site drains through the chest tubes into this bottle. There should be 25 to 50 cc graduations marked on this bottle so that the amount of fluid lost can be accurately determined and appropriate blood replacement instituted.

WATERSEAL BOTTLE, LABELED NO. 2

Air that has been evacuated from the chest is conducted down the long slender tubing in this bottle to exit under water. The air rises to the surface of the water and is suctioned away. A reverse flow of air back into the patient is prevented by the "water seal." Normal respiratory pressures are applied to the drainage system if this bottle is not connected to the suction control bottle. It is then a simple water-seal drainage system.

SUCTION CONTROL BOTTLE, LABELED NO. 3

The amount of negative pressure that is applied to the entire system is controlled in this bottle. Air is drawn from outside the system down the air inlet tube and is suctioned away. The amount of suction that is applied (usually measured in centimeters of water) is determined by the height of the water level above the bottom of the air inlet tube. Increased amounts of suction pressure can be achieved by lengthening the height of this column of water. Even if high-*flow* vacuum is applied, the suction *pressure* cannot exceed this amount as long as the air inlet tube is unobstructed.

When greater suction pressures are desired, and the height of the water column in the suction control bottle cannot produce them, occlusion of the air inlet tube (as by adhesive tape) can provide this increased pressure. The degree of suction applied by the vacuum source is then transmitted directly to the system. Inserting a hypodermic needle through the tape forms a safety valve—moderate suction is obtained with a No. 18 needle, high suction with a No. 20 needle, and very high suction with a No. 22 needle. Alternately, greater suction pressure can be achieved by substituting mercury for the water in the suction control section of the system (particularly useful in the disposable plastic pleural drainage systems; see later).

CONNECTING TUBING

The tubing between the fluid collection bottle and the waterseal bottle should make a high enough loop so that high negative intrapleural pressures (as are developed with deep breaths, sneezing) will not cause siphonage of the water seal back into the fluid collection bottle.

VACUUM SOURCE

The vacuum applied to the system is often provided by the action of a piston pump (e.g., Stedman pump), which is a relatively low-flow system. In newer hospitals, central (wall) vacuum sources provide a high-flow system.

Large volume leakage of air from the lung is transmitted through the system to the suction bottle. If a low-flow vacuum source is unable to handle this leak, air will accumulate within the chest (pneumothorax). A high-flow system (as provided by a wall vacuum) can keep up with this air leak and the system will remain functional.

The three bottle drainage system is prepared with aseptic technique as follows:

1. Add sterile water to the suction control bottle sufficient to provide an appropriate amount of suction (normally 10 to 15 cm water). Water is also added to the second bottle so that the waterseal tubing is at least 1 cm below the water surface. A small amount of fluid added to the fluid collection bottle will help prevent clotting of

blood on the bottom of the bottle and will help facilitate subsequent cleaning.

2. Assemble the connections as indicated in Figure 8–14, making sure the height of the tubing between the fluid collection and water seal bottles is enough to prevent the sucking back of the waterseal.

3. Make sure all stoppers and connections are air tight and cannot come loose.

4. Connect the patient's chest tubes to the fluid collection bottle.

5. Evacuate the air from within the three bottle system before unclamping the patient's chest tubes.

More recently, compact, disposable, plastic pleural drainage systems have been devised and manufactured (Fig. 8–15). Appropriate baffling prevents water from flowing from one section to another.

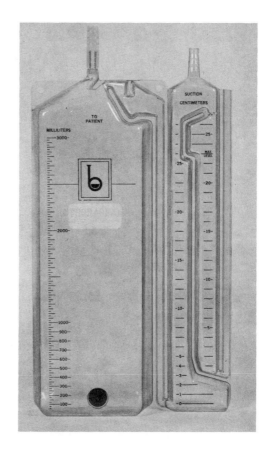

Figure 8–15. Disposable plastic pleural drainage system. The fluid collection chamber is on the left, the suction control is on the right, and the water seal chamber is in the center.

Appendix A

FLUSHING MANIFOLD

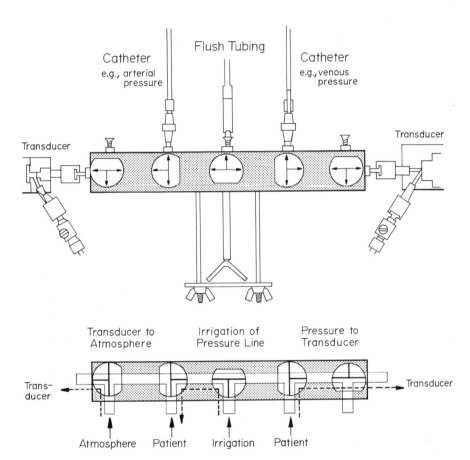

The top diagram depicts a typical arrangement for monitoring two pressures (e.g., arterial and venous) from a single patient. The flush tubing is located in the center so that it can be used to flush either monitoring line. The bottom diagram depicts the arrangement for connecting the transducer to atmospheric air; it is for obtaining a zero (*left*), for flushing one of the monitoring lines (*center*), and for connecting the monitoring line to the transducer (*right*).

Appendix B

PRESSURE TRANSDUCER (Refer to Fig. 8–3)

The transducer is prepared for use in the following manner:

1. The transducer is connected to the male-female Luer assembly of one end of the flushing manifold.

2. By means of an attached three-way stopcock, the sidearm of the transducer is opened to air.

3. A heparinized solution of 5 per cent dextrose in water, Ringer's Lactate, or saline is gently flushed through the chamber in order to evacuate all the air. The solution will exit from the sidearm and its stopcock.

4. Flushing is stopped, the sidearm is closed off, and the manifold flow is arranged so that the pressure catheter is directly connected to the transducer.

Appendix C

ECG PREAMPLIFIER

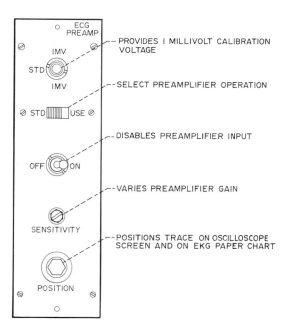

1. Turn on the power supply switch and the oscilloscope and/or the strip-chart recorder.

2. Set the STD-USE switch to STD.

3. Turn ON-OFF switch to OFF.

4. Adjust the POSITION control to the center of the oscilloscope screen or strip-chart recorder paper.

5. Turn ON-OFF switch to ON.

6. Press and hold the 1 millivolt switch and adjust SENSITIVITY control until the desired calibration is reached (10 small vertical divisions on ECG paper).

7. Turn ON-OFF switch to OFF.

8. Set STD-USE switch to USE and the ON-OFF switch to ON. The preamplifier is now ready for operation.

CARRIER (PRESSURE) PREAMPLIFIER

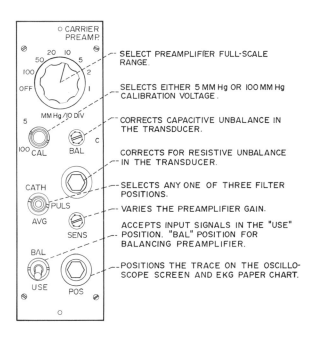

Balancing the Preamplifier

1. Set the ON-OFF switch on the power supply to ON.

2. Set the USE-BAL switch to BAL.

3. Set the ATTENUATOR to OFF (full counterclockwise position).

4. Set the SENS control to the full clockwise position.

5. Set the CATH-PULS-AVG switch to PULS.

6. Center the trace on the cardioscope or the strip-chart paper with the POSITION control.

7. Set the ATTENUATOR to the ×100 position and adjust the C-BALANCE control for a minimum output (minimum deflection).

8. Adjust the R-BALANCE for minimum output.

9. Repeat the C and R-BALANCE adjustments until minimum output is obtained.

10. Turn the ATTENUATOR switch, increasing the sensitivity one step at a time. Check that there is no deflection under "no signal" conditions. If any deflection occurs, and as soon as the deflection is observed, adjust the R-BALANCE control to recenter the trace (zero signal setting) before proceeding to the next step on the ATTENU-ATOR.

11. Return the ATTENUATOR switch to OFF.

12. Set the USE-BAL switch to USE.

Calibration and Operation

1. The calibration voltage (often provided by pumping sphygmomanometer air against the transducer) is applied to the preamplifier through the source. Therefore, the transducer must be connected to the preamplifier input for proper calibration.

2. Calibrate the preamplifier as follows:

   a. Set the monitor to a zero reference level (usually center scale) with the preamplifier POSITION control.

   b. Set the ATTENUATOR to the desired full-scale range.

   c. Switch and hold the CAL switch to either the 5 or 100 mm Hg position.

   d. Adjust the SENS control for the desired deflection with either of the calibration voltages applied to the preamplifier.

   e. Return the CAL switch to the center position.

The preamplifier is now ready for operation.

Appendix D

BEDSIDE MONITORING UNIT

CARDIAC SURGERY PHYSIOLOGIC MONITORING

DATA DISPLAY

Physiologic Parameter	Meter Read-out	Oscilloscope	Recording	Alarm Condition	Audio Signal
Arterial pressure					
Systolic		✓	✓	Pressure > 190 mm Hg Systolic or < 50 Diastolic mm Hg	On alarm condition
Diastolic					
Mean	✓				
Pulse pressure				pulse pressure < 15 mm Hg	
Central Venous Pressure (CVP)	✓				
Left Atrial Pressure (LAP)	✓			> 25 mm Hg	
Electrocardiogram Heart rate	✓			Rate >140 or 160 beats per min	
Wave form		✓	✓		On QRS
Temperature	✓				
Plethysmograph (ear, nose, or finger)		✓	✓		
Electroencephalogram		✓	✓		

CENTRAL MONITORING SYSTEM

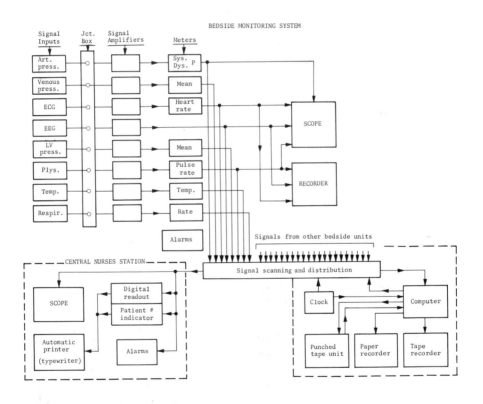

CHAPTER 9

Cardiopulmonary Resuscitation

By ALBERT D. HALL, M.D.,
and RICHARD G. SANDERSON, M.D.

Introduction

Because the nurse is frequently the first person to encounter a patient who has a cardiac arrest, it is essential that she be able to diagnose the condition and to carry out resuscitation procedures. This chapter is meant to describe the essentials of the procedures taken in cardiopulmonary resuscitation.

Cardiac arrest is the sudden and unexpected cessation of cardiac output. This can be due to cardiac asystole, ventricular fibrillation, or profound cardiovascular collapse. Unless it is known that the patient is in the terminal phases of an incurable disease, it can be assumed that the condition is reversible and resuscitation feasible. Although there have been individual successful resuscitation efforts extending back several centuries, it was only recently recognized that it is possible to sustain life by manually compressing the heart to provide circulation while the lungs are being artificially ventilated to oxygenate the blood. Current nonoperative resuscitation techniques have evolved and become generally utilized because of the introduction of external cardiac compression (1960), electrical defibrillation (1947), mouth-to-mouth air insufflation, and control of metabolic and pharmacologic derangements.

The primary initial event leading to cardiopulmonary arrest may be either circulatory or pulmonary. When one system ceases to function adequately, the other rapidly fails; therefore, resuscitation generally must provide for support of both circulation and respiration. When circulation suddenly ceases, evidence of inadequate cerebral perfusion is seen within 30 to 40 seconds. This is manifest by loss of consciousness, gasping respiration, and finally apnea and dilatation of the pupils.

In hospitalized patients, such circulatory arrest occurs most frequently in association with myocardial infarction, hemorrhage, electrolyte imbalance (hyper- or hypokalemia), drug toxicity (digitalis), hypersensitivity reactions (serum, penicillin), CNS trauma, effects of anesthetic drugs, heart block, intracardiac manipulation (cardiac catheterization), or in relation to cardiac operations. In each instance, prompt artificial resuscitation of circulation and ventilation can lead to restoration of spontaneous function. This is known in Europe as "reanimation."

Cardiac arrest induced primarily by inadequate oxygenation of blood can be more insidious in its clinical appearance. As progressively more hypoxic and acidotic blood is circulated, only subtle manifestations of the impending cardiac standstill or ventricular fibrillation may be initially recognized. A restless and hyperventilating patient must be considered hypoxic until proven otherwise, since he may well be in a state of precardiac arrest. The major conditions that lead to such hypoxia in the hospitalized patient include airway obstruction, regurgitation of gastric contents, CNS depression from any cause, neuromuscular paralysis from trauma, disease, or drugs, and lack of oxygen in the inspired air as may occur with failure or disruption of mechanical ventilators.

Prompt diagnosis and expeditious mobilization of an organized team is the key to successful resuscitation. Since delay of two or three minutes can lead to irreversible cerebral damage, it is crucial that time is not wasted unnecessarily in the attempt to confirm that the patient has a cardiac arrest. Evidence of profoundly inadequate ventilation or perfusion is sufficient indication for initiation of resuscitative measures. The precise diagnosis of cardiac standstill, ventricular fibrillation, or profound cardiopulmonary collapse need not be differentiated initially. It should not be assumed that cardiac arrest is an absolute diagnosis that need be confirmed by prolonged observation of the patient before the call for help is sounded and the resuscitation is begun.

The nurse who suspects that a patient is in a precardiac arrest has ample justification to call the cardiac arrest team, since such a team (composed of cardiologists, surgeon, anesthesiologist, ECG technician, and others) is in a unique position to provide instant multidisciplinary consultation, a reservoir of manpower, and the supplies and equipment necessary to effect a resuscitation.

Although all the elements of resuscitation may not be required in every case, patients who have suddenly deteriorated are given the benefit of maximum professional care when the nurse calls the cardiac arrest signal early, rather than too late. The nurse should not be criticized for "hitting the panic button" prematurely. Many more patients can be resuscitated before cardiac arrest occurs by appropriately administered assisted ventilation, by correction of metabolic disturbances, or by use of pharmacologic agents for control of arrhythmias or other cardiac disturbances. Liberalization of the use of the cardiac arrest team is encouraged to increase its effectiveness and to reassure nurses who are criticized for calling "when the patient didn't need us."

Choice of the Patient

Modern techniques of cardiopulmonary resuscitation (CPR) have been proven to be quite successful, and these techniques should be utilized in all patients who might reasonably be expected to resume a normal existence when the resuscitative effort succeeds.

However, vigorous resuscitation efforts do not have to be applied to every patient who suffers a cardiac arrest. Some patients who are in the terminal stages of an incurable disease—terminal cancer, end-stage disease of the kidney, liver, heart, or cerebrovascular systems—should be allowed to "die with dignity." To resuscitate them would only be to return them to a painful, uncomfortable existence in which there would be no hope of a worthwhile survival. The decision as to which patients are not to be resuscitated should not be left to the nurse alone, for this responsibility lies primarily with the physician. Both the nurse and the physician have information and points of view about a dying patient, and it is not unethical or medically inappropriate for them to discuss the eventuality of resuscitation when the patient enters into the terminal phases of his disease.

These comments should not be construed as a restraint in applying resuscitative techniques to the vast majority of patients who would benefit from the procedure. By all means, if there are any questions about the applicability of CPR, or if the patient is not well known to the attending personnel, every possible effort should be extended to these patients.

Recognition of Cardiac (or Pulmonary) Arrest

Emphasis is placed once again upon the urgency of the situation. Recognition of an arrest must be prompt and presumptive. Valuable time should not be lost in a lengthy confirmation of the absence of pulses or respiration. Rather, the CPR "team" should be mobilized when there is a reasonable suspicion that an arrest has occurred; it is far better to call for help for a moribund patient than to allow a delay which might prevent his recovery.

Many seriously ill cardiac patients are cared for in the setting of a coronary or an intensive care unit. Such a patient is often monitored by both the electrocardiogram and a heart rate meter with alarm systems. A cardiac arrest may appear on the monitoring oscilloscope — as ventricular fibrillation or asystole — or it may first be detected when the audio signal sounds for low heart rate. Although many times such an alarm signal is triggered by excessive patient motion, an ECG lead coming loose or by other artifacts, each such alarm must be thought of as "the real thing." The nurse goes immediately to the bedside and checks the patient for an arrest.

In the event the patient is not being monitored, the nurse must make an immediate clinical appraisal of the patient's cardiovascular status. In the patient who has no observable respiratory excursions of the chest, the absence of breath sounds from the nose or mouth can best be detected by placing the ear directly over the nose. Respiratory obstruction (as from aspirated vomitus) should be suspected if the patient is moving his chest but no air is moving through his nose or mouth. Cyanosis of the skin is not a reliable sign of respiratory or cardiac arrest, as many patients can exhibit peripheral cyanosis during periods of hypoxemia or low cardiac output in the absence of an arrest.

When the nurse suspects a cardiac arrest she should first attempt to arouse the patient. This can be done by striking a blow to the sternum with the heel of the hand—a maneuver which will occasionally restore respiration and cardiac activity. She should immediately check for dilatation of the pupils and search for a palpable central (i.e., carotid or femoral) pulse (Fig. 9–1). Pupils will dilate within 45 seconds after effective cardiac output has ceased, but irreversible brain damage usually does not occur for another three to four minutes. This interval is critical and the circulation must be restored during this time if permanent central nervous system damage is to be avoided. Often the exact time of the cardiac arrest is unknown, reducing even further the short interval during which successful CPR can be accomplished.

The absence of a palpable carotid or femoral pulse is a more

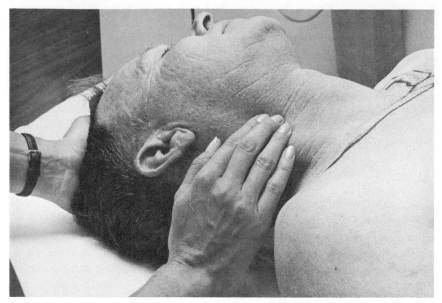

Figure 9–1.   Palpation of the carotid pulse. The index, middle, and ring fingers of one hand press inward on the anterior neck just inside the sternocleidomastoid muscle and about three fingerbreadths below the angle of the patient's jaw.

reliable sign of an arrest than absent peripheral (radial or dorsalis pedis) pulses. Patients with peripheral arterial occlusive disease or with low cardiac output may lack the peripheral pulses yet still have palpable femoral or carotid pulsations. Listening for heart sounds may be somewhat misleading, as the heart may still be beating without any appreciable output of blood. Resuscitation should be started whenever central pulses are absent, even if the heart is contracting feebly; the brain must be protected from anoxia.

The ABCs of Cardiopulmonary Resuscitation

AIRWAY

Obstruction to the passage of air is a very common precursor to cardiorespiratory arrest. In a patient who is unconscious (as in a severe stroke) or who is awakening from deep anesthesia, airway obstruction may be caused by the base of the tongue falling backward against the posterior wall of the pharynx (Fig. 9–2). Another common cause of an obstructed airway is the aspiration or regurgita-

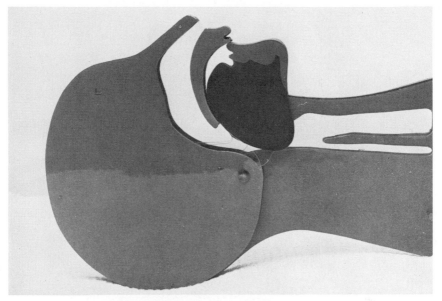

Figure 9-2. Model of the head and neck, showing airway obstruction by the base of the tongue. Note that the head is resting on its occiput, causing mild flexion of the neck. In this position, the tongue obstructs the airway completely.

tion of food, vomitus, or a foreign body into the posterior oropharynx or upper respiratory tract.

When a suction apparatus is available, these materials may be aspirated from the pharynx (and trachea) through a large-bore tubing. When no suction is available, obstructing materials in the oropharynx can be removed by turning the patient's head to one side, and swabbing the hypopharynx and oral cavity with two or three fingers wrapped with an absorbent material.

Most airway obstructions can be easily reversed by any maneuver which separates the flaccid tongue from the posterior wall of the pharynx. The two most easily performed maneuvers are hyperextension of the head and anterior displacement of the jaw bone (mandible). Hyperextension of the head is best accomplished by lifting the patient's neck while forcibly applying downward and backward pressure on the forehead. In this way, the patient will come to rest "on the top of his head," the head will be hyperextended at the junction between the top of the vertebral column and the base of the skull, and the tongue will be raised off the posterior pharyngeal wall, thus relieving the obstruction (Fig. 9-3).

Anterior displacement of the mandible can easily be accomplished by inserting the thumb into the mouth at the corner, hooking it behind the teeth or gum margin, and lifting upward. Alternatively,

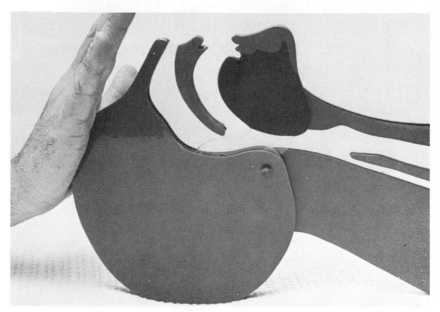

Figure 9–3.   Model of head and neck, held in extension. Simple hyperextension of the head on the neck has caused the tongue to be lifted off the posterior pharyngeal wall, relieving the airway obstruction.

the hands are placed at the angles of the patient's jaw (on both sides) and the mandible is forcibly elevated anteriorly. This latter method is particularly useful if mouth-to-mouth inspired air resuscitation (see the section on breathing) is to be used, as the thumbs of the hands may also be pressed against the patient's nose, preventing air loss from this area.

Once an open airway has been established (by the techniques discussed before), the placement of a nasopharyngeal or oropharyngeal tube may be useful to maintain its patency. These tubes are often available in special care units and can be used as an adjunct in preventing the tongue from slipping backward against the posterior pharyngeal wall. Further, these tubes provide an unobstructed route for air passage when a tightly fitting face mask is applied and ventilation is accomplished through it.

Finally, an orotracheal or nasotracheal tube provides the most definitive way of delivering air to the patient's tracheobronchial tree. These tubes, placed through the mouth or nose, pass beneath the tongue, up into the larynx, between the vocal cords, and then pass into the trachea. They provide an assured, unobstructed route for air to enter directly into the lungs. Further, they usually have attached a circumferential balloonlike cuff, which when inflated will prevent leakage of air up around the tube and will also prevent the passage of food, fluid, or mucus downward into the trachea. The placement of an orotracheal or nasotracheal tube by inexperienced personnel is not recommended, and is usually reserved for an anesthesiologist or other experienced physician.

BREATHING

Once a patent airway has been established, a few ventilations of the patient's lungs should be carried out before external cardiac compression is started. There is little use to restore blood flow to the heart and brain if the blood itself is not oxygenated.

Expired air is a perfectly adequate resuscitating gas if the resus-

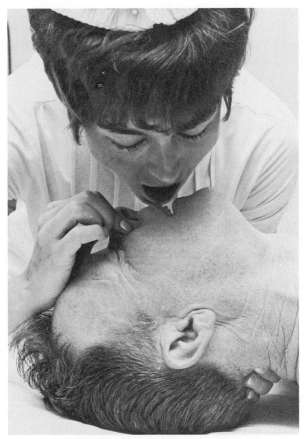

Figure 9-4. Mouth-to-mouth resuscitation. The nurse hyperextends the patient's head, pinches the nostrils, takes a deep breath, and then seals her mouth around the patient's lips as she forcibly inflates his lungs.

citator hyperventilates herself. If her own ventilation is doubled, the oxygen concentration of her expired breath is quite satisfactory (about 18 per cent, as opposed to 20 per cent for room air) and will be effective in oxygenating the patient's blood once blood flow is established.

Expired air ventilation can be accomplished by mouth-to-mouth or mouth-to-nose resuscitation. If the patient's head is held in hyperextension by heel of the hand pressing the forehead backward, and the thumb and index finger occluding the nostrils, mouth-to-mouth ventilation can easily be accomplished (Fig. 9–4). The resuscitator takes a large breath, opens her mouth widely to seal her lips against the patient's mouth, and expires forcibly into the patient until his chest expands. As soon as the "artificial" inspiration is complete, the resuscitator breaks her seal with the patient's mouth, breathes out, and listens to the air which escapes from the patient's mouth. As soon as the patient's exhalation is complete, a new cycle of ventilation is begun. When CPR is first started, the ventilatory cycles are repeated rapidly to "hyperventilate" the patient. Once the lungs are adequately re-expanded by this technique, only 10 to 15 inflations are necessary every minute. If one person is performing the resuscitation alone (before help arrives), two to three inflations are followed by 15 external cardiac compressions (see the section on circulation); this cycle then starts again. When help arrives, the lungs should be inflated after every four to five cardiac compressions.

The technique of mouth-to-nose resuscitation is useful when the patient is edentulous and a good "seal" is hard to effect or when the resuscitator's mouth is much smaller than the patient's. With this technique, the patient's jaw is elevated by pressure upward on the chin and the lips are closed by pressure of the thumb on the lower lip. Hyperextension of the head is equally as necessary as with the mouth-to-mouth technique. The resuscitator's mouth is then sealed around the patient's nose and forceful inflation applied. Exhalation by the patient may be facilitated by allowing the chin to fall back and the lips to open. The cycle is then started again.

In infants, the resuscitator's mouth is usually too large for either the mouth or nose alone. Therefore, the resuscitator seals her mouth around both nose and mouth of the infant. The volume of expired air which is "breathed" into the infant should be less, and can be gauged by his respiratory excursions; the rate of breathing should be increased to 20 to 30 times per minute.

When a face mask and self-refilling reservoir bag is available, they should be utilized, particularly if the bag can be filled with 100 per cent oxygen. These masks are usually equipped with a nonrebreathing valve so that oxygen enters the patient's lungs, but his exhaled air is routed to the room rather than back into the reservoir

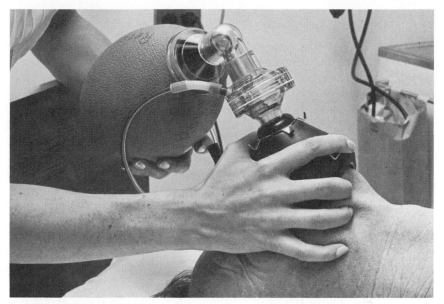

Figure 9-5. Ventilation with the face mask. The nurse presses the mask onto the patient's face with the same hand that lifts the chin, allowing the other hand to compress the reservoir bag. Note the oxygen line entering the inflow system.

bag. The most important consideration of using this technique is to achieve a good seal between the mask and the patient's face. The right-sized mask must be chosen so that it will fit snugly over the patient's nose and chin. Adequate pressure upward on the chin and downward on the face mask will usually effect an adequate seal at the corners of the mouth, even in edentulous patients. With experience, the chin and the mask can be held with one hand and the bag compressed rhythmically with the other (Fig. 9-5). If the resuscitator's hand is too small to easily squeeze the bag, it may be compressed against the patient's head to deliver a volume of gas adequate to inflate the chest.

Ventilation through an orotracheal or nasotracheal tube may be accomplished by mouth-to-tube breathing, but the use of a self-refilling reservoir bag with the tube is much easier and more efficient. The tube cuff is initially inflated with just enough air so that the cuff will barely seal against the trachea with inflation. An excessive volume or pressure in the inflated cuff will cause ischemia of the underlying tracheal mucosa; therefore, the cuff should be deflated at hourly intervals and reinflated with only enough air to prevent excessive leakage.

CIRCULATION

Circulation of oxygenated blood can be achieved by propelling blood from the arrested heart out to the lungs and to the systemic circulation, using external cardiac compression, or less often, open chest massage (internal cardiac compression).

The external method has the advantages that it can be applied immediately, it does not require special equipment or technical surgical skills, and it can be performed by paramedical personnel as well as by doctors and nurses; it is usually equally as effective as the open chest method. Internal cardiac massage is generally reserved for those patients who have previous chest injuries (especially tension pneumothorax or cardiac tamponade), who have a flail chest, or whose chest wall is so thick that effective cardiac compression cannot be produced.

The heart lies just to the left of the midline, about half way between the sternum and the vertebral column. Lateral motion of the heart is limited by the pericardium and by the attachments of the great vessels. There is considerable mobility in the thoracic walls — from the flexibility of the ribs themselves and from the joints between the ribs and the sternum and the interconnecting cartilages. When the sternum is manually depressed by about 2 inches, the heart is compressed against the vertebral column posteriorly, "squeezing"

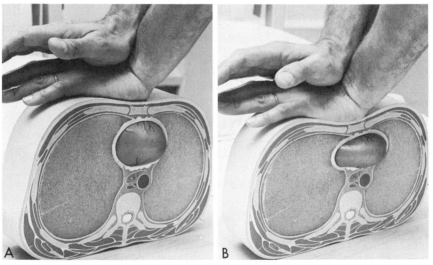

Figure 9-6. "Cutaway" section of the thorax. *A,* The heart lies between the sternum anteriorly and the vertebral column posteriorly. Note that only the heel of one hand is touching the chest. *B,* The sternum is depressed 1½ to 2 inches by the pressure exerted through the extended arms of the resuscitator, compressing the underlying heart against the vertebral column.

blood out of the ventricles into the systemic and pulmonary circulations (Fig. 9–6). When pressure on the sternum is relaxed, the chest wall recoils to its normal position and, in so doing, produces a negative pressure within the thorax, which in turn increases venous return to the heart. With this type of external cardiac compression, blood pressures in the range of 80 to 100 mm Hg systolic and 30 to 40 mm Hg diastolic can be generated, even by a petite nurse. Because of the low diastolic pressure, the mean arterial pressure is lower than normal. Blood flow (cardiac output) with external massage is about 30 to 50 per cent of normal flow.

Effective external cardiac compression requires that the thorax be supported from behind on a hard surface. As most resuscitations are carried out in bed, sternal compression would cause the unsupported bed to "bounce," thereby dissipating the force of the closed cardiac massage. Therefore, a hard surface, such as a metal dinner tray or a bed board, is placed beneath the patient's chest.

Before closed massage is started, the bony landmarks of the anterior chest wall are quickly identified. The position of the sternum is identified by feeling the suprasternal notch (above the manubrium of the sternum) and the xiphoid process at the lower end of the sternum (Fig. 9–7). As the heart is mostly underneath the lower half

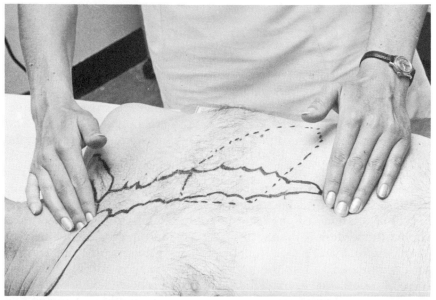

Figure 9–7. Identification of the bony landmarks. The manubrium, body, and xiphoid process of the sternum are outlined on the patient's anterior chest, along with the clavicles and the heart (dotted line). The nurse identifies the suprasternal notch and the xiphoid process before initiating closed cardiac massage over the lower half of the sternum.

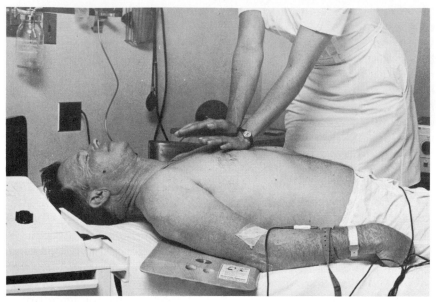

Figure 9–8. Closed cardiac massage. Note the board beneath the patient's chest. The nurse is kneeling beside the patient so that her shoulders are directly over the sternum and their weight can be transmitted directly through her extended arms.

of the sternum, pressure should be applied at the junction of the middle and lower thirds of the sternum. If pressure is applied too far inferiorly, rupture of the liver or spleen may result.

The resuscitator takes a position next to the patient's chest, usually kneeling beside him on the bed (Fig. 9–8). If the resuscitative effort is carried out at arm's length on the level, it is usually ineffective. The heel of one hand is placed at the junction of the middle and lower third of the sternum, with the fingers pointing toward the patient's side. Only the heel of the hand, not the palm or the fingers, should be in contact with the chest wall. The heel of the other hand is then placed over the first hand (Fig. 9–9). The resuscitator's arms are held in a vertical position with the elbows straight, so that the weight of the body can be used to apply the pressure to the sternum. The adult sternum is then rapidly depressed directly downward (not at an angle) by 1½ to 2 inches. The downward pressure is then rapidly released so that the patient's chest may recoil and his heart fill with blood once again. This sequence is repeated 60 to 80 times a minute for most effective circulation. Caution should be used so that excessive sternal pressure is not applied, as rib fractures (often with resultant pneumothorax), trauma to the heart, or laceration of the liver and spleen can result.

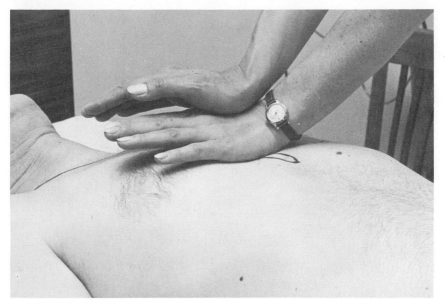

Figure 9-9. Closed cardiac massage, close-up view. Note that the heel of one hand, placed over the lower half of the sternum, is covered by the heel of the other hand. The fingers do not touch the patient's chest wall.

In children, the small chest wall is much more flexible; the pressure applied is much less. In fact, in infants, only the middle and index fingers of one hand or the thumbs of both hands are used to effect sternal depression. The rate of cardiac compression in children should be 100 to 110 per minute.

When the resuscitator is performing CPR alone, she should ventilate the lungs rapidly two to three times in the space of about 5 seconds and then compress the heart 15 times before returning for more quick breaths. When two or more persons are carrying out the resuscitation, one can provide five to six external cardiac compressions for each ventilation by the other resuscitator.

The effectiveness of the resuscitative effort can be judged by feeling for a femoral or carotid pulse. An effective resuscitation should provide an easily palpable pulse. Further, the patient's skin should become less cyanotic, the pupils should then constrict, and the patient will often start to make spontaneous movements of his chest, arms, or legs. Not uncommonly, the patient will ask the (successful) resuscitators to stop their efforts because they are hurting him.

In many institutions, some type of mechanical device is used to assist the resuscitative effort. Closed cardiac massage becomes physically tiring if it is continued for more than 10 to 15 minutes by one

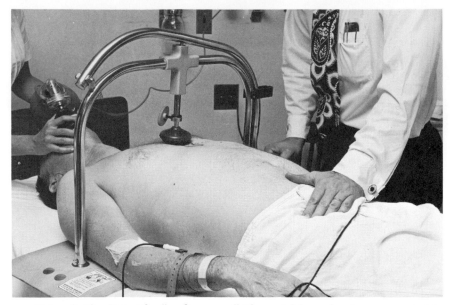

Figure 9–10. Using the "cardiac press." The metal frame has been connected to the board beneath the patient's chest. The handle is depressed with one hand leaving the other hand free to feel the femoral pulse. The patient is being ventilated with a face mask; the ECG leads are attached.

person. Effectiveness of the massage and the reproducibility of the same amount of sternal compression generally decrease as the resuscitator becomes more fatigued.

The *cardiac press* (also known as "the thumper" (Fig. 9–10) will relieve the resuscitator of considerable effort and yet provide the correct amount of sternal compression at the appropriate site. The metal frame is connected to the board beneath the patient, the compressing "knob" positioned over the junction of the middle and lower third of the sternum, and the depth of the compression is adjusted to between 1½ and 2 inches. By depressing the handle of the press, the mechanical advantage of the device will transmit through the compressing knob to the patient's sternum. The effort provided by the resuscitator is much less than with manual closed chest massage and requires only one hand, allowing the other hand to check the effectiveness of the compression (by feeling the femoral pulse).

Other devices for cardiac compression are powered by compressed air and (once adjusted) work automatically; they are particularly useful in cases in which there is a shortage of personnel. In more complicated equipment, respiratory ventilations (through an endotracheal tube) are provided automatically and synchronized with the chest compressions.

Internal cardiac compression is a significantly more extensive undertaking, requiring a scalpel blade, scissors, and rib spreaders. An endotracheal tube or tight-fitting mask is also required to provide adequate ventilation once the thorax is opened. The cardiac nurse will not be asked to perform open massage, but she should know the essentials so that she might assist a physician with this maneuver.

The chest is opened through a thoracotomy incision, usually placed anteriorly. In the postoperative cardiac surgical patient, the previous incision is simply reopened. The ribs are then held apart, preferably with a rib spreader. As the lung is retracted to the side, the pericardium is opened longitudinally, exposing the underlying heart. If the patient's heart is small, one hand can be used to provide cardiac massage. With a large heart, two hands are necessary to apply pressure—first to the apex and then sequentially toward the base of the heart, forcing blood out into the great vessels. The same parameters are used to monitor the effectiveness of open cardiac massage as for closed cardiac massage—pupillary constriction, a palpable pulse, and spontaneous movements.

Definitive Therapy (the DEFs of Cardiopulmonary Resuscitation)

The "definitive therapy" for cardiopulmonary resuscitation requires additional equipment and techniques beyond that used in mouth-to-mouth resuscitation and closed cardiac massage. Drug administration requires a route of access to the blood stream (a large-bore catheter in a vein), electrocardiographic interpretation requires an ECG machine, and fibrillation (ventricular) must be treated by a defibrillatory shock from an external defibrillator.

As soon as the CPR team comes to the patient's bedside, one member immediately establishes a route for intravenous administration of pharmacologic agents. During a cardiac arrest, peripheral veins are decompressed and poorly visible, making percutaneous puncture difficult and unreliable. Therefore, a venous cutdown is quickly performed; the great saphenous vein, as it overlies the medial malleolus at the ankle, is constant in its location and easily accessible (Fig. 9–11). The long plastic catheter is threaded into the vein, and a three-way stopcock is interposed between the catheter and the intravenous administration set so that drugs may be given directly into the venous system.

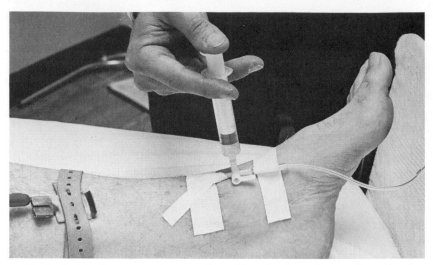

Figure 9–11. Venous cutdown at the ankle. The large bore catheter has been inserted into the great saphenous vein, taped securely in place, and connected through a three-way stopcock to the intravenous administration set.

DRUGS

An arrested heart must be brought to an appropriate metabolic condition if it is to respond to the resuscitative effort. Cardiac arrest quickly leads to hypoxemia and severe metabolic acidosis; these deleterious features must be reversed if CPR is to be successful. Even with effective CPR, cardiac output is reduced below normal and the metabolic abnormalities must be corrected. The prompt and effective administration of drugs to combat acidosis, to strengthen myocardial contractility, and to reduce ventricular irritability is of primary importance if a successful outcome is to be achieved.

Drugs to Combat Acidosis

The rapid fall in blood pH occasioned by a cardiac arrest must be reversed if the patient's heart is to respond to his own (intrinsic) or administered (extrinsic) catecholamines. Sodium bicarbonate is the agent most commonly used to combat the acidosis of cardiac arrest. In adults, a 50 ml dose (4.75 gm or 44.6 mEq) is injected intravenously every eight to 10 minutes during the arrest situation or until arterial blood pH has been shown to return to normal. In children, half this dosage is used. Sodium bicarbonate is also supplied as a 5 per cent solution in 500 ml bottle (about 60 mEq in each 100 ml); continuous intravenous administration of 75 ml every eight to 10 minutes will provide the same buffering effect as the 50 ml ampule of sodium bicarbonate.

Tham-E (tromethamine with electrolytes, known also as tris-hydroxy buffer) is a potent buffering agent which is used to combat severe metabolic acidosis. It has the advantages that it contains only 30 mEq of sodium per liter of the .3 Molar (M) solution (as opposed to 44 mEq of sodium per 50 ml of the concentrated sodium bicarbonate solution), and that it reverses the acidosis very rapidly. However, blood pH must be closely monitored during the administration of Tham-E because of its potency. The drug has the additional disadvantage that it takes a few minutes to prepare; the lyophilized powder is mixed with 1000 ml sterile water for injection to make the .3 M solution. The dosage of Tham-E to correct a given metabolic acidosis is calculated by the following simple formula:

$$\text{Tham-E required (ml of .3 M solution)} =$$
$$\text{body weight (Kg)} \times \text{base deficit (mEq/L)}$$

Drugs to Strengthen Myocardial Contractility

Epinephrine has been found to be a most useful agent because it fulfills two roles. Not only does it strengthen ventricular contractions but it also provides an increased perfusion pressure by its vasopressor effect. Since the cardiotonic effect of epinephrine is produced immediately upon reaching the heart, it should be given as soon as possible, even before an electrocardiogram is recorded. After epinephrine is administered, external cardiac compression will produce a higher pressure, and spontaneous cardiac activity will improve (assuming a reasonable acid-base balance). The route of administration of the drug will depend upon the clinical situation.

Often, a large-bore intravenous drip is not immediately available, or there is considerable delay in establishing a venous cutdown. An immediate effect is required and intracardiac injection of the drug is the quickest route available under these circumstances. In a 10 ml syringe, 1 mg of epinephrine (1 ml of the 1:1000 solution) is diluted with 9 ml of saline. A 3½ inch No. 22 (intracardiac) needle is attached and the intracardiac injection can then be given by either the left parasternal or the subxiphoid route.

In the left parasternal route, the needle is inserted through the fourth or fifth intercostal space, lateral to the sternum, angling the needle slightly upward and backward toward the vertebral column (Fig. 9–12). Suction with the syringe is maintained until blood is aspirated from one of the cardiac chambers (usually the left or right ventricle) and then 5 to 10 ml (0.5 to 1.0 mgm epinephrine) is admin-

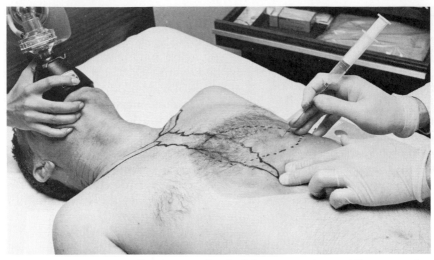

Figure 9–12. Intracardiac injection by the left parasternal route. The intracardiac needle is directed from a point about two inches to the left of the sternum in the fifth intercostal space toward the vertebral column. The flexible No. 22 needle is grasped firmly until it traverses the chest wall; then suction is maintained on the syringe until blood is aspirated from a cardiac chamber.

istered directly into that chamber. The needle is then withdrawn. During the parasternal injection, the pleura and sometimes the left lung itself is punctured; a pneumothorax should therefore be looked for in the postresuscitation care of the patient.

In the subxiphoid injection, the needle is inserted just below the xiphoid process and directed toward the tip of the left scapula (Fig. 9–13). In this route, the needle will pass through the diaphragm to enter the heart (usually the right ventricle). Again, suction is maintained until blood is aspirated, the drug is then given directly into the heart, and the needle is removed. It may be necessary to repeat the 0.5 mgm dose of epinephrine every three to five minutes.

As an intravenous drip, 2 to 4 mgm of epinephrine (2 to 4 ml of the 1:1000 solution) is added to 250 ml of IV fluid. The drip is adjusted to infuse 0.5 mgm every four to five minutes.

Another valuable agent used to strengthen myocardial contractility is isoproterenol (Isuprel), particularly if a bradycardia is present. Usually isoproterenol is given as an intravenous drip, utilizing 1 to 2 mgm of the drug per 250 ml of IV fluid. The drip is adjusted so that 0.1 to 0.2 mgm is infused every four to five minutes. Unfortunately, isoproterenol causes peripheral vasodilatation and may lower the perfusion pressure developed by cardiac compression. Coronary blood flow may decrease under these conditions and therefore a vaso-

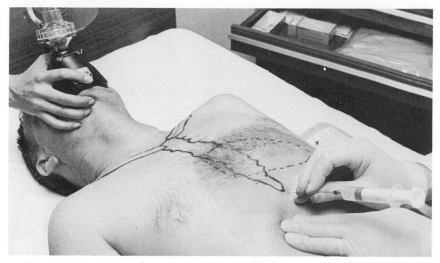

Figure 9–13. Intracardiac injection by the subxiphoid route. The skin surrounding the injection site has been rapidly prepped with iodine. The needle is inserted at a point just beside the xiphoid process and is directed toward the tip of the left scapula.

pressor (levarterenol, phenylephrine, and so forth) may be given simultaneously to raise the perfusion pressure.

Calcium chloride or calcium gluconate may also be useful in stimulating myocardial activity. When hypoxemia and metabolic acidosis are severe, there often is an imbalance of potassium and calcium ions in the heart muscle cells, with potassium "leaking" out of the cell. Calcium is administered in 0.5 to 1.0 gm doses every 10 minutes in order to restore the balance of these ions and to provide increased myocardial contractility.

Drugs to Reduce Ventricular Irritability

During a cardiac arrest situation, particularly when coronary occlusion is the etiology, ischemic areas in the ventricular myocardium may become very irritable. Ventricular fibrillation or ventricular tachycardia may appear repeatedly, starting from one of these irritable foci. The administration of agents to depress these areas will increase the likelihood that electrical defibrillation will be successful and that ventricular fibrillation will not recur.

Probably the most effective and commonly used drug to suppress irritable myocardial foci is lidocaine (Xylocaine). An intravenous injection of 50 to 100 mgm of lidocaine, repeated at intervals of three to five minutes, may suppress the arrhythmia. Often, these "stat" doses are supplemented by an intravenous drip containing 250 to 500 mgm lidocaine in 250 ml of IV fluid. During the arrest, the drip is adjusted to infuse 1 to 4 mgm per minute; when the patient is successfully resuscitated and his condition stabilized (over a period of hours), the drip may then be slowed.

Procainamide (Pronestyl), in doses of 100 to 250 mgm, may be administered intravenously every two to six hours to provide a more prolonged antiarrhythmic effect. Quinidine gluconate, a parenteral preparation given in doses of 100 to 250 mgm, provides a similar control of the myocardial irritability. Occasionally, diphenylhydantoin (Dilantin) or propranolol (Inderal) may be necessary to control the ventricular arrhythmias brought on with the cardiac arrest.

ELECTROCARDIOGRAMS DURING CARDIOPULMONARY RESUSCITATION

Many of the techniques that have been discussed previously can be accomplished without an electrocardiogram (ECG). If the patient was monitored by an electrocardiogram when he arrested, so much the better.

The ECG machine or monitor may be connected to the patient by either plate, needle, or "stick-on" electrodes. As the patient's ECG will probably be compared to his prearrest tracing, the routine limb lead positions should be used to facilitate this comparison. The continuous oscilloscopic display of the patient's ECG is preferable to the brief, intermittent "write-out" obtained by a direct-writing recorder; the combination of the two techniques is ideal. Although isolation circuits are now available in some ECG recorders, many machines will "burn out" if they remain connected to the patient when he is defibrillated.

A patient with the clinical findings of a cardiopulmonary arrest may show either ventricular asystole, ventricular fibrillation, or other ventricular rhythms which are inadequate to produce any appreciable cardiac output (e.g., severe bradycardia, ventricular tachycardia). The descriptions of these patterns have been previously discussed in Chapter 4. No matter which pattern is represented, the techniques of CPR should be carried out until an acceptable ECG pattern is obtained; closed chest massage and artificial ventilation are continued until an effective spontaneous pulse can be palpated.

Ventricular asystole shows a straight or slightly wandering baseline, indicating severe hypoxia or myocardial depression. Drugs to stimulate myocardial contractility are administered as acid-base disturbances are corrected. Under these conditions, the heart will often revert to a severe bradycardia or ventricular fibrillation. The bradycardia can then be stimulated to a faster, more effective rhythm by the administration of isoproterenol and the ventricular fibrillation can then be terminated by defibrillation (see later).

DEFIBRILLATION

If the application of a defibrillating electric shock is to be successful in terminating ventricular fibrillation, the heart muscle must be well oxygenated and near normal in regard to acid-base balance. The fibrillatory ECG pattern should be vigorous, with (relatively) high-voltage oscillations, occurring 400 to 500 times per minute. If the ventricular fibrillatory baseline is wandering in a desultory fashion, defibrillation will probably be unsuccessful.

The electrical shock is applied along the long axis of the heart, and is intended to depolarize every individual muscle fiber completely and simultaneously. Then the highest cardiac pacemaker (usually the SA node) will emerge, initiate a new impulse, and thereby replace the incoordinated fibrillatory activity with a coordinated synchronous pattern, hopefully sinus rhythm. If all fibers are not depolarized, one area may remain irritable and may re-establish ventricular fibrillation in all the fibers.

Various devices have been developed to provide the defibrillatory electrical shock. In general, two types are currently used—the alternating current (AC) and the direct current (DC) defibrillators. In the AC defibrillator, the 110 volt 60 cycle alternating wall current is raised by step-up transformers to an appropriate level. Discharge of this current takes place over 0.25 seconds (15 cycles of a 60 cycle current) and 440 to 880 volts is usually given for external defibrillation. Internal defibrillation usually requires between 120 and 180 volts over 0.1 to 0.15 seconds (six to nine cycles).

With direct current defibrillators, the voltage is stored in capacitors. When the appropriate level is achieved, the capacitors discharge the stored energy very rapidly, usually in 4 to 5 milliseconds (4/1000ths of a second). This type of impulse is thought to be slightly more effective in defibrillation and less damaging to the patient's tissues than is the alternating current defibrillation. External DC defibrillation usually requires between 300 and 400 watt-seconds (or joules) and internal DC defibrillation is usually accomplished with 15 to 40 watt-seconds (joules).

External defibrillation electrodes, usually at least 10 cm in diameter, should be lightly covered with a conductive electrode paste to provide good contact with the patient's chest. The handles of the electrodes are well insulated so that the person performing the defibrillation is protected from the electrical shock. One electrode is

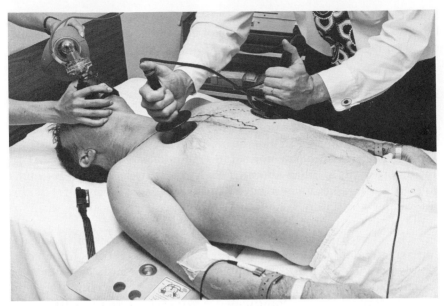

Figure 9–14. External defibrillation. Electrode paste has been applied liberally to the defibrillating paddles, which are positioned across the long axis of the heart—one at the apex and one at the base. Note that the persons defibrillating and ventilating the patient are careful not to contact the bed (the nurse ventilating the patient will momentarily release the face mask and bag as the defibrillating shock is applied). Note also that the ECG machine plug has been disconnected just before defibrillation is performed.

placed over the apex of the heart (usually the anterior axillary line in the left fifth intercostal space) and the other over the base of the heart (the second right intercostal space beside the sternum) (Fig. 9–14). Just before the defibrillating shock is applied, each person of the resuscitating team, including the defibrillator, is cautioned to stand clear of the patient and his bed, so that the electrical shock is not transmitted to them. Contact to the patient is made only through the insulated defibrillator electrodes. The electrodes are pressed firmly against the chest wall and the discharge button (either on the electrodes, on a foot pedal switch, or on the defibrillator itself) is depressed. The patient's skeletal muscles usually have a brief generalized contraction, causing him to "jump" slightly off the bed. A mild erythema is usually seen at the site of electrode application.

Because of persistent irritable myocardial foci or because of inadequate "metabolic" preparation of the heart, the defibrillatory shock may be unsuccessful or only transiently successful. Drugs to depress these irritable foci are then given and the defibrillatory shock repeated until an acceptable cardiac rhythm is achieved.

In internal defibrillation, the electrode paddles, usually flat plates 6 to 8 cm in diameter, are applied directly to the heart itself.

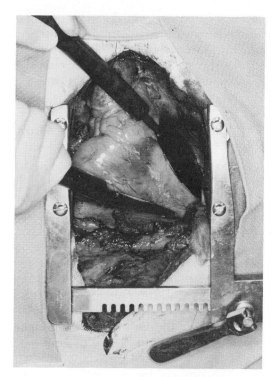

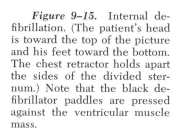

Figure 9-15. Internal defibrillation. (The patient's head is toward the top of the picture and his feet toward the bottom. The chest retractor holds apart the sides of the divided sternum.) Note that the black defibrillator paddles are pressed against the ventricular muscle mass.

Often, gauze sponges soaked in saline are wrapped around the paddles to prevent epicardial burns. One paddle is held on the left side of the heart (next to the left ventricle) and the other paddle is pressed against the right ventricle and atrium (Fig. 9-15). As with external defibrillation, personnel should avoid contact with the patient during the discharge of the electrical shock.

The cardiac nurse is rarely, if ever, asked to perform internal defibrillation; however, many institutions allow qualified and well trained nurses to defibrillate patients externally, even when the physician is not present. If a competent nurse is able to accurately diagnose ventricular fibrillation and eliminate artifact in the arrest situation, she should not be restrained from defibrillating the patient. Often the cardiac nurse is immediately available to the patient when he goes into ventricular fibrillation. In order not to lose the advantage of immediate defibrillation during the very brief "golden period" (before hypoxia, acidosis, and cardiac irritability become fully evident), the nurse should be allowed to defibrillate the patient.

Each institution establishes its own procedures for the nurse in these situations and these guidelines should be fully understood by the nurse starting her work in an intensive care or coronary care unit. Often the medical director of the unit will train the nurses in defibril-

lation by teaching her the correct techniques during elective cardio-
versions on patients with arrhythmias. Once he is convinced that the
cardiac nurse can recognize ventricular fibrillation, can diagnose
cardiac arrest, and can correctly defibrillate, he can then authorize
her to perform defibrillation under emergency arrest situations.

Termination of the Resuscitation

The resuscitative effort is stopped when clinical evidence shows
that it has been either a success or a failure. A successful resuscitation
is evidenced by a resumption of a strong palpable pulse, pupillary
constriction, spontaneous purposeful movements, independent
respiratory effort, and a stable electrocardiogram.

The decision to discontinue the resuscitative effort because of
failure is much more difficult. It is a simple fact that some patients
cannot be resuscitated, even though the resuscitation is correctly
performed and the metabolic conditions are appropriate. Before
stopping, the resuscitative effort should be reviewed for the adequacy
of ventilatory support, the production of a palpable pulse with cardiac
compression, the normalcy of acid-base balance, and the use of the
appropriate cardiac drugs.

The criteria for discontinuing resuscitation (after assuring that
the effort was adequate) include (1) dilated fixed pupils, a flat enceph-
alogram, and cessation of spontaneous respirations or other movements; (2) persistent myocardial failure and inadequate cardiac output
after the heart has been successfully defibrillated; (3) the inability
to defibrillate or to maintain defibrillation; (4) the lack of improvement
in the ECG or pulses after one hour of CPR; and (5) the lack of
response to the administered cardiotonic, vasopressor, or antiarrhythmic drugs.

Although the decision to abandon the resuscitation is difficult,
especially in younger patients, it must be made when the resuscitation has been proven to be unsuccessful. The responsibility for the
decision belongs to the physician, particularly to the physician who
is in charge of the patient's care. He alone can bring together all the
many facets of the patient's condition and the features of the resuscitation in order to arrive at the decision to discontinue the effort.

Postresuscitative Care

When a patient has been successfully resuscitated, the postresuscitative care is extremely important. The patient remains in a

very critical condition, and every effort must be extended to ensure continued improvement and to determine the underlying cause of the arrest. If the patient was not in an intensive care unit when he arrested, he should be transferred to one for the postresuscitative care.

The patient should have careful monitoring—ECG, vital signs, urine output, electrolytes, and arterial blood gases and pH. Cardiac drugs will have to be used judiciously so that blood pressure and cardiac output can be supported and arrhythmias can be held to a minimum. If bradyarrhythmias are troublesome, a temporary transvenous pacemaker can be placed. Adequate continuing ventilation is a necessity if another arrest from hypoxia is to be prevented. If the patient shows signs of central nervous system damage, the use of hypothermia, corticosteroids and anticonvulsive agents may be helpful. Finally, the cause of the arrest must be searched for and treated. Serial electrocardiograms to search for myocardial damage, portable chest films looking for a respiratory etiology, and determinations of serum electrolyte and other chemical constituents looking for a metabolic cause should all be performed. Deficiencies in any of the organ systems should be treated immediately and aggressively to prevent a recurrence of the cardiopulmonary arrest.

Bibliography

Gordon, A. S.: Cardiopulmonary Resuscitation Conference Proceedings. Washington, D.C., National Research Council, 1967.

Jude, J. R., and Elam, J. O.: Fundamentals of Cardiopulmonary Resuscitation. Philadelphia, F. A. Davis Company, 1965.

Stephenson, H. E.: Cardiac Arrest and Resuscitation. St. Louis, Missouri, C. V. Mosby Company, 1969.

SECTION III

Applying the Methods

CHAPTER 10

Nursing Care of the Medical Cardiac Patient

By CAROL CARROLL, R.N. *and* CYNTHIA BECKER, R.N.

Introduction

This chapter is designed to familiarize the registered nurse and related patient-care personnel with the nursing implications of the patient afflicted with medically treated heart disease. The nursing care setting is a coronary care unit (CCU) but the principles of care can be applied to various intensive care units (ICUs). The advent of the CCU has influenced the philosophy and art of the nursing practitioner. Although the nurse has always participated in the return of the patient to health, never before has she initiated diagnostic and therapeutic measures to reverse sudden or subtle lethal processes. The implied responsibility of such nursing actions can frighten the nurse unfamiliar with the concepts of coronary care. It is hoped that through this chapter the clinical role of the nurse in the CCU can be understood and accepted.

Material presented in this chapter will include the selection and education of nursing personnel in the specialized nursing unit, the therapeutic and educational role of the nurse in the patient-family-nurse relationship, the nursing implications in equipment use, the nursing implications in intravenous and drug therapy, and the nurse's role in the physical and emotional complications of the patient with medically treated heart disease.

Selection and Education of Nursing Personnel

The careful selection and education of nursing personnel for a CCU can reduce anxiety in both novice and experienced nurses and can heighten the sophistication of the nursing care in the unit. The use of only registered nurses is highly desirable for the successful operation of the unit. Factors determining the selection of nurses for such a unit include the motivation, the emotional make-up, and the education of each nurse. The motivation of the nurse is indicated by her stated interest in coronary care nursing and by her demonstrated ability in this or other forms of nursing. The emotional make-up of the nurse is, of course, difficult to evaluate. If the nurse can perform competently in stressful situations and is industrious during less tension-producing periods, she is probably well suited for the CCU.

Assessment of the nurse's education is a continual process. Transcripts from schools of formal nursing education and previous professional evaluations can offer clues to the nurse's theoretical and practical nursing abilities. Observation of the nurse as she performs her duties within the coronary care setting is often the best method of evaluation. If, while caring for her patients, the nurse utilizes principles of basic as well as specialized nursing care, if she attends pertinent in-service classes, if she augments formal education with meaningful reading material, and if she gleans nursing information from the care of individual patients, she can be said to be a nurse well educated for the specialized unit.

The Nurse-Patient-Family Relationship

The institution of intensive care settings has offered the nurse the opportunity to establish a realistic therapeutic relationship with her patient and his family. In progressive ICUs, the nurse-patient ratio is often 1:1 or 1:2. In such a setting, the nurse is able to closely observe and quickly report changes in a patient's emotional and physical conditions. Because the nurse has sufficient time to know her patient in his medical, emotional, and social aspects, she can attempt to educate the patient and his family in an individualized manner. Although the various physical, emotional, and socioeconomic factors of each patient overlap and interrelate, each group of factors will be discussed separately for purposes of clarity.

EMOTIONAL CARE OF THE CARDIAC PATIENT

The emotional care of patients in ICUs, while necessarily individualized, can be summarized in general terms. The individual requiring such care is in an anxiety-producing situation not only because of his disease process, but also because of the highly mechanized and procedure-oriented environment of his room or cubicle. The patient is subject to a large number of new, painful, and confusing experiences. The patient and his family are in a situation in which they must answer many questions and in which they are expected, if not coerced, to adhere to hospital and unit policy.

A primary means of reducing anxiety in CCU patients is relief of subjective symptoms. Analgesics and oxygen are given when the patient's condition warrants them. Principles of basic nursing care are, of course, utilized to provide maximum comfort for the patient requiring bed rest or only limited activity. Patient, empathetic, and frequent explanations of equipment, procedures, and medicines can resolve much of the apprehension of an alert and concerned patient. The nurse's voice and manner can be important variables to the patient's emotional state. A calm, organized performance of nursing duties and a low, distinct voice can project a well controlled environment to the patient. During a cardiac arrest or other procedures involving additional equipment and intensive medical and nursing care to an individual patient, visibility in other patient areas should be reduced and a brief explanation given to the other patients.

Throughout the patient's stay, the nurse should be attuned to the patient's behavior as an index of his anxiety. Is the patient restless? Is he diaphoretic? Does he want to see his family or does he want to be "left alone"? Does he talk continuously or not at all? Is he concerned about his disease process and its consequences? Simply watching and talking with the patient and his family can help the perceptive nurse understand the factors causing emotional distress. From this individualized observation and communication, the nurse can establish a therapeutic emotional care relationship with her patient.

In intensive care settings, in which patients can be seen at all times by the nursing staff, it should be remembered that the nursing staff is likewise continually visible to the patient. The patient who understands his disease process and his monitor or other equipment is often reassured by the nurse who vigilantly observes the monitor and who responds quickly to alarm signals and call lights. The nurse who appears lax in her performance can cause increased anxiety in her patient.

CCUs are replete with patients who suffer mild to severe psychologic responses to their prehospital, hospital, or posthospital environment. Apprehension, apathy, depression, denial, and acting-out are only a few of the many behavioral patterns the CCU nurse sees in her patients. Consultation and patient care conferences with members of the departments of psychiatry and psychology can frequently assist the nurse to accept and help the emotionally distressed patient.

PHYSICAL CARE OF THE CARDIAC PATIENT

The treatment of patients with medical heart disease varies with individual physicians and individual CCUs. In general, the care of patients with heart disease has become more flexible. Patients with serious heart disease were formerly required to have complete bed rest for days or weeks. At the present time, patients admitted to most CCUs do require limited activity, but are not necessarily required to stay in bed. Short periods of chair rest are often indicated to improve pulmonary function and also to increase the patient's morale. Bedside commodes and standing weights are often ordered because they require less energy expenditure than do bed pans or bed scale weights. Bed baths, shaving, linen change, and back care formerly prohibited are now given as part of basic nursing care. Patients are generally allowed to feed themselves and perform oral hygiene if they are alert and asymptomatic; the nurse should caution the patient against overexertion.

Patients who spend long periods of time in a recumbent position are in danger of venous stasis affecting the pelvic and leg veins. Because of the possibility of thromboembolic complications, the patient should be instructed to perform isometric leg exercises against a footboard or against the bed mattress. Elastic stockings or bandages are frequently ordered to promote venous return and should be applied in a snug but nonconstricting manner. The leg wraps are to be reapplied at least twice a day and on an "as needed" basis.

Observation and recording of vital signs are an important function of the CCU nurse. In general, nurses working in a CCU are expected to use discretion in monitoring vital signs. The patient suffering arrhythmias, acute heart failure, or shock will require frequent checking of vital signs; the stable uncomplicated patient is usually not awakened or disturbed for routine temperature and blood pressure readings. The use of rectal thermometers is still controversial for patients with heart disease; unit and medical philosophy are the determining factors for the mode of temperature measurement.

The diet of the patient with heart disease depends upon the patient's condition and the physician's medical orientation. Diets may vary from completely regular menus to low-caloric, low-salt, low-cholesterol, and pureed diets. Coffee and tea are often prohibited because of their caffeine and xanthine content. In general, patients in CCUs should have tepid liquids, as temperature extremes can cause a vagal response resulting in arrhythmias. Dietary habits are notoriously difficult to alter, and the patient and his family will require education and support. A dietician can be valuable in educating the patient and his family and in suggesting means of making the diet more palatable.

Socioeconomic and behavioral factors can influence the patient afflicted with heart disease.. If the nurse is aware of living patterns that may harm the patient's hospital and posthospital course, she may be able to offer individualized education to the patient and his family. If stress from the patient's family or employment is thought to have affected the patient's cardiac status, social service workers or vocational counselors may be consulted. The patient should be informed of the influence cigarette smoking, obesity, lack of sleep, sedentary activity, and dietary factors can have on his illness.

Equipment as an Adjunct to Medical and Nursing Care

Because nursing in a CCU implies a broad knowledge of relatively new equipment and new nursing care instruments, the following material will include a summary of equipment common to a CCU and the operation of this equipment. Intrinsic to a CCU is the use of cardiac monitors, preferably a system of centralized monitoring. Such a system entails a bedside cardiac monitor for each patient and a centrally located monitor which carries on one or more oscilloscopes the electrocardiogram of all monitored patients. This monitor arrangement allows the ECG patterns of all patients to be seen quickly and continuously. The individual bedside patient monitor enables medical and nursing personnel to see the patient's ECG as bedside care is given.

Continuous ECG monitoring commences when the patient is admitted to the nursing unit and continues throughout his acute and occasionally his convalescent hospital stay. The oscilloscope provides a constant visual representation of the electrical activity of the heart at a given moment. The clarity of the patient's ECG pattern depends largely on the proper application of the electrodes. The skin is cleansed with alcohol to reduce friction and skin resistance. Sodium-containing "paste" is applied to the electrode and to the underlying skin to further reduce skin resistance. The leads are attached to the skin (often to the skin of the chest wall) by tape or double-faced adhesive applicators. If the leads are placed on the extremities, rubber straps or tape may be used to secure them. Care should be taken that the straps or tape do not interfere with venous circulation. An allowance for "slack" in the wires prevents loss of contact between the skin and the leads. The leads are placed away from areas of voluntary muscle activity to reduce voluntary muscle artifact. In some nursing units, needle electrodes (No. 25, $5/8$ inch metal-hubbed needles) are inserted in the upper arms and thighs. Their application differs from plastic or metal leads in that aseptic technique is used and ECG paste is not used.

The time interval for lead reapplication varies with the type of lead and with the individual patient. Lead reapplication entails the same measures as the original application, but the location of the lead should be varied slightly to reduce skin irritation. Metal and needle electrodes often cause skin irritation and are changed at least every eight hours. Plastic lead reapplication is necessary only once a day unless the patient's skin condition indicates need for more frequent change.

In spite of correct lead application, electrical artifact may appear on the scope. In such a case, the nurse should attempt to ground the monitor and any other electrical equipment in the room. Artifact often results from patient movement or from patient contact with metal surfaces, such as the side rails of the bed. Occasionally reversing the plug in the outlet or moving the plug to another outlet will remove 60 cycle artifact. It is fortunate that most intensive care units are properly grounded and that problems of artifact are minimal.

Most cardiac monitors are equipped with ECG recorders or "write-outs." A legible and accurate write-out is very valuable for patient care. The monitor, while offering a continuous visual indication of electrical cardiac activity, does not provide a permanent record of this activity. Cardiac arrhythmias and artifacts can be transient, sudden, and difficult to discern on the monitor. The write-out can "prove" the existence of the arrhythmia or the artifact. The write-out thus becomes an important tool for intelligent patient therapy. In many CCUs, the write-out begins as an alarm system is sounded (see later). This aspect of the write-out is valuable in that slow or rapid heart rhythms may become apparent to the unit staff members if they did not see them on the scope. It should be noted, however, that the write-out from a monitored chest lead should be used only for interpretation of arrhythmias. Artifactual QRS, ST, and T changes may appear on such a lead, and a conventional ECG (not taken from the monitor) should be obtained for clarification of these other abnormalities.

An alarm system is a necessity for all monitored patients. The impossibility of continuously watching all monitor patterns at all times is well known to CCU personnel. The alarm system, by counting the number of R waves per given time interval, can alert nursing personnel to slow or rapid heart rates, whether or not these heart rates are actually seen. One of the primary responsibilities of the CCU nurse is that of correct placement of the alarm guards. The guards are usually set 20 points above and 20 points below the patient's normal heart rate. This 40 point differential provides a margin for artifacts (counted as R waves) caused by patient movement. In some instances, the patient may have a rapid or slow heart rate, and an increase or decrease of the rate can be life-threatening. In these conditions, the guards should be placed close to the current rate (a total margin of six to eight points) so that a change is immediately indicated.

The electrocardiogram (ECG) provides a graphic recording of the electrical heart activity at a given time and from a given direction (see also Chapter 4). The ECG consists of 12 leads, although there have been several modifications of this lead system. A full ECG provides the interpreter the opportunity of drawing conclusions about the patient's electrical heart pattern as compared to normal heart patterns. While a monitor is valuable for the diagnosis of heart rate and rhythm changes, the ECG provides information helpful in the diagnosis of myocardial infarction or ischemia, pericarditis, ventricular aneurysm, ventricular hypertrophy, and a variety of other heart and lung diseases. An ECG is usually done when the patient is admitted to the hospital, and serial tracings are often ordered. Serial ECGs are indicated, as there may be a considerable time interval between patient symptoms, the heart damage, and alterations in the ECG pattern.

A plethysmograph is a photoelectric cell encased in plastic or metal housing which when placed on the patient's ear lobe or wrist will transmit pulsatile activity to the monitor. The plethysmograph has two major uses. If a patient's alarm continues to sound because of artifact which cannot be eliminated, the plethysmograph may be attached to the patient; the alarm will then be dependent on pulse waves rather than on R waves, simulated by artifact. The plethysmograph is also indicated for use in the patient with a pacemaker. The pacemaker artifact is the impulse "counted" by the alarm system. If, because of failure to capture the ventricle, there is, in fact, no R wave but only the pacemaker artifact, the alarm will not sound. The use of the plethysmograph can obviate this unfortunate situation.

The defibrillator or cardioverter is used for the conversion of certain supraventricular and ventricular rhythms which have not responded to medication, and for the termination of ventricular fibrillation. Depending on medical indications, the termination of supraventricular tachyarrhythmias may involve countershock as the initial medical therapy. In applying countershock for a supraventricular tachycardia, the defibrillator must be synchronized to discharge on the R wave of the complex. Synchronization eliminates the possibility of a (nonsynchronized) charge being administered during the vulnerable period of heart excitability (the terminal portion of the T wave); should the electrical current be discharged at this time, ventricular tachycardia or fibrillation can result (see Fig. 8–6).

Countershock is used for ventricular tachycardia that results in unconsciousness of the patient or for ventricular tachycardia that has not responded to intravenous medication. Countershock is always indicated for the termination of ventricular fibrillation.

Proper defibrillation is achieved by application of sufficient ECG paste to cover the heads of the defibrillator paddles. The paddles then are placed in one of two ways: (1) one over the apex of the heart and one at the base of the heart, or (2) one on the anterior chest and one at the patient's back. Both of these paddle placements allow a current of electricity to pass through the long axis of the heart at the time of discharge, permitting uniform depolarization of all the heart's muscle cells. The patient's normal pacemaker should then take over the electrical activity of the heart. Occasionally, following defibrillation, ventricular tachycardia or ventricular fibrillation may persist. Countershock is repeated until another heart rhythm appears. Should asystole result from defibrillation, closed chest cardiac massage and artificial ventilation are instituted. Isuprel or electrical pacing may be necessary. Determination of the amount of the shock delivered is at the physician's discretion. A policy for defibrillation should be written in all units in which nurses are expected to defibrillate, and the minimum and maximum charges allowed to be delivered should be stipulated.

Several nursing functions are necessary for proper defibrillation. The nurse should advise all personnel to avoid touching the patient and his bed in order to prevent the electric impulse from being transmitted to them, should the paddles be applied improperly. The bed rails should be lowered and avoided during countershock. The nurse should disconnect the ECG machine if it will not withstand a 400 watt-second shock. If the paddles are charged but not used, the power can be dissipated by pulling out the wall plug.

Following successful defibrillation, medical and nursing care is planned to prevent further episodes of ventricular irritability. Some patients complain of skin irritation following countershock and the paddle burn marks are often visible. Application of petroleum jelly to affected areas is usually sufficient for patient comfort.

In describing the defibrillation in the nursing notes, the nurse documents the patient's heart pattern prior to and following countershock. The patient's level of consciousness before and after defibrillation is described. The number of countershocks and the number of watt-seconds are included.

Nursing Implications in Intravenous and Drug Therapy

TECHNICAL ASPECTS OF INTRAVENOUS THERAPY

The patient admitted to a CCU with the diagnosis of medical heart disease is in danger of disturbances of heart rhythm and rate. Because many arrhythmias can cause a precipitous drop in cardiac output, it may be impossible to perform venipuncture for the administration of intravenous medication during the acute arrhythmia period. For this reason it is policy in many CCUs that an intravenous line be kept open should the need arise for intravenous drug administration. In some units the nurses are permitted to insert "scalp vein" needles, straight needles, and indwelling venous catheters. In other units the nurse may be permitted to insert only scalp vein or straight needles, but she is responsible for the daily dressing changes at the entry point of the indwelling venous catheter. As the nurse changes the dressing she cleanses the skin at the site of the needle insertion with alcohol or other antiseptic solutions; she checks the placement of the needle guard and tapes it securely. She securely tapes the tubing remaining outside the patient's vein to the skin, to prevent the tubing from slipping into the patient's vein in the event that the tubing is shorn by the needle. She places a small amount of antibiotic ointment at the needle entry site. The nurse observes all sites of intravenous therapy for infiltration and phlebitis. Indwelling catheters are generally changed every 48 hours to reduce the possibility of infection. If there is any suspicion of infection, the tip of the removed catheter should be cultured. Notation of the date and time of insertion of the catheter on the nursing care plan or nurse's notes is a convenient reminder of the duration of catheter insertion.

The patient in a CCU is not only in danger of complicating arrhythmias; he is also in danger of congestive heart failure. For this reason, the intravenous fluid is often ordered at a rate only to "keep the vein open." Proper regulation of a small drip chamber (60 micro-drops equal 1 ml) can result in maintenance of a patient's intravenous line at only 100 to 180 ml for 24 hours.

DRUG THERAPY

Medications having effects on the cardiovascular system may alter the rate, force, and rhythm of the heart. Therefore, it is essential that the cardiac nurse be knowledgeable of the drug regimen in effect for each of her patients, have documentation of each patient's admission electrocardiogram and the ECG pattern most frequently manifested in the unit, and be able to anticipate and deal with potential changes in the patient's electrocardiogram from the medications being administered.

This section will deal with nursing implications of the medications commonly prescribed for cardiac patients. To avoid redundancy whenever possible, medications will be discussed in groups according to major effects, rather than being presented individually. The reader is referred to Chapter 7 for a more theoretical approach to drug therapy and for presentation of the commonly used dosages of each drug.

Cardiotonic Drugs

Cardiac glycosides (digitalis preparations). Digitalis preparations are most useful in the treatment of congestive heart failure and rapid arrhythmias, such as atrial fibrillation and flutter, paroxysmal atrial tachycardia (not due to digitalis toxicity), and ventricular arrhythmias. These medications act by increasing myocardial contractility (a positive inotropic effect), causing an improved cardiac output, diuresis, and a decrease in heart failure. They also increase vagal nerve stimulation, producing a slowed heart rate, and decrease conduction time through the atrioventricular node, resulting in a slowed ventricular response.

Careful measurement and recording of the patient's fluid intake and output and daily weight are necessary for the assessment of the effects of digitalis preparations. The nurse observes the patient for signs of improving cardiac function, as manifested by less dyspnea and edema, as well as increased urine production. The electrocardiogram is watched for signs of control of the rapid arrhythmia, such as a decreased ventricular response in atrial fibrillation. The amount of diuresis from digitalis and diuretics is recorded every shift; if diuresis is marked and rapid, additional supplementation of potassium may be needed to prevent hypokalemia. Serum and urine electrolyte results are noted. The nurse observes her patient for any of the toxic manifestations listed in Chapter 7; if they are seen, digitalis is withheld and the physician notified. The PR interval is closely observed during digitalis therapy as various degrees of AV junctional delay (heart block) are common manifestations of digitalis toxicity. The nurse is also alert to new or increasing ectopic activity which may be caused by digitalis toxicity and hypokalemia.

Isoproterenol (Isuprel). Isoproterenol is useful in the treatment of heart failure, hypotension, sinus bradycardia, slow atrioventricular junctional rhythms, and advanced degrees of heart block. It increases the rate of electrical discharge at pacemaker sites, enhances conductivity through the atrioventricular node, and increases the heart rate in bradycardia without increasing peripheral resistance.

Because isoproterenol causes increased myocardial irritability which may result in arrhythmias, the patient's ECG is closely monitored by the nurse. She readies antiarrhythmic agents in anticipation of ectopic activity. When ectopics are seen, they are documented by taking an ECG rhythm strip. The nurse either slows or discontinues the intravenous drip (depending upon the number and type of ectopics), takes the patient's vital signs, notifies the physician, and gives antiarrhythmics as ordered. The physician is also notified if the patient's pulse rises significantly, as an increased heart rate may be dangerous, especially to patients with coronary artery disease or mitral or aortic stenosis. The patient's blood pressure should rise with his improving cardiac output, but the peripheral vasodilation from isoproterenol administration may also cause hypotension. Therefore, the blood pressure is closely observed. It is necessary to have the physician make known to the nurse the blood pressure he feels is best for the patient's current condition. Any significant fluctuations from this goal are reported to the physician; the intravenous drip is adjusted by the nurse as necessary. The central venous pressure is also carefully measured, for with an improvement in cardiac output after the administration of isoproterenol, an elevated CVP should return toward the patient's normal level. Besides monitoring the patient's ECG, heart rate, blood pressure, and CVP, the nurse also observes the patient for other signs of improved cardiac function — his urine output should rise, his mental status should improve, and any dyspnea or edema should subside.

Drugs Which Affect the Autonomic Nervous System

Parasympatholytic drugs (Atropine).   Atropine helps to increase the heart rate in sinus bradycardia and improves atrioventricular conduction in acute atrioventricular heart block; it acts by depressing parasympathetic nervous function (a vagal blocking action), thereby permitting an improvement in sympathetic function.

When atropine is given to the patient, he should be informed that he may experience dryness of the mouth, flushing of the skin, or nervousness, so that he will be better prepared to deal with these potential side effects. The nurse must be certain of correct dosage, as atropine is given in small amounts. She observes her patient for an increase in heart rate after it is given.

Sympathomimetic drugs (epinephrine, norepinephrine, metaraminol, methoxamine, and others).   When patients are given sympathomimetic medications, they are closely observed for a lessening degree of shock. Side effects of falling urine production, gradually decreasing blood pressure, and ventricular irritability may be a consequence of ischemic damage to the kidneys, heart, and liver. This damage may have resulted from increased vascular resistance in these organs, and, thus, decreased blood flow; sympathomimetics can cause such ischemia. The degree of shock is determined by frequent measurement of the patient's blood pressure, central venous pressure, and urinary output. Antiarrhythmic drugs are made available in anticipation of myocardial irritability.

It is mandatory that there not be too rapid a blood pressure elevation from too rapid an infusion; patients with coronary artery and cardiovascular disease may be unable to tolerate a rapidly developing hypertension. A high blood pressure may also cause reflex bradycardia, so atropine is made readily available. Metaraminol may have a long duration of action, resulting in a prolonged period of hypertension.

To prevent tissue sloughing, phentolamine (Regitine), 5 to 10 mg in 10 to 15 ml of saline solution, is infiltrated into areas in which sympathomimetics (especially norepinephrine) have extravasated.

Antiarrhythmic Agents (Lidocaine, Quinidine, Procainamide, Propranolol, Diphenylhydantoin)

The patient receiving antiarrhythmic drugs requires frequent observation of his ECG pattern; a decrease in ectopic activity is anticipated. The physician is always notified if there is a significant change of rhythm, especially if this change is associated with a simultaneous fall in blood pressure.

Antiarrhythmic agents have a depressant action on myocardial contractility, thereby lowering cardiac output and predisposing the patient to a lower systemic blood pressure. Therefore, the nurse carefully monitors her patient's blood pressure, and watches for hypotension and bradycardia. Atropine is on hand to treat the potential bradycardia. Vasopressors are made readily available should marked hypotension result, especially after the intravenous administration of procainamide, propranolol, and diphenylhydantoin. The patient is also observed for signs of congestive heart failure.

These medications are often not indicated for patients with depressed AV junctional conduction, or in patients with bundle branch block, as they inhibit conductivity. Large doses of procaineamide may cause atrioventricular block with resultant increase in premature ventricular contractions and greater chances of ventricular fibrillation. Intravenous procaineamide may also have a hypotensive effect. Ventricular fibrillation is also a danger with the use of quinidine. Procaineamide may be used in a situation in which lidocaine is unsuccessful in the control of ectopic activity. Premature ventricular contractions which increase after lidocaine is given are usually due to blockage of conduction, which causes more ectopic activity to compensate for the blockage. Isoproterenol is utilized in this case to improve conduction.

The nurse exercises careful judgment when administering lidocaine via intravenous drip or bolus of 50 to 100 mgm. She obtains physician's orders which clarify the types of situations in which a bolus of lidocaine is to be given, and notifies the physician as necessary before administration. Careful regulation of the lidocaine drip is necessary. Also, a fresh bolus of lidocaine is drawn up each shift and placed at the patient's bedside for emergency use.

If diphenylhydantoin is given intravenously, it must be diluted well and given slowly to avoid causing the patient pain which results from an irritation of the vein. Propranolol is not recommended for use in patients with acute myocardial infarction and obstructive lung disease. Bronchospasm may occur, as this drug produces bronchoconstriction.

Oral doses of quinidine and procaineamide are given punctually at the designated hour (usually every six hours) to maintain a therapeutic level of medication continuously. Increasing ectopic activity often is seen just prior to the time these medications are due to be given; this information is recorded in the nurse's notes.

Diuretics (Mercurials, Thiazides, Ethacrynic acid, Furosemide, Triamterene, Spironolactone)

Diuretics are used in the treatment of edema to increase sodium and water excretion and thereby to reduce circulatory overload.

When diuretics are being administered, the nurse keeps an accurate record of her patient's fluid intake/output and daily weight in order to determine losses or gains in total body fluid. She anticipates arrhythmias which may result from depletion of the potassium level during diuresis; antiarrhythmics are kept close at hand for use in emergency situations. Also, the nurse watches for hypotension and symptoms of thromboembolic episodes; both can result from too rapid a diuresis.

The nurse provides potassium and chloride supplementation as ordered; potassium supplementation may be unnecessary for patients receiving spironolactone or triamterene, for these medications cause only a small amount of potassium loss. The nurse familiarizes herself with the results of her patient's serum potassium and hematocrit values (the hematocrit should not rise too rapidly during diuresis), especially when furosemide and ethacrynic acid are used. Frequent electrolyte determinations are needed, as these two diuretics are rapid-acting and may cause profound changes in blood chemistries. The physician is notified of "stat" results of serum electrolytes as necessary.

Diuresis is begun in the morning, whenever possible, so that the patient is not disturbed during the night by having to void frequently. Intramuscular diuretics are given into nonedematous tissue to promote adequate absorption and the most efficient diuresis. In order to allay anxiety, the patient is told of the impending increased urge to void; a urinal or bedpan is placed within easy reach.

The physician is notified if there is a marked decrease in urinary output; this may indicate kidney failure (diuretics, especially the mercurials, can cause impairment of kidney function).

Anticoagulants

Heparin.   Heparin is the drug of choice when the need for anticoagulation is immediate. It is used for patients with thrombophlebitis, and pulmonary and systemic emboli. It acts by preventing thrombus formation and platelet aggregation. Its use in patients with acute myocardial infarction is still controversial.

In her care of the patient undergoing heparin therapy, the nurse watches for bruising, hematomas, petechiae, excessive bleeding from injection sites, and the presence of blood in the patient's stool, urine, or sputum. She makes sure that a clotting time has been ordered before anticoagulation is begun, and that it is drawn at the same time every 24 hours, usually one half hour before the next dose is given. To effect total absorption, correct technique for the injection of heparin is utilized (this procedure is reviewed in Chapter 7). Subcutaneous administration may result in pain and hematoma formation as well as lack of complete absorption. The intravenous route obviates these objections. To prevent bleeding, intramuscular injections of other drugs are given as infrequently as possible and with careful technique.

The dosage for heparin is now listed in units instead of milligrams. One milligram now equals 120 units and *not* 100 units. In the event of heparin overdosage or serious bleeding, protamine sulfate will reverse the anticoagulation.

Warfarin sodium (Coumadin). Warfarin is useful in long-term anticoagulation to prevent the formation of thrombi in the venous circulation. As part of her interventions, the nurse again observes her patient for the various signs of bleeding mentioned previously. She assumes responsibility for overseeing that prothrombin times are drawn and results are made available to the physician. She recognizes the fact that increased prothrombin time percentages can be noted when the patient is receiving such medications as barbiturates and other sedatives and diphenylhydantoin; decreased prothrombin time percentages may be seen when the patient has taken salicylates, Butazolidin, broad-spectrum antibiotics, quinidine sulfate, and steroids. The nurse also is knowledgeable of the fact that abnormalities of liver and cardiac function lower the prothrombin time and make lower doses of warfarin necessary. Warfarin is neutralized by vitamin K (Aquamephyton).

Antihypertensive Drug Therapy (Reserpine, Hydralazine, Methyldopa, Guanethidine)

The patient receiving antihypertensives requires close observation of his blood pressure. The nurse watches for signs of hypotension, especially when intravenous medications are being used. She notifies the physician when the blood pressure is beginning to lie within normal or desired limits; he may want to decrease the dosage accordingly.

The patient is forewarned of possible side effects of the particular medication he is to receive. His reaction to the drug is carefully noted. He may experience postural hypotension, as manifested by his complaints of dizziness or a lightheaded feeling upon standing or sitting erect. If he has had a long history of hypertension, he may experience these symptoms at a blood pressure which is normal for the average individual, but which is hypotensive for him. To help prevent postural hypotension, the patient is encouraged to sit or "dangle" at the edge of his bed before he stands; this gradual repositioning gives his circulatory system time to adjust to an upright position. "Lying and sitting" blood pressures are often ordered to determine the postural effect of the administered drug.

Nursing Care of the Patient with a Cardiac Arrhythmia

The major rationale for the institution of CCUs is the prevention of complications or death from cardiac arrhythmias. The nurse employed in such a unit must have a thorough understanding of normal and abnormal cardiac rate and rhythm if she is to assume the responsibility inherent in CCU nursing. The following material is concerned with the specific nursing implications in the care of the patient with a cardiac arrhythmia. For a more detailed explanation of these arrhythmias see Chapter 4.

In observing the monitor pattern for cardiac arrhythmias, the nurse must have an understanding of cardiac vectors and must be aware of the normal vector of the lead being monitored. In some coronary care units, three electrodes are placed on the patient's chest. Depending on lead placement, this system can provide a modified lead II or a modified lead V_5 or V_6 pattern. In units utilizing four electrodes (right arm, left arm, right leg, left leg, each of which is placed on or adjacent to the designated extremity and connected to a lead selector box), each of the frontal plane leads can be monitored. The lead selection available with the four electrode system is especially advantageous in that the monitored lead can be changed if the P wave configuration is difficult to discern or if the QRS is changing in a given lead.

In observing the patient for cardiac arrhythmias, the nurse, in addition to frequently *looking* at the monitor, must be aware of (1) the patient's pertinent medical history, (2) his current drug therapy, and (3) his normal cardiac rate and rhythm. The patient's medical history is important not only for the specific heart disease, but also in relation to the presence of other disease processes, such as pulmonary disease, thyrotoxicosis, or renal failure. Drug therapy, as was discussed earlier, can modify cardiac electrical activity either by decreasing abnormal heart rhythms or by causing abnormalities of cardiac function. Many people have chronic arrhythmia problems, such as atrial fibrillation, complete heart block, or six to 10 premature ventricular contractions per minute. In cases of chronic arrhythmias, the nurse should observe the patient for signs of worsening cardiac status, but she need not be unduly anxious about an abnormality which is in fact "normal" (basic) for the patient.

In occasional instances, an arrhythmia cannot be positively diagnosed. In such cases, parameters other than electrocardiographic documentation must be utilized in the treatment of the patient's disorder (e.g., his response to a certain drug regimen). In any case of a changing or new heart rhythm, the arrhythmia is documented by a rhythm strip, a diagnosis is attempted, and the patient's physician is notified.

The nurse recently introduced to the CCU may feel overwhelmed when confronted with the wide variety of cardiac arrhythmias possible in her patients. If the nurse has an understanding of the various portions of the cardiac cycle and the cardiac activity they represent, she is reasonably well equipped to interpret the heart patterns through the following observations: (1) presence (or absence), size, direction, configuration and frequency of the P wave; (2) length of the PR interval; (3) relationship of the P wave to succeeding ventricular complexes; (4) appearance, duration, and frequency of the ventricular complex; and (5) regularity of the ventricular complex.

REGULAR SINUS RHYTHM

Regular sinus rhythm is the normal rhythm of the heart; its usual rate is from 60 to 100 beats per minute. While a pattern of regular sinus rhythm indicates that normal heart rate and rhythm exist, its presence does not preclude the existence of serious disease. It is not unusual for a heart pattern to change suddenly from regular sinus rhythm to a serious rhythm disturbance.

Sinus Tachycardia

Sinus tachycardia is a regular sinus rhythm having a rate between 100 and 160 beats per minute. This arrhythmia can result from any physiologic or emotional stress. At rates over 140, differentiation of this rhythm from other supraventricular tachycardias may be difficult. Carotid sinus massage (CSM) will result in a slowing of a sinus tachycardia with a return to the faster rate when the massage is terminated. If CSM is ineffective for diagnosis, the P waves of the fast rhythm are compared to the P waves of the patient's regular sinus rhythm. If the P waves are identical, the tachycardia is probably sinus in origin. Persistent sinus tachycardia in the diseased heart may result in congestive heart failure, hypotension, or angina on the basis of low cardiac output. The patient may complain of palpitations, angina, or dyspnea. The treatment of this arrhythmia is generally directed at the suspected cause and side effects of the increased heart rate, rather than at the rhythm per se. In caring for a patient with sinus tachycardia, the nurse should attempt to relieve dyspnea or chest pain and closely monitor vital signs. The rhythm should be documented and differentiated from other supraventricular tachycardias.

Sinus Bradycardia

Sinus bradycardia is a regular sinus rhythm with a rate under 60 beats per minute. Although this slow rate may be normal for some individuals, it can be a very dangerous rhythm. This arrhythmia can result from any cardiac disease (especially acute inferior-posterior infarction) or from vagal stimulation caused by drugs (digoxin, morphine sulfate) or by nausea and vomiting. In the patient with heart disease complicated by sinus bradycardia, the slow rhythm may allow an irritable focus to take over pacemaker function and a more serious arrhythmia can result. Sinus bradycardia is differentiated from other slow rhythms by the presence of a normal P wave which initiates each ventricular complex with a constant PR interval. The patient may be asymptomatic or he may complain of weakness, faintness, dizziness, or other signs of reduced cardiac output. Syncope may occur if the patient suddenly stands. Treatment will depend upon the patient's symptoms and the preference of the physician. Atropine may be given orally, subcutaneously, or intravenously on a schedule or on an "as needed" basis. An isoproterenol (Isuprel) intravenous solution (usually 1 to 2 milligrams in 500 ml D_5W) is often kept on "stand by" should the patient's rate decrease significantly. Pacemakers have been used in the treatment of this disorder. Vagotonic drugs such as digitalis or the opiates may be withheld. In caring for a patient with sinus bradycardia, the nurse closely observes the patient for lethargy, mental aberration, signs of congestive heart failure, and other indications of low cardiac output. This rhythm should be documented and differentiated from other slow rhythms, such as atrioventricular dissociation and slow AV junctional rhythms. All vagotonic drugs are held until the physician is notified.

SINUS ARRHYTHMIA

In sinus arrhythmia, the heart rate varies between a slower and a faster heart rhythm. The P wave is normal in appearance as it arises in the SA node. In most cases of sinus arrhythmia, the rate varies with respiration, speeding with inspiration and slowing with expiration. This rhythm is frequently seen with sinus bradycardia and may disappear with a faster basic heart rate; it is generally not indicative of heart disease and is not treated. The nurse should be certain that the slight irregularity of rhythm is not caused by a more serious arrhythmia.

SINUS ARREST (ATRIAL STANDSTILL)

In this arrhythmia, an interruption of heart rhythm occurs as a result of the SA node failing to initiate an atrial impulse. The interval between beats does not necessarily equal a multiple of the normal P-P interval. Atrial standstill results if the SA node fails for two or more consecutive intervals. This heart rhythm is significant, as an ectopic AV junctional or ventricular focus may take over the pacemaker function of the heart. Etiology of this arrhythmia may be carotid sinus massage, vagotonic drugs, or intrinsic cardiac disease. Sinus arrest may also represent an extension of progressive sinus bradycardia. The patient is usually asymptomatic, unless cardiac output is low because of a slow rate or an ineffective ectopic pacemaker. The nurse documents and verifies the arrhythmia; the monitor pattern is closely observed for frequent episodes of atrial standstill, and for the occurrence of AV junctional or ventricular pacemakers. Vagotonic drugs are held until the physician is notified.

WANDERING ATRIAL PACEMAKER

In this arrhythmia, the location of impulse formation wanders through the atria and occasionally to the atrioventricular node. The P wave configuration and PR interval vary in appearance and duration, depending on the site of impulse origin. While this disturbance of rhythm may be normal for some individuals, it may be caused by organic heart disease, increased vagal tone, and digitalis preparations and is commonly seen in patients with chronic lung disease. The arrhythmia may indicate increased atrial irritability and may precede atrial fibrillation or atrial tachycardia. The patient is often asymptomatic and treatment is generally not indicated. The nurse observes the patient for more serious atrial arrhythmias and the doctor is notified before additional vagotonic medications are given.

ATRIAL PREMATURE CONTRACTIONS (APCs)

An atrial premature contraction is the result of activation of one or more ectopic foci in either atria. The beat is premature (i.e., it occurs before the normal sinus beat is due to occur). The P wave of the premature beat may differ from the normal P wave, depending on the location of the ectopic focus. A focus high in the atria may produce a P wave of normal direction, while a focus low in the atrium may produce a P wave with an opposite vector. The PR interval of the premature beat may be shorter or longer than the normal beat, depending upon the location of and the conduction from the ectopic focus. The ventricular complex of the APC is usually the same as the patient's normal sinus complex, although there may be an aberrancy of conduction (see later). An interval termed a *resetting pause* usually follows an APC; this interval is a result of early depolarization of the SA node during the APC. The resetting pause is the time interval between the P wave of the APC and the P wave of the next normal beat; it is usually equal to the normal P-P interval. This pause differs from a compensatory pause (see later) in that it is not exactly twice the normal R-R interval. It is often difficult to differentiate an APC originating low in the atria from an AV junctional premature contraction originating high in the atrioventricular node; in these cases the term *supraventricular premature beat* is used to include both types of beats. Atrial premature contractions can occur in normal individuals; they can be caused by tobacco or caffein-containing liquids. Atrial premature contractions may also be caused by digitalis preparations. Although intrinsic heart disease may cause APCs, the presence of these premature beats is not absolutely diagnostic of cardiac disease. The frequent occurrence of these beats may indicate atrial irritability and may forewarn of more serious atrial arrhythmias, such as atrial fibrillation and atrial tachycardia. Treatment may not be indicated, or quinidine may be used to reduce the atrial irritability. The patient is usually not symptomatic. The nurse reports frequent APCs (greater than six per min) or runs of two to three consecutive APCs to the physician and she observes the patient for atrial tachycardia, atrial fibrillation, or atrial flutter. The arrhythmia is documented and differentiated from other ectopic beats.

Blocked Atrial Premature Contractions

Occasionally an APC is blocked, i.e., atrial depolarization occurs during the absolute refractory period of the ventricle and a ventricular response does not occur. The P wave in such an instance is buried in or near the T wave; a resetting pause follows.

PAROXYSMAL ATRIAL TACHYCARDIA

Paroxysmal atrial tachycardia is a regular rhythm with rates usually between 160 and 220 per minute. The rhythm is irregular only in instances in which there is more than one atrial ectopic focus or when AV junctional or ventricular ectopic beats interrupt the heart rhythm. The PR interval in this rhythm may be longer than usual; in such a case, the P wave may be buried in the preceding T wave and the rhythm may appear to be AV junctional in origin. The most common cause of paroxysmal atrial tachycardia is traumatic emotional experience; less common etiologic factors are coronary artery disease, thyrotoxicosis, and mitral valve disease. It may be difficult to distinguish paroxysmal atrial tachycardia from other rapid supraventricular tachycardias. Carotid sinus massage, when applied to a patient with this rhythm, may abruptly terminate the arrhythmia. If carotid sinus massage produces no change in rhythm, the P wave of the tachycardia is compared to the P wave of the patient's regular sinus rhythm pattern. If the P wave of the faster rhythm differs from the P wave of the slower rhythm, the arrhythmia is probably atrial rather than sinus in origin. Paroxysmal atrial tachycardia may last from a few seconds to several days, and if it is not terminated, coronary insufficiency and congestive heart failure may result.

Patients are often symptomatic with this rapid rate and they may complain of palpitations, "flutter in the chest," or lightheadedness. Dyspnea, cerebral aberrations, angina and other signs of low cardiac output may occur in protracted states. The treatment of paroxysmal atrial tachycardia may at first be carotid sinus massage. If the patient is emotionally distraught, psychologic support and sedation are indicated. Synchronized countershock (if the patient is not in danger of digitalis toxicity) may be administered. Drug therapy, such as digitalis preparations, quinidine, and Tensilon or Aramine may be indicated.

The nurse can attempt to reduce the possibility of this arrhythmia by keeping the patient's environment as free as possible from emotional stress. In spite of relatively stress-free environments, paroxysmal atrial tachycardias will occur, and the nurse has several responsibilities during the acute arrhythmia period. The nurse continues to reassure the patient by affecting a calm and efficient manner. The patient's heart rate, blood pressure, and central venous pressure are monitored closely and the physician is notified at the first signs of congestive heart failure, coronary insufficiency, or shock. The high alarm guard on the heart rate monitor is set within three to four beats of the current rate as an increase in rate can be quite dangerous. Ordered sedatives and analgesics are given immediately. Cardiac drugs and equipment for synchronized countershock should be readily available. Following stabilization or termination of the arrhythmia, the nurse continues to offer reassurance to the patient and again attempts to reduce traumatic emotional stimuli.

Atrial tachycardia with a 2:1 block is often a manifestation of digitalis toxicity, but can also occur as a manifestation of heart disease, quinidine therapy, and hypokalemia. This rhythm appears electrocardiographically as an atrial rhythm that occurs twice as fast as the ventricular rhythm. Digitalis toxicity may manifest as atrial tachycardia with a 2:1 block (a fast atrial rhythm—240 per minute with a ventricular rate of 120 per minute). In this instance, any ordered digitalis is held and the physician is immediately notified. The treatment is usually directed toward the correction of digitalis toxicity and of any accompanying hypokalemia.

ATRIAL FLUTTER

In atrial flutter, the atrial rate is from 220 to 350 beats per minute. The AV node and ventricles are unable to respond to each atrial discharge and a degree of atrioventricular block results. The degree of block at the AV node is often constant from two or three atrial impulses to one ventricular response, thereby producing a regular rhythm. The block may vary, however, and in these cases the rhythm will be irregular. Occasionally a 1:1 atrial flutter occurs and the resulting rapid heart rate constitutes a very serious cardiac arrhythmia. Diagnostic of atrial flutter is a saw-toothed appearance of atrial activity. In cases of 1:1 or 2:1 atrial flutter, the rhythm may simulate atrial or AV junctional tachycardia and differentiation of these rhythms may be difficult. Carotid sinus massage may cause an increase in the block at the AV node (i.e., from a 2:1 block to a 4:1 block) or may cause a regular ventricular response to become irregular, indicating transient or erratic changes in AV conduction. Rapid, untreated atrial flutter can result in congestive heart failure and other complications of low cardiac output. The symptoms in atrial flutter are often related to ventricular rate: the patient with a rapid ventricular rate may complain of a "pounding in the chest," angina, dyspnea, and hypotension, while the patient with a slower ventricular rate may be asymptomatic.

The treatment of this arrhythmia may be drugs (digitalis or quinidine preparations) or may be synchronized cardioversion. Patients in atrial flutter often require large doses of digitalis preparations to control the rate. It is not uncommon that digitalis therapy may change the rhythm from atrial flutter to atrial fibrillation before converting to regular sinus rhythm. The nurse caring for a patient with atrial flutter documents and differentiates the rhythm from other supraventricular rhythms. The physician is notified immediately at the onset of this heart rhythm. The nurse notes the degree of AV block and is alert to increased ventricular response and signs of reduced cardiac output. In cases of a persistent 1:1 or 2:1 flutter, the patient's appearance and vital signs are closely monitored, and appropriate drugs and equipment for cardioversion are made ready.

ATRIAL FIBRILLATION

Atrial fibrillation is a heart rhythm in which rapid chaotic atrial impulse formation (over 350 per min) results in irregular and ineffective atrial contraction. The ventricular response in this rhythm is irregular, as repetitive depolarization of the AV node prevents conduction of many of the impulses. In the electrocardiographic record of atrial fibrillation, the P wave is absent, the baseline is undulating, and the ventricular response is irregular, unless there is independent AV junctional rhythm with atrial fibrillation. In occasional instances, very rapid atrial fibrillation or well controlled atrial fibrillation may appear to have a regular ventricular response, but with caliper measurement a slight discrepancy in R-R interval can be noted.

The causes of atrial fibrillation are the same as those of atrial flutter. The rhythm may occur in normal individuals in paroxysmal or chronic form. The saw-toothed electrocardiographic pattern is diagnostic of atrial flutter, but, in instances of rapid ventricular rate, the rhythm may simulate any of the supraventricular tachycardias. Carotid sinus massage performed upon a patient in atrial fibrillation will usually result in some ventricular slowing. The undulating baseline and absent P waves seen during this slowing lead to a diagnosis of atrial fibrillation.

Digitalis preparations are considered the drugs of choice in the treatment of atrial fibrillation. This rhythm may also be treated with quinidine, after digitalis has slowed the ventricular response and changed the rhythm from atrial fibrillation to atrial flutter. Cardioversion may be utilized before drug therapy or in cases in which the rhythm is refractory to medication.

In observing a patient with atrial fibrillation, the nurse is alert to changes in ventricular rate as an indication of therapeutic response. Here again a rapid ventricular rate can result in complications of low cardiac output; a slow, almost regular ventricular rhythm may be AV junctional in origin and a manifestation of digitalis toxicity. The quivering of the atria leads to stasis of blood and can result in atrial thrombus formation; the patient is observed for signs of pulmonary and systemic embolization.

ATRIOVENTRICULAR NODAL ARRHYTHMIAS (NOW CALLED AV JUNCTIONAL ARRHYTHMIAS)

Atrioventricular Nodal Delay or Block

Atrioventricular conduction defects, also termed *AV block, AV dissociation,* and *heart block,* comprise a group of arrhythmias in which the conduction of sinus impulses to the ventricle is delayed or blocked. Atrioventricular block is classified as (1) incomplete block consisting of first degree and second degree block, and (2) complete or third degree block.

Incomplete heart block. First degree heart block is a delay in conduction between the original sinus impulse and the resulting ventricular activation. First degree heart block may occur in individuals with no known heart disease. Acute infectious diseases, especially rheumatic fever, may cause this type of block. First degree block may also result from drug therapy such as lidocaine and quinidine, digitalis preparations (by means of their vagal effect), coronary artery disease, and congenital heart disease. Electrocardiographically, first degree heart block is diagnosed by the presence of a PR interval of greater than .20 seconds. This interval may be as long as 0.60 seconds in a very slow heart rate. The atrial and ventricular rhythms are equal and regular; every sinus impulse elicits a ventricular response. The patient is usually asymptomatic, unless his heart rate is very slow.

Second degree heart block may take three forms: (1) periodic, (2) constant, and (3) Wenckebach. The causes of second degree block include digitalis toxicity, quinidine toxicity, infectious diseases (especially diphtheria), coronary artery disease, and myocardial infarction. Patients may or may not be symptomatic.

In periodic AV block, periodic failure of atrioventricular conduction exists. This arrhythmia is best understood by example: the first four of a series of five atrial impulses are each followed by a ventricular complex, but the fifth atrial impulse does not elicit a ventricular response. This cycle continues with every fifth atrial complex failing to evoke a ventricular complex. This type of second degree heart block is frequently associated with first degree heart block.

In constant second degree heart block, the ventricle responds only to every second, third, or fourth atrial impulse. The atrial rate is regular, i.e., the P-P interval is constant. The ventricular response may be constant and regular, or may vary from 2:1 to 3:1 or 4:1 conduction; in such cases, the ventricular rhythm will be irregular.

The Wenckebach type of second degree heart block is cyclic in occurrence. This type of heart block differs from periodic heart block in that a gradual lengthening of the PR interval (and often a shortening of the R-R interval) precedes a nonconducted atrial impulse. The number of beats in each cycle may or may not be constant. This type of second degree block is frequently a manifestation of digitalis toxicity, but is also commonly seen in an acute myocardial infarction.

Complete heart block. Complete or third degree heart block is a heart rhythm in which the atrial and ventricular activities are disassociated. The etiology of this rhythm is the same as the etiology of second degree heart block. Electrocardiographically, this rhythm has atrial activity which is not followed by a QRS in any identifiable relationship. The atrial rate and rhythm may be normal (sinus) or the atrial rhythm may be atrial tachycardia or atrial fibrillation. The ventricular rhythm is regular with a rate of 20 to 80. The ventricular pacemaker is located either in the AV junctional tissue or in the ventricle itself. If the pacemaker is AV junctional, the QRS will usually appear normal and the rate usually will be from 60 to 80. If the pacemaker is in the ventricle, the QRS will have the appearance of the QRS of a premature ventricular contraction, and the rate can be from 20 to 60.

Heart block caused by digitalis toxicity, if adequately treated, generally does not affect the patient's prognosis. Heart block resulting from an acute infectious process usually subsides with alleviation of the infection. Patients with a slow heart rate from complete heart block caused by coronary artery disease often experience episodes of dizziness or fainting, but an occasional individual may be able to tolerate the slow rhythm for many years without symptoms. A variable prognosis and significance exists with heart block resulting from myocardial infarction.

The treatment of all degrees of heart block depends upon the etiology of the block, the patient's symptoms, and the clinical judgment of the patient's physician. In cases of AV block due to digitalis toxicity, therapy includes withholding of digitalis preparations and correction of factors predisposing to the toxic state. Supplemental potassium therapy is usually not indicated, and may be contraindicated as potassium inhibits conduction of impulses across the AV node. As mentioned before, successful treatment of acute infection causing heart block generally results in the relief of an AV conduction disturbance. Implantable pacemakers may be indicated for the patient with heart block caused by coronary artery disease. Atropine and Isuprel are often utilized in the treatment of acute and chronic forms of heart block.

Medical treatment of heart block resulting from myocardial infarction remains controversial today. Management of AV conduction disturbances ranges from insertion of a transvenous pacemaker at the first sign of AV delay, to withholding mechanical pacemakers unless the patient is symptomatic from second or third degree block. The rationale for the use of pacemakers at the earliest indications of AV delay is that second or third degree heart block can rapidly develop, can compromise cardiac output, and can lead to serious complications or to death. In opposition to this theory is the opinion that the complications of pacemaker insertion can outnumber the incidence and severity of complications of heart block. Although insertion of a pacemaker in a patient who exhibits acute second or third degree block may be considered a positive action for the patient's benefit, the pacemaker itself may worsen the patient's condition. Pacemakers have been incriminated in the production of ventricular irritability, as evidenced by premature ventricular contractions, ventricular tachycardia, and ventricular fibrillation occurring during and after pacemaker insertion. Perforation of the heart and sudden death may occur if the pacing wire is inadvertently pushed through the free wall of the ventricle (or through the interventricular septum). Phlebitis can result from irritation and inflammation caused by the pacemaker wire. Serious ventricular irritability can result from movement of the electrode within the heart or from faulty pacemaking equipment should the pacemaker discharge its impulse in the vulnerable period. In spite of the controversy surrounding the use of pacemakers, it can be generalized that pacemakers are indicated for patients who have at least second degree block, who have an anterior myocardial infarction with or without an inferior myocardial infarction, and who have one or more of the following: hypotension, cerebral symptoms, congestive heart failure, ventricular rate below 50, and an intraventricular conduction defect. A patient with all of these criteria will, of course, be a very poor risk and may die, even though adequately paced. A patient with complete heart block with none of the previously mentioned symptoms may do well with or without pacing; his heart block may revert to regular sinus rhythm with myocardial healing (three to seven days after the infarction).

The three major types of permanent pacemaker units now in use are the asynchronous, the synchronous, and the demand pacemakers. The asynchronous or "set rate" pacemakers continuously discharge electrical stimulation at a preset rate. This pacemaker will continue to fire whether or not the patient's heart rate is faster or slower than the set rate. The hazard of this type of pacemaker is the firing of the pacemaking impulse during the period of maximum heart excitability; this phenomenon, referred to as R on T, can lead to ventricular fibrillation. At the present time, set-rate (asynchronous) pacemakers are used, if at all, in the patient whose heart rhythm, while basically slow, may be complicated by frequent episodes of ventricular tachycardia. The rationale for a set-rate pacemaker in this case is the attempt to suppress ventricular ectopic foci by the maintenance of a constant and more rapid heart rate. Unfortunately, ventricular tachycardia can occur in spite of the faster-paced rate and can also be a result of the R-on-T phenomenon.

The synchronous type of pacemaker has an atrial and a ventricular electrode. The ventricular electrode is synchronized to fire if atrial activity is not followed by ventricular activity within a short interval (0.16 second). The pacemaker thus allows atrial contraction to contribute to cardiac output. This type of pacemaker requires thoracotomy and thus it is not used for most coronary care unit patients.

The "demand" type of pacemaker is used most frequently for treatment of acute heart block. The demand pacemaker discharges only when the patient's intrinsic heart rhythm is slower than the rate at which the pacemaker is set. Should the patient's heart rate increase above the pacing rate, the pacemaker will not discharge. Because the pacemaker fires only after a specific diastolic pause, stimulation in the vulnerable zone is avoided.

The temporary transvenous pacemaker wire is frequently used for the treatment of acute heart block. It may be in the form of a large-bore bipolar electrode (the size of the wire necessitates a cutdown on an antecubital vein) or as a unipolar floating pacemaking wire which may be inserted via venipuncture with a No. 14 needle.

The pacemaker wire is usually inserted into an antecubital vein and is advanced along the vein to the vena cava, then to the right atrium, and finally to the right ventricle. Because accurate placement of the electrode is vital to proper pacing, the procedure is best performed under fluoroscopy. In cases in which fluoroscopy is not available, the limb leads of electrocardiograph are connected to the patient and the distal portion of the pacemaker wire is attached to the chest lead of the ECG machine. As the electrode enters the right atrium, large atrial and small ventricular complexes are seen; as the electrode enters the right ventricle, smaller atrial and larger ventricular complexes are recorded. The bipolar pacing wire is a grounded system, but the unipolar wire requires grounding accomplished by placing a metal-sheathed suture into the skin and inserting the distal portion of the metal suture into one of the terminals of the pacemaker box. When the wire is adequately positioned, the pacemaker unit is attached to the wire, the milliamperage and rate are adjusted, and the pacemaker unit is activated to assure adequate pacing. The pacemaker unit may or may not be turned on, depending upon the patient's present need for artificial pacing. As soon as adequate pacemaker activity is verified, antibiotic ointment and a dry sterile dressing are applied at the insertion site. The pacemaker unit is then secured to the patient's body by tape or elastic straps.

The majority of patients admitted to CCUs who develop atrioventricular conduction delays or other arrhythmias requiring artificial pacing are treated initially with temporary transvenous demand pacemakers. Should the patient's condition indicate a need for permanent pacing, a permanent pacemaker can be inserted when the patient's clinical status warrants.

Nursing Care of the Patient with AV Conduction Disturbance

The nursing care of the patient who is afflicted with disturbance of AV conduction is influenced by the type of heart block, its etiology, its treatment, and its effect upon cardiovascular function. Although all patients being monitored are observed for signs of AV conduction disturbance, there are several disease processes and drug therapies that can increase the possibility of AV conduction disturbances. The patient with an inferior myocardial infarction is closely observed for AV block, as the blood supply to his AV node may be compromised. Patients receiving digitalis preparations are observed for all types of AV conduction disturbance because of the increased refractory period of the AV node caused by these preparations. Patients receiving myocardial depressant medications, such as Lidocaine, are observed for depressed AV junctional conduction. Patients with a history of right or left bundle branch block thought to be caused by coronary artery disease may manifest degrees of AV block as a result of progressive disease.

Frequent measurement and notation of the patient's PR interval on admission and throughout the hospital course are basic to the early recognition of AV conduction disturbance. The physician is notified of prolongation of the PR interval and ordered digitalis or cardiac depressant drugs are held. At the first signs of second and third degree heart block, the doctor is notified and drug therapy as mentioned before is held. The nurse attempts to diagnose and document the type of second degree block; she observes the patient for signs of low cardiac output and reports these immediately to the physician.

Although many individuals can lead relatively normal lives with complete heart block, the development of this arrhythmia over a period of days, hours, or minutes can severely compromise cardiac output. Low cardiac output in such a patient results from two basic factors: (1) atrial and ventricular activity are separate and atrial contraction does not contribute to total ventricular filling and (2) ventricular response may be so slow as to result in inadequate cardiac output. The patient who changes suddenly from a regular sinus rhythm to a complete heart block may have a Stokes-Adams attack; he may become unconscious and death may ensue owing to asystole or ventricular fibrillation. The nurse in the CCU must therefore be observant not only of early signs of AV conduction disturbance but also of the sudden development of second and third degree block. The patient with AV delay is always observed for signs of low cardiac output and for irritable ectopic foci (escape beats) that may become active during the long ventricular diastole.

Nursing Care of the Patient Requiring Artificial Pacing

In observing patients with pacemakers, the nurse must be aware of several terms and their meanings.

The pacemaker *artifact* is an impulse which is recorded electro-cardiographically as a vertical line and which indicates that the pacemaker is "firing." The pacemaker artifact is always immediately followed by a QRS complex if pacing is adequate.

The term *capture* indicates that the pacemaker has discharged an impulse and has immediately activated or captured the ventricle. A noncaptured beat indicates that the pacer has discharged but has not activated the ventricle.

In certain instances, one of the patient's own inherent pacemaker sites (atrial, junctional, or ventricular) may fire and activate ventricular depolarization. In these cases, the QRS will usually be different from those of the pacer-stimulated impulses.

Fusion beats in the patient with a pacemaker occur when the pacemaker fires almost simultaneously with the patient's intrinsic ventricular depolarization. The resulting complex may appear as a pacemaker artifact followed by a normal QRS complex or a pacemaker artifact followed by a QRS complex, part of which resembles the pacing QRS complex and part of which resembles the patient's normal (basic) QRS complex. Fusion beats may occur when the patient's intrinsic heart rate and the rate of pacemaker firing are equal.

Nursing care during the positioning of a transvenous pacemaker requires (1) an explanation of the procedure to the patient, (2) careful monitoring of the patient's heart rhythm with preparation for treatment of arrhythmias, and (3) general considerations of nursing care during a cutdown or venipuncture. The patient requiring a pacemaker will be apprehensive and will require a detailed explanation of the procedure. He is often quite fearful that he will need the pacemaker permanently; the nurse can explain to the patient that the pacemaker is often only a temporary measure and that with the return of normal AV conduction the need for external pacing will cease. The patient is often fearful that his heart cannot function without a pacemaker; the nurse can explain that the pacemaker (if it is a demand pacemaker) fires only when the patient's own heart rate is slow.

Passage of a bipolar pacing wire requires a cutdown tray with antiseptic and local anesthetic solutions. A unipolar pacing wire can be inserted into any large superficial vein by means of a venipuncture with a No. 14 needle. For either type of pacing wire, an external pacemaker unit with a battery and a spare fully charged battery should be available. If the wire insertion is to be performed under fluoroscopy, preparations for the use of this equipment are made. If the wire is to be placed "blindly" (by electrocardiographic evidence of pacemaker position), the properly grounded electrocardiograph is connected to the patient. A cable with an alligator clip on both ends (one clip to the electrocardiograph chest lead and one clip to the distal pacemaker wire) is made available. The patient is monitored continuously throughout the procedure for evidence of myocardial irritability and other complications of pacemaker insertion. A bolus of Lidocaine and a defibrillator are readily available in the event of dangerous ventricular rhythms. When the pacemaking wire is thought to be in the superior vena cava, the cable with the alligator clips is connected from the pacemaking wire to the chest lead of the electrocardiograph. The pacemaker wire is then positioned properly, tested for adequacy of pacing, and the cutdown site is closed.

Following successful implantation of the pacemaker, connections from the pacemaker unit to the wire are secured and checked frequently, as arm motion can dislodge tenuous connections. Careful observation should be made of the patient's intrinsic heart rate and rhythm and of the adequacy of pacemaker performance in the event the intrinsic rhythm becomes slower than the demand rate setting. A QRS must follow every pacer artifact to prove adequate capture.

The occurrence of ventricular premature contractions is noted and reported to the physician, as they may be the result of the pacemaker irritating the ventricle. If the pacer has been placed prophylactically and turned "OFF," the nurse observes the patient's status for need of pacing: (1) development of symptoms from high degrees of atrioventricular block, (2) significant bradycardia with or without symptoms, (3) frequent or increasing periods of sinus arrest, and (4) development of symptoms of low cardiac output.

If the pacemaker is turned "ON," the nursing observations will vary with the type of pacemaker utilized. The patient with an asynchronous pacemaker is observed for R-on-T phenomenon as well as for stimulation from ectopic foci. The nurse observes the patient with a synchronous pacemaker for accurate pacing as indicated by a pacemaker artifact or ventricular complex following each atrial discharge, depending on the delay at the AV node. The patient with this type of pacemaker is also observed for rapid atrial rates. The patient with a demand pacemaker is observed for proper firing and capturing of the ventricle. The nurse is aware of the rate at which the pacemaker is set and notes whether or not the demand pacemaker fires when the patient's intrinsic rate is lower than the demand rate.

ATRIOVENTRICULAR JUNCTIONAL RHYTHMS

Junctional Premature Beats

Atrioventricular junctional premature beats originate from an ectopic focus in the atrioventricular junction tissue. These beats, which usually have a normal (basic) QRS configuration, stimulate the atria in a retrograde fashion. The relationship of the P wave to the QRS complex depends in part on the location of the ectopic focus in the atrioventricular junctional tissue. An ectopic focus high in the atrioventricular junction tissue may fire the atria in a retrograde manner and the PR interval may be normal or short; the P wave may be inverted or flattened. Such an ectopic beat is indistinguishable from a low atrial premature contraction and therefore both types of beats are referred to as *supraventricular premature beats.* The P wave of a low junctional premature contraction may follow the QRS and may show delayed conduction to the atria. In all junctional premature beats, a resetting pause follows the beat. The physician is notified of junctional premature contractions occurring frequently (more than over six per minute) or in runs, as they may indicate irritability of atrioventricular junction tissue and may precede atrioventricular tachycardia or more serious arrhythmias.

Atrioventricular Junctional Rhythm

The rate of atrioventricular junctional rhythm can be from 40 to 80 beats per minute. The site of the pacemaker in the atrioventricular tissue may be high or low, as with junctional premature contractions. *Coronary sinus rhythm* is a term used to describe a junctional rhythm originating from a focus high in the atrioventricular junctional tissue. Atrioventricular junctional rhythm may occur in normal individuals and as a result of carotid sinus massage. Causes of transient or permanent junctional rhythm include digitalis and quinidine administration and organic heart disease. The physician is notified of the occurrence of atrioventricular junctional rhythm and ordered digitalis or quinidine is held pending a reorder.

Atrioventricular Junctional Tachycardia

Atrioventricular junctional tachycardia may occur at rates of 120 to 200 beats per minute. The rhythm is regular and the appearance of each complex is similar to a junctional premature contraction. As with that of junctional premature contractions, the site of origin of the tachycardia will determine the configuration and timing of the P wave. Because P waves are often not discernible in an atrioventricular junctional tachycardia, this rhythm is often best referred to as a supraventricular tachycardia. Atrioventricular junctional tachycardias have etiology, treatment, and prognosis similar to those of atrial tachycardia. The nurse notifies the physician at the onset or increase of this tachycardia and observes the patient for signs of congestive heart failure or other symptoms of low cardiac output.

INTRAVENTRICULAR CONDUCTION DEFECT

An intraventricular conduction defect is defined electrocardiographically as a QRS which is prolonged over 0.1 second. This type of conduction defect may be peripheral and may not fit the criteria of a right or a left bundle branch block. Intraventricular conduction defects may result from drug administration (digitalis, quinidine, Pronestyl or Lidocaine), coronary artery disease, ventricular distention, congenital heart disease, and infectious myocarditis. The nurse continually observes the patient for widening QRSs, especially when the previously mentioned drugs are being given. The physician is notified of any new changes in QRS duration over 0.1 second, or of any change in the direction of the QRS complex.

VENTRICULAR PREMATURE CONTRACTIONS (VPC)

Ventricular premature contractions (see also in Chapter 4 under Ventricular Premature Beats) are the result of the discharge of an irritable focus located anywhere in the ventricular myocardium. P waves are not present with a ventricular premature contraction unless the atria are fortuitously depolarized before the VPC or depolarized in a retrograde manner (see later). The ventricular complex of a ventricular premature contraction is wide because the ventricle is depolarized via slow muscle fiber to muscle fiber conduction rather than via the normal rapid ventricular conduction (Purkinje) system.

The T wave of a ventricular premature contraction is often opposite the direction of the QRS complex, indicating abnormal repolarization. A compensatory pause equal to twice the patient's normal R-R interval follows the VPC, except in the instance of retrograde conduction of the atria or in arrhythmias with irregular atrial and ventricular rhythms, such as atrial fibrillation. The compensatory pause occurs because ventricular premature contractions usually do not depolarize the atria and thus the sinus pacemaker continues to fire on time (the first sinus impulse following a ventricular premature contraction will usually not activate the already refractory ventricle). Ventricular premature contractions can often be differentiated from atrial premature contractions and junctional premature contractions by the absence of a conducted P wave, by a wider than normal QRS, and by a compensatory (rather than resetting) pause. Differentiation of a ventricular premature contraction from an aberrantly conducted atrial premature contraction or junctional premature contraction is thought to be impossible by some electrocardiographers.

Types of Ventricular Premature Contractions

Unifocal ventricular premature contractions are ventricular ectopic beats arising from one focus. These ventricular premature contractions have the same direction and configuration in any given ECG lead and have a fixed coupling interval to the previous sinus beat (the coupling interval being the time interval between the end of the T wave of the sinus beat and the beginning of the ectopic beat).

Multifocal ventricular premature contractions are ventricular ectopic beats arising from two or more foci. Because each of the foci will stimulate the ventricle from a different direction, the vector of the ventricular premature contraction will vary. Multifocal ventricular premature contractions generally indicate a higher degree of myocardial irritability.

Reciprocal beats occur as the result of the retrograde activation of the atria by ventricular premature contractions. The activated atria may conduct impulses to the AV node and ventricle if they are no longer refractory from the ventricular premature contraction. If the ventricle is refractory, a nonconducted P wave is seen following the ventricular premature contraction (reciprocal beats may also occur with atrial premature contractions and junctional premature contractions).

Interpolated ventricular premature contractions may occur between two sinus beats without disturbing the normal R-R interval. This type of ventricular premature contraction is seen in slower (60 to 70 per minute) sinus rates.

Ventricular premature contractions occurring during the relative refractory period of the ventricle (before repolarization is complete) indicate a strong ectopic focus. This type of ventricular premature contraction is significant in that the stimulus may occur during the period of maximum cardiac electrical vulnerability and may trigger ventricular tachycardia or ventricular fibrillation (the R-on-T phenomenon).

Ventricular bigeminy is an arrhythmia in which each sinus beat is followed at a fixed coupling interval by a ventricular premature contraction. This arrhythmia is frequently a manifestation of digitalis intoxication, although it may be seen with any organic heart disease.

Causes of ventricular premature contractions include any organic heart disease, digitalis intoxication, hypoxia, electrolyte and acid-base disturbances, cardiac depressant medications (such as quinidine, lidocaine, and Pronestyl), epinephrine, isoproterenol, caffeine, and amphetamines. Some individuals have premature ventricular contractions for years with no symptoms and no apparent heart disease.

Patients may have no symptoms from ventricular premature contractions. Others may complain of missed beats or chest or neck pain caused by the more forceful ventricular contraction following the premature one.

The significance of premature ventricular contractions depends upon their etiology, their frequency, and their relationship to the T wave of the previous beat. Ventricular premature contractions occurring in the individual with recent myocardial infarction are dangerous and require immediate treatment because of the electrical irritability of freshly infarcted cardiac tissue. Frequent ventricular premature contractions (more than six per minute), bigeminy, multifocal, ectopic beats occurring during the T wave of the preceding beat, or two or more consecutive ventricular premature contractions can lead to ventricular tachycardia and ventricular fibrillation.

Treatment of VPCs

The treatment of ventricular premature contractions will depend upon their etiology. In general, acute episodes of ventricular premature contractions (as with myocardial infarction) are treated with antiarrhythmic agents, such as lidocaine, quinidine, and Pronestyl. Digitalis-induced ventricular premature contractions are treated by withholding further digitalis preparations, by the administration of supplemental potassium, and by intramuscular or intravenous Dilantin or other antiarrhythmic drugs, VPCs thought to be caused by hypoxemia are treated by raising the patient's arterial oxygen content.

Ventricular premature contractions occurring with congestive heart failure may be treated with digitalis preparations. Occasionally, ventricular premature contractions are caused by cardiac depressant medications, such as lidocaine, quinidine, and Pronestyl. The depressant action of these drugs is thought to produce ventricular premature contractions by suppressing one or more areas of the myocardium which then do not depolarize with the rest of the ventricle. At a critical point following the normal depolarization, the "suppressed" focus will depolarize, and a premature ventricular contraction results. This type of premature ventricular contraction is treated by withholding the suppressant medication.

The nursing implications in the care of the patient with premature ventricular contractions are many. The nurse is aware of the pertinent medical history of the patient and his previous arrhythmic status. The onset or increasing frequency of ventricular premature contractions is reported immediately to the physician. The relationship of the ventricular premature contraction to the preceding T wave is always noted. The patient with myocardial infarction is closely observed for ventricular premature contractions, as ventricular tachycardia and ventricular fibrillation may occur suddenly and with little warning in these patients. Digitalized patients are closely observed for unifocal and multifocal ventricular premature contractions. Runs of two or more ventricular premature contractions in a row are always dangerous and the nurse must be well prepared to give appropriate medication immediately. The patient being treated for ventricular premature contractions by any of the cardiac depressant medications is closely observed for ventricular premature contractions which may result from these drugs. A patient with hypoxemia or acid-base disturbances is likely to have irritable myocardium; the underlying cause should be treated and the patient closely observed for ventricular premature contractions and other arrhythmias. The nurse notes suppression or cessation of ventricular premature contractions but is always alert for recurrent episodes of ventricular irritability.

VENTRICULAR TACHYCARDIA

Ventricular tachycardia results from the rapid discharge of a single focus (occasionally there may be more than one focus) in the ventricular myocardium. The rate is from 140 to 220 beats, but may be as low as 100 per minute. The rhythm, while often appearing to be regular, is slightly irregular. This tachycardia does not respond to carotid sinus massage. The causes of ventricular tachycardia are the same as the causes for ventricular premature contractions; in addition, general anesthesia may precipitate this arrhythmia. The rhythm appears electrocardiographically as a rapid heart action with wide, slightly irregular QRS complexes. P waves may be seen in the ECG, but their appearance bears no relationship to the ventricular complexes unless they are retrogradely conducted from the ventricle. If the patient has been in atrioventricular disassociation, P waves may appear in a regular fashion but they are slower than the ventricular tachycardia. Ventricular tachycardia is defined by some as two or more consecutive ventricular premature contractions but, more generally, six or more consecutive ventricular premature contractions constitute ventricular tachycardia or "a run of ventricular tachycardia." The hemodynamic effects of ventricular tachycardia are generally considered to be quite serious as cardiac output is usually reduced, leading to low tissue perfusion. Some authors report that ventricular tachycardia may have relatively benign hemodynamic effects (in normal hearts), depending on the site of the ventricular focus. It can be assumed that ventricular tachycardia of any duration is a very serious arrhythmia as it often severely compromises cardiac output and may lead to ventricular fibrillation and death. The treatment of ventricular tachycardia is similar to the treatment of ventricular premature contractions if the patient is conscious. If the patient suffers a syncopal episode during the tachycardia, countershock is indicated.

The patient may be asymptomatic from ventricular tachycardia if his cardiac output is not appreciably altered. In the majority of cases, patients are symptomatic, and often profoundly so, with signs of shock, dizziness, chest pain, dyspnea, and confusion.

The nurse in the CCU must, of necessity, be able to cope with this serious arrhythmia. When this arrhythmia is noted on the cardiac monitor, the nurse first checks the patient and monitoring system to be certain that the ECG pattern is not a result of artifact. The patient is observed immediately for signs of syncope and shock. If the patient is still conscious, the physician is notified immediately and anti-arrhythmic medications are given as ordered. If the patient is not conscious, direct current countershock is performed. Many CCUs have written policies concerning the administration of a lidocaine bolus for all patients having ventricular tachycardia. This type of policy is of great help to the patient who suddenly experiences ventricular tachycardia with no significant warning and for whom time-consuming telephone calls may be hazardous. The nurse should be aware of the number of times lidocaine is injected and the amount of milligrams which the patient has received during an episode of ventricular tachycardia. A lidocaine intravenous "drip" is frequently necessary after administration of the bolus to maintain blood levels of the medication. The patient is observed closely thereafter for increased ventricular irritability or additional ventricular tachycardia.

VENTRICULAR FIBRILLATION

Ventricular fibrillation is the most serious of all cardiac arrhythmias. The ventricular myocardium is twitching in an irregular and rapid manner and this chaotic heart activity results in an extremely low or nonexistent cardiac output. Electrocardiographically, this rhythm appears as a rapid and irregular baseline with bizarre ventricular configurations. The causes of ventricular fibrillation are similar to those of premature ventricular contractions and ventricular tachycardia. Ventricular fibrillation may also occur as the terminal event in debilitating diseases, such as carcinoma, renal and hepatic failures, or as the result of an electric shock. The patient experiencing ventricular fibrillation will become rapidly unconscious and may have agonal respirations.

The treatment of ventricular fibrillation is always DC countershock. In the event that defibrillation is unavailable or unsuccessful, closed chest cardiac massage and artificial ventilation are immediately instituted to maintain adequate tissue perfusion. Often, acid-base balance must be returned toward normal with buffering agents before defibrillation will be effective. Several DC countershocks may be necessary to terminate ventricular fibrillation and the nurse must be prepared to administer these shocks promptly. The severity of this arrhythmia justifies the need for every CCU nurse to be proficient in defibrillation procedures as well as cardiopulmonary resuscitation.

Nursing Care of the Patient with Respiratory Disease Related to Cardiac Disease

Cardiac disease may be complicated by disturbances in respiratory function. These respiratory disorders may be directly or indirectly related to the existing cardiac abnormalities. Pulmonary edema, for example, can be categorized as a respiratory disorder directly related to cardiac pathology, and emphysema can be classified as being indirectly related to cardiac disease. Any concomitant respiratory disease process, though, is detrimental to the cardiac patient when it compromises adequate oxygenation of blood circulated by the debilitated heart.

The problem to be discussed in this section is respiratory insufficiency—failure of the lungs to adequately exchange gases in order to meet metabolic demands of the body. Clinical manifestations or findings of respiratory insufficiency will first be presented. The subject of concern will be the manner in which these findings are seen in several respiratory disease states which may accompany cardiac disease. The various disease states will be described with a presentation of their respective signs and symptoms. Major emphasis will be directed to the appropriate interventions and observations which should be made by nursing personnel in the intensive coronary care setting. In general, the nurse's role is to protect the patient from the effects of oxygen deficiency and to initiate measures to maintain adequate ventilation for the patient.

CLINICAL MANIFESTATIONS OR FINDINGS OF RESPIRATORY INSUFFICIENCY—ASSESSMENT OF THE PROBLEM

Hypoxia

Hypoxia, or the inadequate supply of oxygen to body tissues, can be the result of any one of the following causes:

1. Arterial-venous shunting. Venous blood bypasses a number of alveoli, failing to exchange its waste products for oxygen, and then dilutes the arterial stream with this unoxygenated blood.

2. Hypoventilation.

3. Problems of diffusion across the alveolar-capillary membrane.

4. Ventilation-perfusion disorders. A disproportion exists between blood flow distribution and ventilation.

Early signs of hypoxia are tachycardia, hyperventilation, and hypertension. These compensatory mechanisms result from the effect of hypoxia on the sympathetic nervous system, causing it to become more active and leading to vasoconstriction and increased peripheral resistance. Restlessness, anxiety, confusion, and cyanosis often accompany the mechanisms listed before. It must be stressed, though, that the presence or absence of cyanosis is often difficult to assess, and the patient may be experiencing a severe degree of hypoxia before cyanosis becomes evident.

In chronic or advanced stages of hypoxia, the sympathetic nervous system response fails, and a decreasing heart rate and hypotension ensue. The patient experiences disturbances in seeing and hearing and often has chest pain.

Hypercarbia

Hypercarbia, or carbon dioxide retention, produces the following effects: various degrees of circulatory failure, hypertension, and cerebral depression (ranging from mild sedation to deep coma) caused by a local depressant effect on the function of brain tissues. From stimulation of the autonomic nervous system, there is an increase in cardiac output and heart rate. The signs and symptoms the patient manifests are a combination of these two interacting effects of depression and stimulation. Muscle twitching, visual defects, increased cutaneous blood flow with erythema and diaphoresis, cardiac arrhythmias, and drowsiness progressing to severe coma and respiratory arrest may be seen.

Hypotension

Hypotension associated with marked peripheral vasoconstriction brings about cold, clammy, pale skin, tachycardia, and a thready peripheral pulse.

Dyspnea

Hypoxia may also cause dyspnea or difficult and labored respiration. The role of the nurse is one of continual anticipation and assessment of the manifestations of respiratory insufficiency. The nature of the patient's respiration should be evaluated in terms of its rate, type, rhythm, quality of excursion of the chest, relationship between inspiration and expiration, chest sounds, and resulting color of skin and mucous membranes. If the patient is found to be experiencing respiratory distress, a quick check of his level of consciousness, airway patency, and quality of respiration takes priority. Interventions are geared to the severity of the respiratory insufficiency. The patient in mild distress may benefit from the administration of oxygen via nasal prongs, catheter, or face mask; from elevation of the head of his bed to a semi-Fowler's or Fowler's position; and from reassurance until the physician is able to assess the underlying problem. The patient in severe distress requires a patent airway and resuscitative measures. In either type of situation, the nurse's first response is to attempt to determine the cause of respiratory insufficiency. She tries to alleviate the situation and calls for assistance from nursing and medical team members as necessary (see later in this Chapter for a more detailed discussion of the management of acute respiratory failure).

DISEASE PROCESSES

Pneumonia

Pneumonia is an infection of the alveolar spaces of the lung caused by bacterial, viral, rickettsial, or fungal infectious agents. Microorganisms reach the lungs via the respiratory passages or via the blood stream, become lodged in the alveoli, and proliferate. Their metabolic products initiate an inflammatory process. Edema fluid is poured into the alveolar spaces, and becomes a vehicle for the spread of the inflammation to other alveoli, lobules, and lobes of the lungs.

In assessing this problem, the patient is interviewed and observed. He frequently gives a history of an upper respiratory infection, shaking chills, and sharp pains in his chest. He complains of a cough with pinkish to rusty, thick, purulent sputum, headache, dyspnea, delirium, and painful respiration.

Physiologic measurement of the problem reveals rapid respirations (25 to 45 per minute), temperature elevation (101 to 105° F), rapid pulse (100 to 130), and sometimes a pleural friction rub.

Medical interventions consist of the administration of appropriate antibiotics once the causative bacterial organism is identified, the symptomatic treatment of viral pneumonia, and the control and removal of secretions.

The nurse, during her interventions, exercises clean technique to protect other patients and herself from contamination. Fluids are forced to hydrate the patient. Water is also delivered to the mucous membrane to topically thin the secretions. This is accomplished by the administration of mist from ultrasonic aerosol generators, and by the delivery of aerosolized water 10 to 15 minutes before each intermittent positive pressure breathing treatment. Bronchodilator therapy also facilitates sputum production. Dry gases should never be inhaled for prolonged periods of time, as they dry secretions and irritate the airways.

Removal of secretions. This is accomplished by encouraging the patient to cough and expectorate sputum. Endotracheal or naso-tracheal aspiration is indicated when the patient is unable to satis-factorily expectorate and when secretions block his airway. The method of aspiration is as follows:

1. Depending on the status of the patient, delivery of 100 per cent oxygen may be needed prior to and after each aspiration.

2. Clean technique is used. The nurse washes her hands before and after the procedure, uses gloves, and utilizes either sterile, dis-posable, plastic suction catheters or catheters stored in an antiseptic solution.

3. A size 14 to 16 French catheter is inserted into the trachea via the nose or mouth while the patient's tongue is held forward and his head is facing the opposite direction of the bronchus to be aspirated. The patient is encouraged to cough or take a deep breath while the catheter is being advanced.

4. No suction is applied during the catheter insertion. The loca-tion of the catheter is checked by listening for breath sounds from the external tip of the catheter. If there are no breath sounds, or if the patient did not cough when the catheter was introduced, there is a good chance the catheter is in the upper esophagus instead of in the trachea.

5. Five to 10 ml of sterile saline solution may be injected through the catheter to stimulate an effective cough and to liquefy and loosen secretions.

6. The catheter is attached to the suction apparatus, is with-drawn while intermittent suction is applied and while continuous rotation of 360 degrees of the catheter tip occurs. No more than 5 to 7 seconds should elapse during the aspiration, as inhaled air or oxygen will also be aspirated.

7. The oropharynx is aspirated.

8. The patient is reassured during the procedure.

9. Asepsis is promoted if the suction catheter is never reinserted into the lungs after it has been introduced into a container of unsterile solution used to unclog the tubing.

Postural drainage. Postural drainage of the bronchial tree aids in the removal of secretions by producing a simple gravity mechanism and by aiding the cough reflex. The position used should not be so uncomfortable as to cause the patient distress. The bronchi and trachea should be lower than the segment of lung to be drained, and the thorax should be lower than the hips so both bases of the lungs can be cleared. Coughing is encouraged as positions are rotated from side to back to side in order to evenly drain the various bronchial areas. Goals of postural drainage are further enhanced by 10 minutes' inhalation of heated aerosolized water mist and 10 minutes of intermittent positive pressure breathing, sometimes with bronchodilator therapy. Both are done before the drainage is begun. Physiotherapy by "cupping" and percussing of the chest wall during drainage helps to mobilize secretions.

Intermittent positive pressure breathing (IPPB). IPPB is advantageous in several ways. It helps to mobilize secretions in patients with or without respiratory failure and improves the expansion of terminal airways. Also, it is an effective means of delivering bronchodilators.

The nurse observes the patient on bronchodilator therapy, utilizing isoproterenol or phenylephrine, for side effects of these medications—diaphoresis, tremors, palpitations, tachycardia, and cardiac arrhythmias—and notifies the physician when they occur. Bronchodilator therapy is dangerous in patients with hypertension or coronary, cerebral, and peripheral vascular disease. Aminophylline is sometimes used for its bronchodilatory and diuretic effects. Since secretions increase at night and cause increased airway resistance, bedtime bronchodilator treatment and IPPB when the patient awakens during the night provide easier breathing for the patient.

When, despite coughing and suctioning, secretions are retained and obstructive atelectasis continues, bedside bronchoscopy may be indicated. This procedure allows viewing of the pathologic process, aspiration of secretions, and delivery of oxygen simultaneously through the side arm of the bronchoscope. It also stimulates vigorous coughing; the postbronchoscopy period is a valuable time for clearing atelectasis.

During bronchoscopy, a topical anesthetic for the oropharynx and vocal cords is often utilized to prevent laryngospasm. The patient should be sitting at a 30 degree angle with his head tilted back over the head of the bed or a pillow. Because of the nature of the procedure, the patient needs an explanation of the reasons for it, and must be reassured and comforted.

If the patient continues to manifest signs of respiratory insufficiency despite the previously mentioned medical and nursing measures, he may require endotracheal intubation. Intubation is definitely indicated when the patient obviously (or potentially) cannot maintain his own airway; this is the primary initial treatment in respiratory arrest. Tracheostomy is usually performed only electively when ideal facilities are available.

Endotracheal intubation promotes the following:

1. Establishment and maintenance of an airway.

2. Prevention of aspiration by separating the trachea from the upper gastrointestinal tract.

3. A pathway for effective removal of tracheobronchial secretions.

4. Facilitation of a closed system for the most effective delivery of IPPB treatments.

Only cuffed endotracheal tubes should be used, and the cuff should be inflated with several milliliters of air prior to insertion to test it for air leakage. The intubation procedure is explained to the patient as applicable, and reassurance is given. A topical anesthetic is employed as necessary. Because of the danger of tracheal wall necrosis, the cuff is deflated every hour for five to 10 minutes. Double-cuffed endotracheal tubes also help to decrease this danger.

The technique for suction through the endotracheal tube is modified slightly from nasotracheal suction. It should be performed in direct relation to the amount of the patient's secretions.

1. Administer 100 per cent oxygen for several breaths prior to and after aspiration, as needed.

2. With sterile technique, aspirate from the tube.

3. Aspirate the oropharynx using clean technique, so that secretions above the cuff will not drop into the lungs.

4. Deflate the cuff.

5. Aspirate from the tube a second time, with a sterile catheter (different from the oropharyngeal one).

6. Reinflate the cuff until the respirator "triggers."

The number of milliliters of air needed to inflate the cuff just barely to occlusion should be recorded.

Frequent auscultation of the chest by the nurse is advised to be sure the patient is adequately ventilating both lungs and to rule out the possibility that the tube has dislodged and become misplaced.

The major complications of endotracheal intubation are damage to the vocal cords and edema of trachea and larynx. The patient is carefully observed after removal of the tube for signs of airway obstruction resulting from severe edema. In addition, continual assessment of the patient's total respiratory status is important after extubation.

While intubated, the patient requires reassurance that he will be able to communicate with the nursing staff. Pencil and paper and a bell for him to ring help him to communicate his needs. Sedation may be needed to allay his anxiety, but this is used with caution because of its respiratory depressive effects.

The indications for a tracheostomy are similar to those already cited for endotracheal intubation. Tracheostomy is performed when maintenance of an airway is needed for greater than 36 hours, when an endotracheal tube is not tolerated by a conscious patient, and when an endotracheal tube is contraindicated because of pre-existing pharyngeal or laryngeal obstruction from other causes.

The fresh tracheostomy incision is observed for evidence of excessive bleeding and is protected from contamination. If a metal tracheostomy tube has been inserted, the inner cannula is removed every two hours for cleaning with a detergent solution, is rinsed with sterile water, and is reinserted immediately. The physician is notified if there is difficulty in replacing the inner cannula. An additional tracheostomy tube should always be kept at the bedside.

Adequate humidification is mandatory, as once the trachea is opened, its natural wetting function is lost. The patient often loses his cough reflex and requires suctioning to remove secretions. Instillation of 5 to 10 ml of sterile saline solution through the tracheostomy tube just prior to aspiration helps to moisten secretions. This instillation should not be done excessively, though, because it may cause additional damage to the mucosal surface of the tracheobronchial tree. Aspiration is done only in relation to the amount of the patient's secretions. As with the intubated patient discussed before, the patient with a tracheostomy benefits from much comforting and from the use of a bell and writing utensils to communicate his wishes.

Inhalation therapy equipment is changed at regular, frequent intervals to ensure aseptic technique for the delivery of gases into the lungs. Water nebulizers are especially prone to be excellent media for gram-negative organisms; they should be rinsed out thoroughly with sterile water or a dilute acetic acid solution each time before they are refilled and should be replaced with new sterile equipment at least once daily.

Left-Sided Congestive Heart Failure

Congestive heart failure is the state of insufficient cardiac output to provide for the body's metabolic needs. The left ventricle fails owing to myocardial damage from various disease processes. The ventricle is unable to contract as efficiently as needed, leading to the situation of "forward failure." Blood volume increases in the left ventricle with resulting increased systolic and diastolic volumes, and the ventricle is unable to empty itself completely during systole. Hypertrophy of the ventricular wall ensues. Because of incomplete emptying, the pressure in the ventricle during diastole is elevated; this increased pressure is transmitted into the left atrium and pulmonary venous circulation, causing "backward failure." This vascular engorgement often leads to acute pulmonary edema, which, in turn, causes an increase in pressure in the pulmonary arterial system; the right ventricle then must exert higher pressures to overcome this increased vascular resistance. Decreased renal blood flow from the poor cardiac output causes less efficient glomerular filtration, a falling output of sodium, chloride, and water, with resulting fluid retention. Increased tissue and blood volumes thus further worsen the circulatory congestion.

In assessing this problem, the nurse first observes the patient. He may give a history of or may manifest dyspnea, orthopnea, paroxysmal nocturnal dyspnea, cough with or without hemoptysis, wheezing, distended neck veins, anxiety, anorexia, and nausea. He frequently sits upright to facilitate respiration.

Secondly, physiologic measurement reveals a central venous pressure which often is elevated, and a rise in pulmonary arterial pressure. Rales in both lungs, tachycardia, gallop rhythms, and cardiac arrhythmias are often seen. An enlarged, tender liver, ascites, and edema of the feet, sacrum, and flanks may be present.

Medical interventions may consist of the administration of diuretics to control edema and to decrease sodium and water retention, digitalis and isoproterenol to increase myocardial contractility, and morphine to allay anxiety and to decrease tachypnea. Intake of sodium and fluid is restricted. Rest and limited activity are ordered because metabolic demands are lessened.

If pulmonary edema exists, the following measures are taken:

1. The patient is reassured and made comfortable; the head of his bed is elevated.

2. Digitalis is given to increase myocardial contractility.

3. Aminophylline is sometimes used to decrease bronchospasm and to improve cardiac output.

4. Morphine is administered to allay anxiety, to decrease tachypnea, and to reduce pulmonary edema.

5. Enriched oxygen mixtures are delivered via positive pressure breathing apparatus, mask or nasal prongs.

6. Rapid-acting diuretics (ethacrynic acid, furosemide, or a mercurial diuretic) are given intravenously.

7. A rapid decrease in the intravascular volume in severe pulmonary edema is promoted by the use of rotating tourniquets or phlebotomy.

Prophylactic anticoagulation decreases the incidence of pulmonary embolization resulting from thrombi formed in slowly circulated venous blood. Antiembolic stockings or Ace bandages help to prevent venous pooling, and isometric exercising of the lower limbs improves muscle tone around veins and speeds venous return.

The nurse intervenes by making the patient as comfortable as possible and by creating a restful environment. She understands the mechanism of action of the diuretics being administered, recognizes the signs and symptoms of electrolyte imbalance, and is familiar with the normal values of serum and urine electrolytes. In particular, she is constantly alert for changes in serum potassium.

The patient receiving diuretics is potentially prone to develop hypokalemia, a situation hazardous to the critically ill. Signs of hypokalemia may consist of neuromuscular disturbances (paresthesias, hyporeflexia) and cardiac abnormalities (arrhythmias, increased sensitivity to digitalis.) The ECG commonly shows the following: prolonged PR interval, tall P waves, widened QRS complexes, flat or inverted T waves, prominent U waves, and depressed ST segments.

Findings of hyperkalemia include areflexia, muscular or respiratory paralysis, and paresthesias. Bradycardia, hypotension, ventricular fibrillation, and cardiac arrest may occur. The ECG may show tall peaked T waves, depressed ST segments, a prolonged PR interval, a diminished-to-absent P wave, and a widening of the QRS complex with prolongation of the QT interval.

Other nursing interventions in a patient with congestive heart failure include:

1. Whenever possible, diuretics are given starting in the morning instead of near bedtime to avoid disturbing the patient's sleep because of diuresis.

2. A baseline ECG is obtained for later reference before digitalization is begun.

3. The patient is observed for such side effects of morphine as nausea, vomiting, and depressed respiration.

4. Auscultation of the chest determines the rate at which rales and gallop rhythm are decreasing after treatment is begun.

5. Proper care is taken of edematous skin to prevent skin breakdown resulting from poor circulation.

6. Antiembolic stockings or Ace bandages are applied so as not to constrict circulation and are removed once every eight hours. The patient is asked to uncross his legs while he reclines in bed.

7. The patient on anticoagulation therapy is observed for signs of bleeding. All stools are tested for occult blood. Intramuscular injections are avoided when possible.

8. Dextrose (5 per cent) in water to keep the IV open is de-

livered at the slowest rate possible to the cardiac patient in order to prevent pulmonary edema from excessive fluid administration.

9. If rotating tourniquets are indicated, blood pressure cuffs inflated to less than the patient's systolic blood pressure may be utilized. They are rotated every 15 minutes. Tourniquets, though, may be of little value if marked edema or venous distention is present.

10. If phlebotomy is indicated, 100 ml of blood is removed every five to 10 minutes. It is usually contraindicated in the presence of shock.

Right-Sided Congestive Heart Failure

In this case the problem is right ventricular enlargement and failure resulting from the backward failure associated with left heart failure or from pathology in the lungs. Pulmonary congestion and hypertension increase the workload of the right ventricle; inadequate systolic emptying produces increased right ventricular diastolic pressure and rising atrial and peripheral venous pressures.

Medical interventions are geared toward correction of hypoxia, hypercapnia, and respiratory acidosis and toward decreasing pulmonary vascular resistance so the right ventricle can recover. Any electrolyte or acid-base abnormality complicating right ventricular failure during acute respiratory failure is corrected. Digitalis, rest, diuretics, salt restriction, and phlebotomy are indicated as in the situation of left heart failure.

Nursing activities are similar to those initiated for the patient experiencing left heart failure. Phlebotomy is indicated here, though, for a slightly different reason. Polycythemia and increased blood viscosity may be present because of the compensatory mechanism of a body reacting to chronic lung disease. Polycythemia increases the workload of the right ventricle and thus must be minimized. It also creates the danger of intravascular thrombosis with possible embolization.

Pulmonary Embolization and Infarction

Pulmonary embolization is the lodging of a blood clot in a pulmonary artery; pulmonary infarction is the death of a portion of lung tissue resulting from occlusion by a lodged embolus. Both are brought about by the creation of thrombosis in veins of the lower extremities in the pelvis, or in the right side of the heart. Fragments of thrombosed material break loose and are carried by the blood stream to the pulmonary artery. Occlusion of the pulmonary artery leads to a generalized spasm of pulmonary arteries and veins and to pulmonary hypertension. Overloading and dilatation of the right side of the heart, along with decreased filling of the left ventricle, creates a lowered cardiac output, decreased peripheral circulation, and congestive heart failure.

Symptoms the patient experiences depend on the circulatory impact of the embolus and on the size and location of the infarction. The embolic process may be undetected clinically or severe shock may ensue. Often, there is a sudden onset of acute chest pain accompanied by acute dyspnea, jugular venous distension, and gross hemoptysis. Pleuritic pain may last for several days. Tachycardia, fever, tachypnea, and hypotension are frequently manifested along with the patient's subjective complaints.

Control of the circulatory reaction to the embolism is one of the most important of the medical interventions. Oxygen, digitalis and levarterenol are administered as needed to treat hypoxia, heart failure and shock. Anticoagulation with heparin therapy is initiated immediately to prevent further embolization. Appropriate treatment of any cardiac arrhythmias (usually supraventricular tachycardia, atrial fibrillation, or atrial flutter) is instituted. Pain medication is administered. Occasionally, inferior vena cava ligation is performed for patients who have recurrent emboli despite anticoagulant therapy. Thrombophlebitis is treated if present. Depending on the patient's status, surgical embolectomy may be indicated.

The patient receiving anticoagulants is carefully observed by the nurse for signs of bleeding. Anticoagulants decrease the possibility of parts of thrombi breaking off into the circulation and prevent further thrombus formation. Any signs of thrombophlebitis (inflammation of part of an extremity, along with an increase in pulse and temperature) are reported to the physician. The nurse comforts the patient and attempts to allay his anxiety.

Cardiogenic Shock

Cardiogenic shock is the most serious of the cardiac disease processes affecting the respiratory system. Myocardial damage from whatever cause impairs cardiac contractility and results in a sharply reduced cardiac output, congestive heart failure and systemic hypotension. Usually, both the systemic and pulmonary circuits are affected. The decreased perfusion of peripheral tissues leads to the accumulation of lactic acid and the decreased blood flow to the lungs leads to a lowered oxygen supply for the body. The resultant metabolic acidosis and hypoxemia compound one another in a vicious cycle of cardiac deterioration unless aggressive medical treatment intervenes and breaks the cycle.

The patient may manifest cold, clammy skin, restlessness, and confusion sometimes progressing to a comatose state. Physiologic measurement and observation reveal rapid, thready peripheral pulses, a low or unobtainable blood pressure utilizing an external sphygmomanometer, falling urine output, low or normal central venous pressure (may be elevated if right heart failure is present), and a decreased arterial oxygen tension, often less than 60 mm Hg.

Medical interventions attempt to increase cardiac output. Oxygen is administered and IPPB by face mask or endotracheal tube may be necessary to help reduce pulmonary edema. The central venous pressure or arterial pressure is monitored, and intravenous fluids are delivered if the central venous pressure is normal or low. Isoproterenol is given to increase cardiac output by its positive inotropic and chronotropic effects; it also decreases peripheral vasoconstriction. Metaraminol and levarterenol may also be used to increase cardiac output, but they also increase peripheral vascular resistance. Digitalis is administered if there are clinical signs of congestive failure. Arterial blood gas studies are performed to determine the degree of hypoxia and acidosis present. Sodium bicarbonate is employed to counteract the existing metabolic acidosis.

The nurse continually observes the patient's vital signs, level of consciousness, central venous or arterial pressure, skin color and warmth, urine output, and so on. She is especially aware of the numerous pathophysiologic causes for potential cardiac arrhythmias, which are ever present in this critical situation.

The Nurse's Role in Cardiopulmonary Resuscitation

The nurse functioning in the intensive coronary care setting is one of the persons most likely to discover a patient in cardiopulmonary arrest. She must, therefore, be capable of assessing the situation quickly and intervening in an intelligent, calm manner during this critical situation. Effective resuscitative efforts on her part will be enhanced by a review of the following outline of nursing practices.

Today, most intensive care units are equipped with a mechanical alarm system which is triggered when the heart rate rises or falls beyond predetermined levels. The alarm may serve as the first indication that something is amiss. The astute nurse never depends solely upon this auditory means of assessment; instead, she vigilantly watches the cardiac oscilloscope.

On the oscilloscope, cardiac arrest is noted by the presence of either chaotic electrical activity (indicative of ventricular fibrillation) or a flat tracing (indicative of cardiac asystole). Once either of these patterns is noted, the nurse immediately verifies its validity by observing the patient. Often the ECG artifact resulting from the patient's activity or the flat tracing from a loosened electrocardiographic lead may mimic the cardinal oscilloscopic manifestations of cardiac arrest. If the patient is then found to have a deathlike appearance (unresponsiveness, apnea, cyanosis, dilated pupils, no pulses), the nurse assumes the occurrence of cardiopulmonary arrest, notifies another nurse in the unit, and notes the time of arrest, never leaving the patient for any reason.

She begins cardiopulmonary resuscitation, which is performed urgently but smoothly, and which is never stopped until the physician in charge decides whether or not the resuscitative measures have been successful. Time is of the utmost concern in the prevention of brain damage, which occurs within three to five minutes after oxygen is withheld. Thus, during resuscitation, it is mandatory that nursing and other medical personnel function as a team to avoid confusion and to improve efficiency. Only a core team of workers is necessary: an internist or resident physician (the patient's physician who is responsible for making the final decisions in the course of resuscitation), an anesthesiologist or well trained inhalation therapist, a nurse (two, if possible), and a surgeon. Excess onlookers should be encouraged to leave the area to provide maximal working space in rooms which frequently are quite small.

Until the physicians arrive, the nurse manages the resuscitation herself. Regardless of the cause of the arrest, a sharp blow with her hand to the anterior chest is occasionally helpful in initiating spontaneous respiration or cardiac function. Little time should be wasted, though, in assessing its effectiveness. If no change in the patient's condition is immediately apparent, resuscitation is begun.

If ventricular fibrillation was noted on the oscilloscope screen, the nurse's first intervention is to establish a patent airway while the second nurse is bringing the defibrillator into the area (it is obvious to mention here that if the patient had not been monitored prior to his arrest, he should soon be attached to some mode of assessing his cardiac activity). She then defibrillates the heart. (The nurse in the intensive care setting should be trained to defibrillate, since precious minutes may be lost while she waits for a physician to do this. In any case, her role in relation to defibrillation should be properly clarified beforehand by the institution of her employment.)

The procedure for defibrillation is as follows:

1. Conductive paste is applied to the paddles in an amount which will prevent burning of the patient's chest. Dribbling of paste across the chest is avoided. Too much paste may fly outward from the paddles during the application of the electrical shock, causing a current to cross above the chest wall.

2. The handles must be insulated and dry, and all equipment coming in contact with the patient must be grounded. If necessary, the ECG machine and cardiac monitor are unplugged just before the discharge to prevent damage to this equipment.

3. The paddles are applied so that the current will run along the long axis of the heart. If they are applied on the anterior chest wall, one paddle is placed over the base of the heart (second right intercostal space) and the other over the ventricular apex (usually the sixth left intercostal space in the anterior axillary line.) Paddles must be firmly applied.

4. The usual voltage for external direct current defibrillation is 200 to 400 watt-seconds. Usually the maximum amount of voltage is given with each shock, although some physicians think the first shock should be given with a smaller voltage; then the voltage is gradually increased with each successive defibrillation.

5. Current should never be discharged until all personnel are at a safe distance from the patient. The nurse must assume responsibility for the prevention of injury to the staff. No one should be in contact with the patient or his bed.

6. The cardiac monitor or ECG machine is utilized to determine the effectiveness of the initial shock. The patient may require subsequent shocks and maintenance of acceptable cardiac rhythm with such antiarrhythmics as lidocaine.

7. The patient may regain consciousness soon after defibrillation, once his cardiac output has improved. He will need an explanation and reassurance about what has happened to him.

8. Equipment is properly cleaned, dried, and returned to its designated location after use.

For the patient who has arrested as a result of asystole, the nurse performs artificial ventilation and external cardiac massage until a cardiac rhythm is re-established. Since cessation of respiration may have contributed to the cardiac arrest, the nurse first attempts to remedy the situation by clearing the airway, inserting a plastic oral or rubber nasal airway, and initiating respiratory therapy. She performs mouth-to-mouth or mouth-to-nose ventilation until a manual resuscitator bag and face mask are available. Oxygen at high flow rates is then delivered to the patient.

The airway is opened by exerting a maximal backward tilt of the head and by displacing the mandible forward. Patency of the airway

TABLE 10–1. Phases of Resuscitation*

Therapeutic Goal	Measures Taken	Decision By
Phase I — Emergency Reoxygenation of the Central Nervous System		
Establish airway	1. Tilt head backward, clearing pharynx	M.D., R.N., Lay person
	2. Displace mandible forward	M.D., R.N., Lay
	3. Insertion of pharyngeal tube	M.D., R.N., Lay
	4. Endotracheal intubation	M.D.
	5. Cricothyroid membrane puncture	M.D.
	6. Tracheostomy (usually later)	M.D.
Establish breathing by intermittent positive pressure ventilation	1. Mouth-to-mouth or mouth-to-nose breathing	M.D., R.N., Lay
	2. Mouth-to-adjunct-tube breathing	M.D., R.N., Lay
	3. Use of bag mask or bellows	M.D.
	4. Use of mechanical oxygen-respirator if patient is intubated	M.D.
Establish circulation	1. External cardiac compression	M.D., R.N., Lay
	2. Internal cardiac compression (still required in some patients)	M.D.

Essential Therapy	Measures Taken	Decision By
Phase II — Restoration of Spontaneous Circulation		
Stimulate circulation (elevate B.P.)	Drug: vasopressor	M.D.
Correct metabolic acidosis	Drug: sodium bicarbonate	M.D.
Establish heart beat	1. Drugs: Epinephrine, calcium chloride, calcium gluconate	M.D.
	2. Pacemaker — most effective in Stokes-Adams syndrome	M.D.
	3. Defibrillator; for ventricular fibrillation (AC or DC current)	M.D.
Maintain blood volume	1. I.V. fluids	M.D., R.N.
	2. Cut-downs to supply I.V. fluids	M.D., R.N.
Phase III — Long-term Resuscitation		
Reduce body temperature if neurological changes appear	Hypothermia	M.D.
Intensive care		
Adequate ventilation	Tracheostomy	M.D.
	Prolonged artificial ventilation	M.D.
	Adequate suctioning	M.D., R.N.
Maintain fluid and electrolyte balance	Carefully administered I.V. fluid and drugs	M.D.
Reverse causative agent of arrest	Monitoring with careful observation for additional arrests. Proper use of drugs and equipment if further symptoms occur	M.D.

NOTE: In some situations nurses will be expected to make some of the decisions delegated to the doctor in this outline. Each nurse must clarify the policies of the employing institution before assuming the responsibility for these decisions.

*From Modell, W., Schwartz, D. R., Hazeltine, L. S., and Kirkhom, F. T., Jr.: Handbook of Cardiology for Nurses. 5th ed. New York, Springer Publishing Company, Inc., 1966.

is maintained by removing foreign materials or secretions with a cloth or suction apparatus. The nurse readies the endotracheal intubation tray, which is equipped with a laryngoscope and endotracheal tubes of various sizes; she assists with the intubation by checking the endotracheal tube cuff for air leakage and by lubricating the tube.

As an airway is adequately established, the work of maintaining the circulation ensues. Femoral and carotid pulses are checked as an indication of the quality of the cardiac output. If they are absent, external cardiac massage is continued.

The techniques and theoretical considerations of cardiopulmonary resuscitation were presented in Chapter 9 and will not be duplicated here. However, Table 10–1 on the phases of a resuscitation will serve to orient the cardiac nurse to her responsibilities.

It is the nurse's responsibility in dealing with an arrest to note the time of arrest, the time and amount of medications administered, the therapeutic procedures performed, and the patient's subsequent response. Also, she documents the electrocardiographic events during the resuscitation. It is often helpful to obtain a rhythm strip from the "memory loop" of the cardiac monitor so that documentation of the patient's cardiac rhythm just prior to his arrest is available.

Once spontaneous cardiac and pulmonary activity resume, the patient requires the utmost of nursing care. Frequent observation is made of his vital signs, electrocardiogram, level of response, and so on. Prevention of complications is the most important nursing goal. Any subtle changes in the patient's status, such as increasing myocardial irritability, decreasing urinary output, or deteriorating level of response, are reported immediately to the physician.

During the arrest, other patients in the unit are protected from viewing upsetting procedures by having their curtains drawn. A nurse in the unit makes sure that the other patients' needs are met at this time. Too frequently it is the most spontaneous response for a majority of nurses to help with the arrested patient, often at the expense of other patients' nursing care. But patients, especially when they feel the stress of the emergency situation, have needs which become paramount at this time. Their reactions to the emergency will be highly individualized; the nurse responds to their questions and behavior at a level appropriate to the patient's apparent ability to cope with the situation. Often a simple explanation of the fact that one of their fellow patients has become very ill and is receiving intensive medical treatment will suffice. Some patients are able to ask whether or not the patient has died; if he has, many times an affirmative answer along with an explanation that the patient had been very ill will satisfy the patient's curiosity. A reminder that he is receiving the best of medical care frequently helps to allay some of his fears about his own condition. Other patients are not able to verbalize questions such as these; it is a test of the nurse's judgment to be able to deal with her patient's subjective response to stress and death. She helps him deal with his feelings only as soon as he is ready. In any case, it is not appropriate for the nurse to deny the fact that an emergency has occurred in the unit.

Bibliography

Goldman, M. J.: Electrocardiography. Los Altos, California, Lange Medical Publications, 1966.

Hurst, J. W., and Logue, R. B.: The Heart. New York, McGraw-Hill Book Company, 1969.

Lyght, C. E. (ed.): The Merck Manual. 11th ed. Rahway, New Jersey, Merck & Co., Inc., 1966.

Phipps, W. J., and Barker, W. L.: Respiratory Insufficiency and Failure, Concepts and Practices of Intensive Care for Nurse Specialists. Philadelphia, The Charles Press, 1969.

Sedlock, S., Scheinman, M., Morrelli, H., and Griffeath, H.: Drug Sheet for Coronary Nurses. Regional Medical Program, Area I, July 1970.

Smith, J. W. (ed.): Manual of Medical Therapeutics. 19th ed. Boston, Little, Brown and Company, 1969.

CHAPTER 11

Nursing Care of the Surgical Cardiac Patient

By Stephanie A. Sedlock, R.N.

The Preoperative Phase

After the patient has been admitted to the hospital, the period before surgery is utilized to make an accurate diagnosis and to evaluate the need for surgical intervention. If surgery is indicated, the patient's physical status may need improving, and during this preoperative period it is possible for the nurse to (1) know the patient so emotional support can be given, (2) establish a baseline for postoperative evaluation and care, and (3) do preoperative teaching to make the patient a "vital link" in the "team."

Getting to know your patient

Getting to know the patient is a very crucial phase. Once you learn what the patient is like and he learns what you are like, together you are able to begin working out present problems, developing inner resources, and preparing for the forthcoming surgery.

460

Establishing a Meaningful Rapport

It takes more than one visit the night before surgery to develop a meaningful rapport with the patient. Therefore, the nurse will be able to accomplish more if she sees the patient on several occasions. Establishing a meaningful rapport is synonymous with becoming a friend who is real and genuine, one who cares. This type of relationship will open communications which will allow the patient to disclose his feelings and uncertainties. Once these feelings are brought to the surface, it is possible for both the nurse and the patient to work with them. The nurse with a "bedside manner" that has a ritualistic, formal manner may block communication and prevent a meaningful relationship from developing.

Helping the Patient Learn the Patient Role

Once communications are opened, a trust develops and the nurse begins to learn what the patient is like as an individual. We are all individuals and hospitalization tends to depersonalize patients; for this reason, it is important to recognize and encourage the patient to be an individual and to maintain his integrity and self-image. In order to do this, he will need help in learning his role as a patient, and the nurse will need to learn more about his emotional patterns.

Previous hospitalizations do not seem to provide the kind of familiarity which makes a patient comfortable within the hospital environment. If the patient is to become a "vital link" in his care and be under less tension, the nurse will need to teach him about his environment and what is expected of him. The patient needs more orientation, as the hospital is a special world of unfamiliar phenomena, and different personnel with specific and varying functions.

The patient should first be oriented to his immediate surroundings so he can meet the personnel on the floor, learn the meal hours, his current regimen of treatment and testing, and the visiting hours. From here the nurse can expand her orientation to include the special procedures and tests, what the patient will experience with each one, and why these tests are necessary. Since medicine has a language all its own, the sooner this problem is countered by explanation of medical terminology, the better. Also, it may be helpful to introduce the patient to other patients on the medical floor who have had surgery or who are awaiting it, as it is comforting to know that other people have similar fears, and it is encouraging to see a patient who has successfully recuperated from surgery. Patients with similar problems tend to group together, and through an *esprit de corps* they give each other a great deal of help and support. Many times the ability to help someone else will give a patient a sense of worth, and a real feeling that others need him. To isolate preoperative patients from postoperative patients on the assumption that the preoperative patient will be frightened or will receive incorrect information is erroneous. The patients' "grapevine" is very expedient and constantly functioning. Thus, it is best to encourage the patients to learn from each other and if your lines of communication are good, you will be able to correct misconceptions the patient has learned.

If the patient learns what is expected of him, and realizes how important his cooperation is in his subsequent care, he will be an active participant. In order to promote full participation and maintain open communication, it is important for the nurse to constantly meet the needs of the patient and provide support and guidance. Trust can be broken easily in this stressful period, if the patient is not given adequate support.

The Patient's Attitude Toward Surgery

To understand and to be of assistance to the patient preparing for surgery, it is necessary to know why surgery is being done, and who or what has influenced the patient to make this decision. This information will help to determine the patient's attitude toward his forthcoming surgery. If the cardiac problem has developed over a long period and the patient has reached a point where decompensation has made it impossible to comfortably carry on the activities of daily living, he realizes he is seriously ill and may look forward to surgery as a means of making him a healthy person again. If the onset of the disease is acute as opposed to being chronic, the patient does not have much time to mobilize psychologic forces to deal with the threat of cardiac surgery.

The patient will have a smoother postoperative course if he is looking forward to relief of his symptoms. In addition, he will have a fuller life, as opposed to being threatened by a loss of the "crutch" his disease could provide for manipulating people and getting special attention. Insight into this situation might be gleaned by learning if the patient made the decision for surgery on his own, or was forced into it by his family. A patient who has used his illness as a "crutch" will be less able to help those attending him and may not want to get well.

Previous experience with a serious illness or major surgery will help determine a patient's present attitude and fears. If his previous encounters with the hospital have been pleasant experiences, he will have a more positive attitude. If they were unpleasant experiences, he may be bitter or have an overwhelming fear of pain or death. These feelings are not unique to the patient, and are usually also felt by the family. It is essential to help the patient and family verbalize these fears so they can be openly dealt with in a healthy manner. This process may take time, as it is easier for some patients to sublimate or deny fear. If the nurse opens channels in which intense feelings like fear of death can flow, it is important for her not to be threatened by these feelings and turn the patient off with a comment like, "Oh, don't worry. You'll be just fine." Many times the patient only needs a good listener and can work these fears out by himself once he has been able to talk about it. On the other hand, he may just need more information to clarify misconceptions he has about his disease and surgery.

How Does the Patient Meet a Crisis Situation?

The nurse can be of more help if she is able to determine how the patient meets crisis situations. People have a tendency to develop certain patterns of meeting crisis situations that are more effective for them, and thus these patterns are used over and over again. Cardiac surgery can pose a crisis situation in the life of the patient and his family owing to the high mortality rate, the pain, the isolation, and the expense that is involved. If the nurse can learn the patient's past patterns of behavior in similar situations, she will be more helpful to the patient and his family.

Sometimes it is difficult to determine what method the patient uses to deal with stress, and even if the nurse is able to put a name to the method, unless she has had special psychologic preparation it may be impossible to plan specific therapy for the patient. What is more important at this time is letting the patient know that you care for him and that you will be there to give him support. The nurse should find out what strengths the patient has for meeting this crisis situation and make it possible for him to utilize them. He may find strength from any or all of the following: (1) himself, owing to a great ego strength or from being used to being a "loner," (2) strong bonds with his family who need, love, and depend upon him, (3) deep religious beliefs that may be present all the time or may develop in times of crisis, or (4) a trusting, meaningful relationship he has with a "significant" person, who may be either the doctor or the nurse.

As the time for surgery nears, whatever method the patient is using to meet the crisis, it will become more intensified. If he is not dealing effectively with this situation, he may be anxious, withdrawn, glib, or joke inappropriately. This behavior can be a clue that he will

need more emotional support postoperatively. Patients usually depend upon a "significant" person for strength; thus, the nurse should
plan on providing and supporting this "significant" person for her
patient. She can help by finding a clergyman for counseling, allowing
the family to stay at the bedside for longer periods of time or encouraging more patient contact for the member of the team who has good
rapport with the patient.

The nurse should remember that not all patients need or want
emotional support at this time. There are patients who have very
healthy ways of dealing with stress, and would prefer to receive
accurate information so they can determine what they will need and
how they will approach the problem. To them, the thought of surgery
may not cause stress and anxiety, as they have successfully worked
this situation out. In this case, the patient's individuality should be
respected and supported.

ESTABLISHING A BASELINE

Establishing a baseline is the key to providing good care and to
preventing complications. A baseline can only be accomplished by
having a thorough knowledge of the patient. In the preoperative
period, the nurse should seek out information that will provide her
with knowledge regarding the present status of the patient, his cardiac
problem, the severity of his illness, and any injuries or diseases
(past or present) which might complicate his recovery. This information can be obtained by attending the cardiac medical-surgical rounds
in which the patient is evaluated, by reading the chart and reviewing
the special test data, and by the nurse personally examining the
patient. Essentially this involves a process of data collection which
can be formulated into a plan of action at a later time.

The information that can be obtained from the chart and from the
nurse examining the patient will be presented here as a guide. The
rationale behind the evaluation of these systems will be expanded in
the acute postoperative phase and in other sections of this chapter.
As the nurse gets used to reviewing the chart and examining the
patient, the meaning and importance of this preoperative review will
prove its worth in the postoperative and convalescent periods.

Information from the Chart

Information from the chart will supply the following pertinent
data:

What brought the patient to the hospital?
1. What is the problem relating to the proposed surgery?
2. How has this problem evolved?
   a. Gradual deterioration.
   b. Acute deterioration, with urgent surgical intervention needed.
3. What are the expected complications and mortality from this surgical procedure.

What is the present status of the patient?
1. ECG
   a. Arrhythmias?
   b. Bundle branch blocks?
   c. Hypertrophy patterns?
2. Cardiac catheterization data
   a. A high left ventricular end-diastolic pressure indicating left ventricular failure?
   b. Direction of shunting and whether it is in the atria or ventricles.
   c. Cardiac output or cardiac index, as an indication of the heart's ability to meet the needs of the body.
   d. Elevated pulmonary artery or right ventricular pressures which might indicate overloading of the lungs, as with mitral valve disease.
   e. High AV oxygen difference?
3. Pulmonary function tests
   a. Are the lungs able to maintain a normal ventilation as evidenced by a normal arterial P_{O_2} and P_{CO_2}?
   b. Is there anything to indicate the patient will need additional or prolonged respiratory support?
4. Laboratory values: (Are the following normal?)
   a. Electrolytes, especially potassium and sodium.
   b. Hematocrit and hemoglobin.
   c. Clotting mechanisms: platelets, prothrombin time, Lee and White time.
   d. Evidence of kidney malfunction as seen by:
      A low urinary creatinine clearance
      A high serum creatinine
      A high blood urea nitrogen
5. Has the physician's history and physical examination revealed any of the following:
   a. Chronic lung disease as evidenced by:
      Increased A-P diameter of the chest
      Previous chronic pulmonary disease, i.e., asthma, tuberculosis
      Lengthwise ridging of the finger nails (except the thumb)

Bronchiastesis, or emphysema
Fixed expansion of the lower rib cage
b. Arteriosclerotic changes
Pulses of less than 4 plus quality
Discolored, shiny, tight skin over the lower legs
c. Liver damage or engorgement
Abnormal liver function studies (SGOT, BSP)
Liver below the rib margin
Pulsatile liver
Previous history of heavy drinking or alcoholism
d. Previous history of myocardial infarction
How recently has this occurred?
Is there any residual damage?
Ventricular aneurysm
Conduction defects
Ruptured papillary muscles

Nursing Evaluation of the Patient

Present status of cardiac and respiratory systems
1. Blood pressure
   a. Is it the same in both arms?
   b. Are the values normal for the patient at this time?
   c. Where is it best heard?
   d. Is there any evidence of pulsus alternans or pulsus para-doxicus?
2. Pulse and heart beat
   a. Where are the pulses best felt, and what is their quality in the periphery?
   b. Is there any deficit between the apical rate and the pulse rate in the peripheral pulses?
   c. Where can the heart be best heard? Pulmonic, aortic, tricupid or mitral area?
   d. Are there any obvious murmurs or gallops that can be detected?
   e. What is the basic rhythm, and are there any ectopic beats?
3. Chest and respirations
   a. What is the rate and quality of respirations?
   b. How much are respirations affected by changes in position from supine to sitting?
   c. What do the chest sounds indicate?
      Evidence of chronic lung disease — decreased breath sounds, wheezing, or rhonchi.
      Evidence of congested lungs — fine rales and wheezing.

d. In which areas are the lung sounds best heard?

e. How effectively can the patient cough and raise deep mucus?

f. Is there any evidence of respiratory embarrassment?

4. Temperature

a. What is the normal temperature for this patient?

b. Is there any afternoon or evening temperature spiking which might indicate infection?

5. Periphery

a. Color of nailbeds, ear lobes, lips, and buccal mucosa

b. Rate of capillary filling

c. Edema: where present and to what degree?

d. Bruising or petechiae?

Residual effects from injuries or diseases

1. Strokes

a. Any weakness or paralysis?

b. Asphasia or speech difficulties?

c. Impairment of mental capacity?

2. Joint involvement from arthritis, fractures, or bone malformation

a. Limitation of joint mobility?

b. General positions which would provide the best rest.

3. Diabetes

a. How is it presently controlled?

b. What complications have evolved from it?

c. Tissue necrosis or ulceration?

4. Sensory defects

a. Problems with vision?

b. Hearing defects?

PREOPERATIVE TEACHING

The preoperative teaching will be most effective when it is based upon information gathered from evaluating the emotional needs of the patient, from reviewing the chart, and from the nurse's examination of the patient. The teaching should be geared to the level of the patient's comprehension, and determined by how much he desires to know. A child will require simple explanations and exposure to the equipment and personnel. Children usually do better if they are not shown the recovery room which can be overwhelming and frightening, especially if there are patients in it at the time it is seen. Children seem to benefit more when they meet the people who will care for them, and when they are exposed to the equipment they will be using, such as the oxygen mask, the respirator, and the oxygen tent.

Adults usually want more factual information; however, there are times when a patient may be so frightened that he cannot face the thought of the postoperative period, and may not want detailed descriptions. His main concern may be more with the control of pain and knowing that someone familiar will be there to help him.

When beginning the preoperative teaching, find a place that is quiet and free from interruption and plan it at a time when the family can attend. In this way, the family will know what the patient is being taught and how they can participate in his care. Due to stress, a patient and family might not be able to remember what they are told. For this reason, repetition and the use of written material in the form of pamphlets or booklets should be utilized, as they will be helpful references when something has been forgotten. Since the patient is dealing with so many people at this time, it may also be helpful for the nurse to write down the names of the primary physicians and nurses who will be providing most of the care for the patient.

An explanation of the general course of postoperative events is a good way to begin the introduction of the patient and his family to the postoperative period. They should know where the recovery room is located; what type of visiting privileges are allowed; the expected length of stay in the recovery room; and how the recovery room patterning will vary from the ward routine. Then the patient can be oriented to the specific presurgical preparation, which may include baths two to three times a day with a bacteriostatic soap like pHisoHex; the use of special nose drops to kill bacteria in the nose and nasal pharynx; learning how to cough effectively; and the use of the respirator with IPPB several times a day. The night before surgery, the patient will be without fluids or food from midnight to the morning of surgery. The morning of surgery he will receive injections to make him sleepy and to dry his secretions. He will be taken to the operating room where anesthesia will block his memory until he awakens in the recovery room.

Now it is appropriate to present detailed explanations of the physical aspects of care which will be encountered in the postoperative period. The more pertinent aspects of care to be discussed follow.

General Nursing Routines

The need for frequent vital signs, turning, suctioning, and stripping of chest tubes should be presented as part of the *normal* routine and not as an indication that the patient is in danger. The rationale for these routines and what the patient will experience is explained to alleviate fear and to gain cooperation. Since the need for vital signs and treatments is so essential, sleep will be intermittent and limited until about the third or fourth day when the patient is discharged from the recovery room, unless complications have occurred.

Special Equipment

ECG monitors. If the patient understands that the monitor displays the electrocardiogram, that a sound may be issued with each heart beat, and that there is a tendency for false alarms to occur with movement or when an electrode comes loose, he will not be frightened when these things occur.

Urinary catheters. Urinary catheters are routinely inserted the morning of surgery, or while the patient is under anesthesia in the operating room. These seldom cause discomfort unless they are not secured well to the leg with tape, allowing tension to develop on the catheter. Sometimes the presence of the catheter within the bladder or blockage of the tubing will give the patient a desire to void. If there is no evidence of blockage, bladder spasms may be present and they can be treated with antispasmotic medicines.

Endotracheal tubes. A patient can be frightened to awaken with an endotracheal tube in his nose or mouth that prevents him from talking. Even if there is no strong indication preoperatively for the use of these tubes, their function and the sensations the patient will experience are crucial points which need emphasizing.

The endotracheal tube will cause pain only when the patient suddenly moves his head, and usually he will experience a sensation of fullness in his throat and a desire to swallow or gag. It is necessary to emphasize the importance of this tube, and to help the patient learn how to "think around" its existence and the discomfort it causes. If the patient has a very sensitive gag reflex and "bucks" the respirator, it may be necessary to remove the tube early, sedate the patient heavily, or perform a tracheostomy.

A positive approach as to the usefulness of the endotracheal tube is most essential. The patient needs to understand that it will allow him to rest by taking over respirations or making them less of an effort, and that it will allow direct suctioning of the lungs, and save him the energy of excessive coughing. The patient should understand that he will not be able to talk with the tube in place, but the loss of his voice will return when the tube is removed, and the hoarseness and sore throat that follows will disappear within a few days.

Respirators. Although the patient has been oriented to the respirator preoperatively, when it is used continuously there is more of a need to have complete chest relaxation so there will be less resistance for the respirator to overcome. The respirator then can do all the work of breathing when the rate is preset. If the patient finds it hard to breathe with the respirator, he will be comforted to know that the staff is on the alert for respiratory problems and are especially trained to correct them.

Once the patient is off continuous respiratory assistance with an endotracheal tube and onto intermittent therapy, he usually will need another demonstration of the correct use of a face mask or mouthpiece. Even though he will be tired, the importance of the respiratory therapy now lies with the ability of the patient to use the respirator and to cough effectively. If he understands in advance that this is his most important job and the point at which he is most vital in assisting with his own care, he can be encouraged and coaxed to help even when he is tired and in pain.

Coughing

If the nurse is unfamiliar with teaching the proper method of coughing, the help of an inhalation therapist or a physical therapist may be beneficial. They may already be part of the cardiac team and may routinely be utilized in preoperative teaching.

The process of effectively raising mucus begins with full, deep expansion of the lungs. This is why the respirator is routinely employed, and why preoperative teaching of coughing and deep breathing is necessary. The following methods can be utilized in eliciting good lung expansion and coughing.

1. Have the patient put his hands on the lateral, lower portion of his ribs and breathe so he can either see or feel his hands move upward and outward.

2. Teach the patient to take a deep breath and hold it for a second before expiring. This will allow better gaseous exchange and will open more alveoli.

3. Place the patient before a mirror so he can see the need for outward movement of the ribs, as opposed to upward motion of the shoulder girdle.

4. To encourage deep breaths, hold a piece of tissue paper about a foot away from the patient's mouth and tell him to exhale with pursed lips, as if it were a candle.

5. To produce an effective cough, have the patient take a deep breath, tighten his abdominal muscles, and force the cough out with an open throat.

6. If the patient has difficulty coughing, tell him to keep inspiring in one long breath until he cannot tolerate it any longer, or until it causes him to cough.

There are some patients who have never been able to cough well and, even with good instruction, will not be able to cough effectively. This fact should be acknowledged, and the patient should be told of the need for endotracheal suctioning and how he can best cooperate.

Pain

Pain is a primary concern of patients about to undergo surgery, with good reason. Usually people have the ability to avoid unnecessary pain, and once it has occurred, they are independent enough to use medicines and prescribed analgesics to control the pain. A major surgical procedure causes pain that is difficult for the patient to comprehend owing to its magnitude, duration, and exact location. A subsequent fear of the unknown may result unless patients are fully prepared for their encounter with this pain. The estimation of their pain in relation to a specific type of surgical incision and procedure cannot be accurately predicted, but it can be approximated by the patient's previous history and ability to tolerate other painful experiences. Even if this pain threshold cannot be determined, the presence of pain should be honestly acknowledged, and the availability of narcotics to alleviate or diminish the severity of the pain should be emphasized. If the patient is aware that the initial pain medicine may not be adequate, he should be made to realize that procedures and medications can be adjusted according to his needs. If hypotension or respiratory depression occur which would limit the amount of narcotic used, and he is informed of this, he will still be able to maintain a trust in the people who are caring for him. Honesty and concern for the patient should prevail at all times and should be expressed to the patient!

Dreams and Hallucinations

Narcotics, lack of uninterrupted sleep, excessive fear, or cerebral microembolism can cause some patients to experience frightening, unreal dreams, or visual and auditory hallucinations. Unless these reactions are gross, patients may go through the acute postoperative period having experienced these phenomena without relating them to the staff. Thus, if the patient is not alerted that he may experience these things and is not encouraged to let the staff know that they are occurring, he may have a fear of going insane and may compound the problem by not talking about it. The onset of hallucinations may necessitate moving the patient out of the recovery room into a room in which the noise level is less and adequate sleep can be sought more effectively.

Patient Mobility

The degree of patient mobility will depend upon the type and intensity of monitoring and the placement of catheters and leads. If certain anatomic locations are routinely used for these devices, the patient can be told of them ahead of time. It usually is adequate at this time to inform the patient that he may be asked not to bend a leg or arm sharply or to limit a full range of motion in a joint owing to the placement of catheters. Then immediately after surgery, the nurse can specifically point out the catheters and leads and demonstrate to the patient how much freedom of movement he will have with each. This instruction will allow fuller cooperation owing to the patient's ability to be an active, decision-making participant.

In summarizing, it should be remembered that teaching in the preoperative period involves many things that are unfamiliar to the patient. For this reason, the nurse will be most effective if she begins the teaching process a week or more before surgery. This will allow enough total time for frequent, short teaching periods to determine if the patient understands what he has been taught and for questions by the patient and the family. Repetition is a good teaching tool, so frequent visits are needed in order to answer the many questions that will arise at a later time and to clarify answers previously given by the nurse but perhaps not fully understood.

Acute Postoperative Phase

If only one point is made in this chapter, it is the fact that *without a sound baseline, it is impossible to anticipate and observe the subtle changes that indicate the trend of the patient's condition.* If the nurse has not carefully assessed the patient preoperatively and in the initial postoperative period, if she has not explored every possible nook and cranny which can provide pertinent information, then she is in a poor position to offer preventive care and may be capable of assisting *only* in times of crisis.

In establishing a baseline, the first thing the nurse does is to carefully observe, examine, and listen to the patient. The observed signs give evidence as to the present status of the patient and, to be fully comprehended, they should be correlated with theoretical information. To merely describe and to report these phenomena without comprehension is not enough. Therefore, the development of this section will be done in a way to correlate theory with the nurse's observations and her plan of action.

At the time the patient is admitted to the recovery room, there is a feeling of tension and urgency. The physicians are tired from surgery, and the nurses are tense in anticipation of receiving the patient. When the patient arrives, the mood may swing from one of urgency and confusion to one of joviality and relief that the surgery has been successfully completed. In either case, it is essential that the patient not be forgotten. Although attention must be temporarily directed to the technical aspects of connecting the various lines and monitoring devices, the emphasis should not shift from the patient to these tasks. The nurse can prevent this occurrence if she has previously defined and differentiated her responsibilities from those of the other members of the team. This delineation of responsibilities should free the nurse so she can begin examining the patient and taking vital signs as soon as the patient is admitted to the recovery room. If the nurse waits until the various lines and monitoring devices have been connected, precious time has been lost and pertinent problems may go unnoticed. The nurse who has previously determined her nursing functions and has set them in order of priority will act more effectively at this stressful time.

Immediate evaluation of the patient is important as the patient has been unmonitored during the trip from the operating room to the recovery room. The team moving the patient has been in motion, leaving little opportunity to check vital signs or to closely observe the patient. Because of this temporary absence of monitoring, only the patient's general appearance has been used as an index of his condition. Thus, when he is received in the recovery room, the nurse should be prepared *within the first 15 minutes to establish an immediate baseline.* Although this immediate baseline only provides a superficial skimming of pertinent organ systems, it should reveal any gross problems and provide enough information to build a fuller picture of the patient.

ESTABLISHING AN IMMEDIATE BASELINE

General Appearance

A quick look at the patient from head to toes tells you (1) his color (pale, mottled, cyanotic, pink, or flushed) and (2) his level of alertness (comatose, deeply asleep, easily awakened, or restless). These signs reflect the level of oxygenation, adequacy of blood replacement, depth of anesthesia, and evidence of cerebral insult.

To be sure that this quick look will be adequate, extra covers should be removed so that most of the body is visible. If the patient is well covered, the nurse will not be able to ascertain (1) if the lines are patent, (2) if bleeding is present on dressings or around catheters, (3) if there is subcutaneous crepitus around the chest tubes, (4) if there is abdominal distention, or (5) if there are areas of bruising.

Ventilation

Whether the patient's respiratory status is normal or has been aided by a tracheostomy or an endotracheal tube, the question is, "Is ventilation adequate?" At this time the nurse needs to determine if both lungs are being well ventilated, and whether or not there are secretions which need removing. By (1) carefully observing the exposed chest as to the depth, rate, and equality of respiration on both sides of the chest; (2) putting her hand over the airway to estimate the quantity of air flow; (3) listening to both sides of the chest for breath sounds; and (4) carefully observing the color of the lips, ear lobes, and nail beds, the nurse will find any major ventilatory problems.

Cardiac Function

The main responsibility of the cardiac surgical nurse is to clinically evaluate the patient's cardiac output. The tools available in this situation are (1) her hands (to check peripheral pulses to determine if they are full or thready, weak or strong, and where best present), (2) the stethoscope (are the heart sounds clear or muffled, soft or loud?), (3) the blood pressure (is it normal for the patient at this time, is it easy or hard to hear?), and (4) the electrocardiogram (what is the rate and rhythm?).

Cerebral Function

Since the brain is so vital and has such high oxygen requirements, any embarrassment to the circulation is immediately reflected in the brain and deserves prompt treatment. To evaluate the cerebral function, the nurse should check (1) the patient's level of consciousness (is he alert, somnolent, or comatose?), and (2) if there is any evidence of localized cerebral embolism (can he move all extremities, is he hypersensitive to stimuli?). If any of these signs are abnormal, the pupils should be checked for response to pain and stimulation. By using these criteria of evaluation, the immediate baseline has been established, and any gross or life-threatening problems should have been disclosed.

NURSING CONSIDERATIONS

Cardiac Function

When the nurse evaluates the patient's cardiac status, she is primarily determining the effectiveness of his cardiac output by her clinical observations and by the measurements she routinely takes.

The term *cardiac output* generally remains unfamiliar to nurses, as they have had little experience in applying it to patient care. The cardiac output is the quantity of blood in liters that is ejected from the heart per minute. An average-sized adult at rest will have a cardiac output of approximately 5.0 L per min. The stroke volume and the heart rate are the main components of the cardiac output as seen in the following formula:

$$\text{Cardiac output} = \text{heart rate} \times \text{stroke volume}$$

As the formula indicates, whenever the stroke volume or the heart rate changes, the cardiac output is directly altered. If either the stroke volume or the heart rate decrease, the cardiac output will drop, and the opposite will occur if their values increase. Since the nurse is at the bedside taking vital signs, replacing blood losses, recording intake and output, and observing changes in the patient and in the vital signs, she is in a position to effectively evaluate the

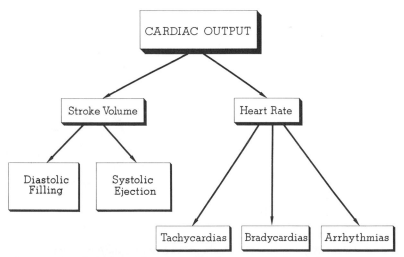

Figure 11–1. Component features of cardiac output. The cardiac output is determined by the stroke volume and the heart rate. The main components in the stroke volume are the diastolic filling and the systolic ejection, whereas the heart rate is affected by tachycardias, bradycardias, and other arrhythmias.

patient's cardiac status and, hopefully to prevent deterioration in his condition. To understand how the performance of these tasks can alter the patient's cardiac status, it is helpful to categorize cardiac output as shown in Figure 11–1.

Stroke volume. The amount of blood that is ejected each time the ventricles contract is the stroke volume. It is affected by the diastolic filling and the systolic ejection of blood from the ventricles. Either one of these components can be markedly altered owing to the trauma of cardiac surgery, as the myocardium has been manipulated and incised, and the correction of the pathologic lesions has suddenly changed pressures and rates of flow within individual chambers. The circulating blood volume has also been changed due to the use of hypothermia and heart-lung by-pass which can cause pooling of blood in various organs and vasoconstriction.

DIASTOLIC FILLING OF THE VENTRICLES (Fig. 11–2A). If the ventricles are to be filled adequately, two things must be present: (1) a high atrial filling pressure with an atrial contraction and (2) a relaxed, distensible ventricle.

A high atrial filling pressure is necessary to open the mitral and tricuspid valves so the ventricles will fill adequately. If the atrial pressure is low or the atrial contraction is absent, there will not be adequate force to move enough blood from the atria into the ventricles. Thus, the amount of blood available for systolic ejection will be limited.

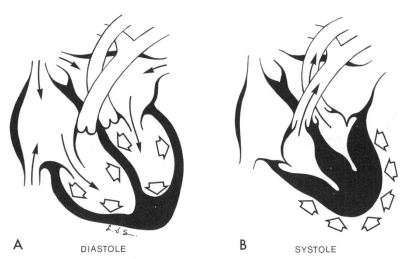

A   DIASTOLE   **B**   SYSTOLE

Figure 11–2. A, Diastole. Ventricular filling occurs during diastole and is dependent upon a good atrial filling pressure and distensible ventricles. B, Systole. During systole, blood is ejected into the pulmonary and systemic arterial systems. This phase is dependent upon a strong ventricular contraction that can overcome outflow resistance.

The atrial filling pressures will be less effective when the following are present: (1) inadequate blood replacement with a low circulating blood volume, (2) an absence of atrial contraction to aid in delivering blood to the ventricles (i.e., atrial fibrillation or flutter, junctional or ventricular rhythms), and (3) lack of synchronized beating between the atria and the ventricles (i.e., AV dissociation, premature ventricular contractions, and advanced heart block).

The ventricles are relaxed during diastole and distend easily when blood enters. There are some conditions that can impair ventricular distensibility—(1) fibrotic myocardial infiltration from diffuse coronary artery disease or myocardiopathies, (2) constrictive pericarditis, (3) cardiac tamponade, and (4) severe myocardial hypertrophy. All these conditions will limit the amount of blood entering the ventricles and thus will drop the stroke volume.

SYSTOLIC EJECTION OF BLOOD FROM THE VENTRICLES (Fig. 11-2B). During systole the ventricles contract, ejecting blood into the pulmonary and systemic arterial systems. If enough blood is to be delivered into these systems, it is necessary to have strong ventricular contractions that can overcome outflow resistance.

Some of the more prominent postoperative problems that can weaken the force of the ventricular contraction are hypoxia, acidosis, hypokalemia, myocardial infarctions, and overdistention of the ventricles. The nurse should check to see if any of these conditions are present if she suspects by clinical observation that the myocardium is failing. If the myocardium is failing, the clinical changes are those of a low output syndrome with signs of shock. The underlying cause will need treatment, but at this time the physician might desire to use inotropic drugs like Isuprel or digitalis preparations which would strengthen the myocardium.

The ventricular contraction will also be weakened when the ventricles become overdistended from excess fluids or blood. This problem can occur over a short period of time if the IV line is left open, or it can take place over a period of days. If the formula cardiac output = stroke volume × heart rate is again reviewed, there seems to be a contradiction to the fact that an increase in the circulating blood volume would lower the cardiac output. It seems more reasonable that by giving more fluids, the stroke volume and thus the cardiac output would increase. This fact is true only to the extent that the excess fluid does not stretch the ventricles so much that they weaken and are incapable of emptying completely with each contraction. If overdistention occurs, the systolic emptying of the ventricles will be incomplete, there will be less space for diastolic filling, and thus less blood will be ejected.

Starling's Law in essence says that the myocardium, with its elastic properties, can provide a larger ejection of blood when it is fully stretched, but this maximal force of ejection will reach a "critical" point beyond which the muscle fibers are so overstretched that they weaken and cannot completely empty the ventricles during systole. With each successive filling the ventricle distends more, as it has not completely emptied from the previous ejection. This law can be compared to a balloon and its inherent elastic properties. If a balloon is blown up repeatedly with larger amounts of air each successive time, it reaches a "critical" point at which it becomes flabby and does not deflate rapidly or completely. Beyond this "critical" point, the balloon (and also the heart) becomes weakened and less effective.

The nurse should pay particular attention to the patient's pulse pressure, which is the difference between the systolic and diastolic blood pressure. The pulse pressure indicates how much pressure the left ventricle is able to generate in overcoming the outflow resistance in the aorta. Whenever the systolic and diastolic pressures come close together, this is a good indication that the cardiac output is falling. Therefore, whenever the pulse pressure is less than 40 mm Hg, the ventricle may be weakening, and the patient must be watched for signs of a falling cardiac output. For instance, if the blood pressure is 140/80, the pulse pressure is 60 mm Hg. If the blood pressure changes to 120/90, the pulse pressure is 30 mm Hg and the patient may be getting into trouble.

Heart rate.   Changes in the heart rate and rhythm can lower the cardiac output. Heart rate problems encountered by the cardiac patient in the postoperative period include bradycardias, tachycardias, and other arrhythmias.

Bradycardias are potentially caused by direct suturing through the conduction system, edema from suture lines near the conduction system, hyperkalemia, myocardial infarction, vagal stimulation, digitalis and other drug toxicities, and acidosis. Tachycardias are potentially caused by fever, pain, stress, hypovolemia, anemia, alkalosis, hypoxia, infection, hypokalemia, and hypocalcemia. Other arrhythmias and ectopic beats are potentially caused by hypoxia, alkalosis or acidosis, hypokalemia or hyperkalemia, hypocalcemia or hypercalcemia, myocardial infarction, myocardial irritability owing to incisions and suturing in the heart, drug toxicities, and monitoring lines, valvular prostheses, or pacing wires within the heart.

BRADYCARDIAS.   Whenever the ventricular rate is less than 60 beats per minute, a bradycardia is present. When the heart rate drops, the stroke volume will need to increase if the cardiac output is to remain the same. The stroke volume can be increased by (1) sympathetic discharge to strengthen the force of contraction so more blood can be ejected with each beat, or by (2) retaining sodium and water to increase the circulating blood volume and thus increase the stroke volume. The increased sympathetic activity will increase the stroke volume within a very short period of time, while the retention of sodium and water to increase the stroke volume will take days. The ventricle may not be able to tolerate a larger diastolic filling volume and may not therefore generate a sufficient contractile force to eject all the blood. The problems due to a bradycardia can eventually result in a lowered cardiac output with inadequate coronary perfusion resulting in myocardial ischemia.

The nurse should be alert to bradycardias under the following conditions.

1. Surgery in which the suturing has been done near the AV node or the common bundle of His (e.g., repair of tetralogy of Fallot, ventricular septal defect correction, or an atrial septal defect correction low in the atria) which may prevent conduction of impulses from the atria to the ventricles, resulting in a pacemaker with a lower inherent rate taking over.

2. Digitalis preparations, due to their action of slowing conduction between the atria and the ventricles, can cause bradycardias when toxicity is developing. The nurse should observe for changes which may indicate digitalis toxicity as related in the electrocardiogram: (1) prolongation of the PR interval which could progress to first degree heart block, (2) premature ventricular contractions, or (3) slowing of the ventricular rate below 60 beats per minute, and (4) paroxysmal atrial tachycardia with block.

3. The vagus nerve which primarily innervates the heart at the SA and AV nodes can slow the heart rate whenever it is stimulated. If the patient is endotracheally suctioned, retches, vomits, or bears down as if having a bowel movement (Valsalva maneuver), the heart can suddenly slow. It is useful for the nurse to observe the monitor for these changes in heart rate when the patient is performing activities that can stimulate the vagus nerve.

TACHYCARDIAS. A tachycardia is present when the ventricular rate is over 100 beats per minute. Tachycardias are of particular concern as they lessen the diastolic filling time, decreasing the time for perfusion of the coronary arteries. They also greatly increase the oxygen requirements of the heart. All of these would put an extra burden on a heart that is healing and adapting to new hemodynamics.

The onset of a tachycardia deserves prompt treatment owing to its deleterious effects. Whenever a tachycardia develops, the nurse should check to see if the cause is one she can correct, such as fever, pain, or hypovolemia. If the potential causes of tachycardia are absent, then additional help will be required to diagnose the etiology of the problem.

OTHER ARRHYTHMIAS AND ECTOPIC BEATS. This classification has been included under heart rate to deal specifically with irregular rhythms and arrhythmias in which an atrial beat does not precede each ventricular response. The arrhythmias that do not have a

P wave preceding each QRS (e.g., atrial fibrillation, atrial flutter) can cause a decrease in the diastolic filling of the ventricles owing to the absence of an atrial systolic thrust to aid in filling the ventricles. If these same rhythms occur at higher rates, the diastolic filling time is also decreased. With rhythms like second and third heart block in which an atrial systolic thrust is available, it may not occur synchronously with relaxation of the ventricles, thus decreasing the filling pressure from the atria. The overall result will be a drop in the cardiac output as with bradycardias and tachycardias.

If the patient has an arrhythmia that is difficult to identify owing to a questionable absence of P waves, it is possible to make a "salt bridge" out of a long CVP line whose tip is in the right atrium. To do this:

1. Attach the patient to an ECG machine.

2. Fill a glass syringe with a metal hub with normal saline. Insert the syringe in the CVP line, and fill the CVP line with the normal saline.

3. Attach one end of an alligator clamp to the metal end of the "V" or precordial lead from the ECG machine, and the other to the metal hub on the glass syringe that is attached to the saline-filled CVP line.

4. Take a tracing from the ECG machine on "V". If P waves are present, they will be much bigger in amplitude than the QRS.

5. Be sure the patient is well grounded while doing this procedure.

It is not uncommon for patients with cardiac lesions to have been in atrial fibrillation before surgery or to develop it after surgery. This arrhythmia can sometimes be controlled with the administration of digitalis and quinidine.

The arrhythmias that are potentially dangerous and may cause death are given in the following list.

1. Ventricular tachycardia can lead to ventricular fibrillation. The onset of ventricular tachycardia is often preceded by frequent premature ventricular contractions, especially ones that land near or in the "vulnerable" zone of the preceding T wave. Lidocaine is the drug of choice with ventricular tachycardia, although cardioversion and Pronestyl may be used. If ventricular fibrillation occurs, defibrillation and cardiopulmonary resuscitation are indicated.

2. Second degree heart block (especially the Mobitz Type II) and third degree heart block may suddenly lead to asystole, ventricular tachycardia, or ventricular fibrillation. For this reason, some surgeons will implant pacemaking wires in the heart before surgery is terminated. The nurse should have specific instructions on the operation of the pacemaker, when to use it, and how to evaluate its

performance. If a pacemaker is not in place and these types of heart block develop, a physician should be notified in anticipation that drugs such as Atropine and Isuprel which accelerate heart rate may be utilized.

Now that the pertinent components affecting the cardiac output have been reviewed, the question is how can the nurse effectively evaluate the patient's cardiac status. The ability to do this will vary with the nurse's experience and with the equipment that is available to her. The equipment may be as minimal as a blood pressure cuff, or it may include the monitoring of ECGs, arterial and venous pressures, and other highly sensitive parameters pulmonary artery and left atrial pressures and blood gas analyses. Regardless of the situation, it is important to remember that the *nurse is the most important component of the monitoring equipment.* The mechanical equipment merely records the data and cannot ascertain its importance or formulate a plan of action to correct the problems that arise.

Hopefully, the nurse will have seen the patient preoperatively and will know his "norms" in appearance, color, pulses, blood pressure, heart rate, rhythm, and chest sounds. If the vital signs and blood replacement are checked with the anesthesiologist to see what trend they took during the operation, the nurse will be able to determine what is *now* normal for the patient.

Methods of determining the effectiveness of the cardiac output. The various sites of the measurements and signs the nurse will be observing and measuring fall into two categories: (1) core and (2) peripheral. Core parameters are centrally located with the body and are usually more objective as they are directly measurable. The peripheral parameters are located outside the body and deal more with subjective changes, as they are not clinically measurable and depend upon powers of clinical observation.

CORE MEASUREMENTS. Core measurements include (1) blood pressure, (2) central venous pressure, (3) pulmonary artery pressure, (4) left atrial pressure, (5) heart rate, and (6) urinary output.

Blood Pressure. The systolic blood pressure normally is 90 to 140 mm Hg and has a diastolic pressure approximately 40 mm Hg below the systolic pressure. The blood pressure is easily audible and each beat should be heard. Changes in blood pressure readings which indicate problems are as follows:

   a. A systolic pressure below 90 mm Hg, unless present preoperatively.
   b. A pulse pressure less than 40 mm Hg.
   c. Difficulty in hearing the blood pressure.
   d. A pulsus paradoxicus. After the blood pressure cuff has been pumped up and the first systolic beat is heard as the mercury column falls, listen to hear if the blood pressure disappears on inspiration

and returns on expiration. If this phenomenon occurs, note the interval in millimeters of mercury over which the pulsus paradoxicus has occurred. If it is heard over more than a 10 mm Hg interval, it is considered indicative of left ventricular failure or pericardial constriction. If a patient had a blood pressure of 140/90 and a pulsus paradoxicus between 140 and 110, this would be significant, as the pulsus paradoxicus is 30 mm Hg.

e. A pulsus alternans. After the first systolic beat has been heard as the mercury column falls, listen to hear if one beat is loud and the next beat is soft or absent. Then notice how many points of mercury the pulsus alternans has occurred over. If it occurs over a 10 mm Hg interval, it is significant and may indicate left ventricular failure if tachycardia is not present. For example, with a blood pressure of 120/70, if the pulsus alternans occurs between 120 and 100, it has occurred over a 20 mm Hg interval.

Central Venous Pressure. The central venous pressure is a reflection of the circulating blood volume, the pumping action of the heart, and the vascular tone. If an accurate measurement is to be made, the tip of the catheter must be located in the right atrium or in a vessel near the right atrium (i.e., venae cavae, innominate, subclavian, or iliac veins). Placement of the catheter tip in a peripheral vein will not provide an accurate central venous pressure.

Although the normal central venous pressure is 2 to 7 mm Hg (3 to 10 cm H_2O), this value will vary greatly depending upon the condition of the patient, the tone of the vessels, and the amount of volume replacement that is required. The trend of the central venous pressure measurements is more important than the individual numbers, and should be correlated with other clinical data. What may be a very high central venous pressure in one patient, may be a necessary central venous pressure in order to provide high enough filling pressures in another patient.

The nurse should be aware that an elevated central venous pressure can be due to an increased blood volume, right heart failure, cardiac tamponade, vasoconstriction, massive hemothorax, tension pneumothorax, a high pressure on the respirator, and tenseness or bearing down by the patient. A low central venous pressure can be caused by a low circulating blood volume or by vasodilation.

To ensure that the central venous pressure monitoring system is patent and functioning accurately it should have the following characteristics: (1) it should fluctuate with respirations, (2) IV solutions should easily run through it, and (3) blood should be able to be withdrawn from it. The latter is the most important, as a catheter that has slipped out of the vein into the chest cavity will have the first two characteristics, but cannot have blood withdrawn from it.

Pulmonary Artery Pressure. The pulmonary artery pressure

is valuable in detecting left ventricular failure and pulmonary hypertension before it progresses to right ventricular failure with a resultant rise in the central venous pressure. This measurement is more valuable than a central venous pressure in evaluating left ventricular failure as it is closer to the left ventricle. Earlier detection of problems will allow earlier preventive treatment.

The pulmonary artery line can be inserted at the time of surgery, or after surgery it can be inserted through a vein and with the assistance of fluoroscopy can be "floated" into the pulmonary artery. The normal value for the pulmonary artery is a systolic pressure of 20 to 22 mm Hg, a diastolic pressure of 8 to 10 mm Hg, and a mean pressure of about 13 mm Hg. The pulmonary artery pressures indicate problems when they are elevated and not when they decrease in value. As the left ventricle fails, fluid will back up and eventually fill the lungs. When the pulmonary artery mean pressure rises above 40 mm Hg in a patient who previously has had normal pressures, there is danger that pulmonary edema and right ventricular failure are developing.

Left Atrial Pressures. Left atrial monitoring lines are inserted at the time of surgery and their pressures are probably a more sensitive and accurate means of reflecting signs of left ventricular failure than pulmonary artery pressures, as the left atrial lines are next to the left ventricle. The normal left atrial pressure is 5 to 10 mm Hg, and when this pressure begins to rise and the blood pressure begins to fall, the left ventricle may be failing, causing a backup of fluid and increase in pressure in the left atrium. Many times, the patient will be "loaded" with additional fluids in order to increase his left atrial pressure and diastolic filling volume, thus increasing his cardiac output. This additional fluid stretches the ventricular muscles optimally (Starling's Law), and by increasing the left atrial pressures, increases the cardiac output.

These lines are potentially hazardous to the patient and must be guarded zealously by all. Any air or foreign matter that enters these lines can immediately enter the arterial system, resulting in a cerebral insult, or damage in other parts of the arterial system.

Heart Rate. Since the heart rate is one of the major components in determining the cardiac output, it is necessary for the nurse to determine the rate, rhythm, and strength of the heart beat. The most accurate method of determining the heart rate is by taking an apical pulse with a stethoscope either at the "mitral" area (in the fifth intercostal space, midclavicular line on the left chest) or at the "aortic" area (in the second to third intercostal space adjacent to or overlying the right side of the sternum). If the heart rate is routinely counted from the cardiac monitor without listening to the heart, the nurse will miss important changes in the heart sounds and will not be able to determine the effectiveness of the heart beat as it is transmitted to the periphery. Even though the nurse may be able to visualize a normal-looking ECG pattern on the monitor, this electrical activity of the heart does not necessarily indicate that the myocardial contraction has been forceful enough for blood to reach the peripheral tissues. To determine the effectiveness of the heart beat, a simultaneous rate should be counted apically with one from a peripheral pulse. If the count at the peripheral pulse is less than the apical count, the heart is not strong enough to cause a pulse to be felt with each beat in peripheral locations — a pulse deficit.

Urinary Output. The urinary output can be considered a core measurement, as it is dependent upon the cardiac output to produce a high enough arterial pressure to adequately perfuse the kidney so filtration of urine can occur. If hydration is adequate and no renal damage is present, the kidneys normally will produce 20 to 60 cc of urine per hour. If the urinary output drops, there is good reason to assume that the cardiac output had also dropped, especially if there is no concurrent increase in the specific gravity. Careful monitoring of hourly urine outputs from a urinary catheter is important if this information is to be correlated with other measurements.

PERIPHERAL MEASUREMENTS. Peripheral measurements consist of (1) skin color, (2) skin temperature, (3) skin moistness, (4) capillary filling, and (5) peripheral pulses.

Skin Color. The color of the skin is determined by the status of the capillaries near the surface of the skin, by the amount of oxygenated hemoglobin, and by the quantity of blood that is flowing through the capillaries. If the skin vessels become vasoconstricted or the cardiac output drops, the blood flow may decrease enough to cause the skin to become cool, moist, and cyanotic.

If the skin vessels vasodilate increasing the amount of blood that is circulated through the peripheral capillaries, the skin becomes warm and pink. When the hemoglobin is poorly saturated with oxygen, the superficial skin becomes cyanotic, as compared to the normal pink color with fully saturated hemoglobin. Total absence of arterial blood flow or severe anemia will cause pallor.

The nail beds, lips, buccal mucosa, and ear lobes are good peripheral areas for observing the level of oxygenation and cardiac output, as these areas are richly endowed with capillary beds that are near the surface and easily visible. Changes in skin color may reflect problems, but usually occur later, so they should be used to verify other earlier changes. The following changes in skin color may indicate problems.

Cyanosis or duskiness may occur from low cardiac output, inadequate oxygenation of the blood, peripheral vasoconstriction to shunt blood back to core, peripheral vasoconstriction due to cold, and polycythemia with poorly saturated hemoglobin. Pallor may be due to inadequate blood replacement, hemodilution from overhydration or anemia, and obstructed arteries as with arterial emboli. Flushed or reddened skin may occur from fever, allergic reactions, and reactive hyperemia from inadequate tissue oxygenation.

Skin Temperature. Skin temperature will rise as the peripheral vessels vasodilate and will fall as the peripheral vessels vasoconstrict. Either one of these processes can occur depending upon the body's internal temperature, the body's temperature regulating mechanisms, and the ambient temperature. A good indication that the cardiac output has fallen and that compensatory mechanisms are in effect is seen when the skin becomes cool, moist, and slightly cyanotic or mottled. At this time, the sympathetic nervous system has released norepinephrine in the periphery to close down these vessels, shunting as much as 5 to 10 per cent of the blood in peripheral vessels back to organs that are vital for survival and have higher metabolic requirements, i.e., brain, heart, and liver. Skin has a low metabolic need which allows a decrease in blood flow to the skin without causing tissue injury.

Skin Moistness. Normally skin is dry, but when there is overactivity of the sympathetic system with vasoconstriction as in shock or with vasodilation as in fever, skin moisture will range from mild perspiration to one of gross diaphoresis. It is possible to lose 500 cc or more fluid through the skin under normal conditions within a 24 hour period. Skin moistness is classified as part of insensible fluid loss, and even though it cannot be measured accurately, these losses need to be replaced.

Capillary Filling. To determine the rate of capillary filling either a finger or a toe is compressed until it turns white, then it is observed and timed until the original color returns. If the blood supply to this digit is slow, the rate of capillary filling will also be slow. The normal rate of capillary filling is quite rapid (2 to 3 seconds) making the differentiation of high cardiac output states difficult by this parameter. Usually, considerable clinical experience is needed to determine if the capillary filling is adequate.

Peripheral Pulses. The peripheral pulses are usually rated from 1 plus to 4 plus. The higher the number, the better the quality of the pulse. Preoperative examination will determine the quality of the pulses and where they are best felt. The quality of the peripheral pulses will deteriorate with a low cardiac output, moderate to severe arteriosclerotic changes, or with arterial emboli. The further the pulse is from the heart, the better the correlation with the heart's ability to perfuse these peripheral tissues. The cardiac surgical nurse should know the anatomic location of these pulses and should routinely check them to determine peripheral perfusion. In palpating pulses, the nurse should gently place her fingertips over the area of the artery, and slowly press down until she can palpate the artery. It is possible to press on the artery too hard initially and thus obliterate the pulse, leading the nurse to believe that the artery is not palpable.

The following pulses should be checked: (1) radial, (2) dorsalis pedis, and (3) posterior tibial. If these pulses are poor or absent, the nurse should check pulses that are closer to the core, such as the (1) carotid, (2) brachial, (3) popliteal, and (4) femoral.

A normal pulse should be full, easily palpable, equal to the same pulse on the opposite side, and rated 4 plus in quality. If peripheral perfusion is hindered, then the pulses will become (1) thready, (2) weak, (3) intermittent, or (4) absent.

Case presentation. In order to put the preceding discussion of nursing considerations into perspective, the following case presentation will be helpful. This study represents one of the more common problems that the nurse caring for a postoperative cardiac patient will be likely to encounter.

Mr. George has just returned to the recovery room after open heart surgery. He is intubated and on controlled respiratory support. His skin is cold, and his extremities are mottled with thready, intermittent pulses. His vital signs are

Temperature	95°F;
Pulse	80 and regular;
Blood pressure	110/60 mm Hg;
Central venous pressure	8 mm Hg;
Urinary output	100 cc per hour;
Chest drainage	100 to 150 cc per hour, which is being replaced with whole blood.

The orders of the next eight hours regarding fluid and blood replacement are (1) 500 cc D_5W with 20 mEq potassium chloride, and (2) replace the chest drainage with whole blood, cc for cc.

During the next few hours the following changes have occurred with Mr. George:

Temperature	101°F;
Pulse	115 and regular;
Blood pressure	90/60 mm Hg;
Central venous pressure	3 mm Hg;
Urinary output	20 cc the last hour;
Chest drainage	25 cc the last hour.

Mr. George's skin is warmer with less mottling, but his pulses remain thready and intermittent. He responds sluggishly to verbal commands. The nurse realizes that Mr. George is getting into difficulty not only from the changes in the preceding measurements but also from decreasing alertness, diaphoresis, and mottling. The nurse suspects the following from the information she has obtained:

1. The drop in blood pressure, the narrowing of the pulse pressure, and the rise in pulse indicate a low cardiac output with the compensatory mechanisms of shock.

2. The decrease in urinary output (without a rise in specific gravity) is a sensitive index that there is a decrease in the cardiac output.

3. The vasodilation due to the increased temperature may have unmasked a fluid deficit that was hidden by vasoconstriction from a low temperature, causing a falsely high central venous pressure and blood pressure. The vasodilation enlarged the vascular space, causing the circulating blood volume previously occupying it to become inadequate in filling this larger vascular space.

4. A drop in the central venous pressure from 8 mm Hg to 3 mm Hg indicates less circulating blood volume. This decrease in the circulating blood volume could be caused by pooling in organs, an enlargement of the vascular space from vasodilation, or a fluid loss greater than the fluid or blood replacement.

5. The sudden slowing of chest drainage is unusual and might indicate clotting of the chest tubes, or pooling of blood within the thoracic cavity.

From the preceding information, the nurse has decided that the problem is one of hypovolemia probably owing to vasodilation and pooling of blood within the thoracic cavity. In order to justify her decision before calling the physician, she decides to:

1. Check the CVP line for patency and accuracy:
    a. Can you withdraw blood through the line?
    b. Does it fluctuate with respirations?
    c. Does taking the patient off the respirator change the value?
    d. Is "zero" positioned at the level of the right atrium, or is the machine balanced?
2. Check the patency of the chest tubes:
    a. Does the blood in the chest tubes fluctuate with respirations or with the heart beat?
    b. Are there clots visible in the tubing?
    c. Is the chest suction working properly?
3. Check to make sure that blood is not pooling in the chest:
    a. Gently roll the patient from one side to the other.
    b. Independently strip each chest tube.

After completing these observations, the nurse has found that the CVP is accurate, the chest tubes are patent, and the patient has pooled 250 cc of blood which the nurse was able to remove by rolling the patient to the side of his thoracotomy. After replacing this blood loss as ordered, the patient's vital signs returned to normal, his pulses were fuller, and the cyanosis and mottling began to disappear. The urine output increased to 40 cc per hour, and the patient was more alert.

If Mr. George's vital signs had remained low after this additional blood replacement, the doctor should have been notified and probably would have changed the orders to give enough blood and fluids to keep the CVP and blood pressure at levels to adequately perfuse the patient.

Pulmonary Considerations

The pulmonary and cardiac systems cannot function independently of each other and sustain life. Although the primary function of the lungs is to oxygenate blood and remove carbon dioxide from the body, these functions are dependent upon an adequate cardiac output to bring enough unoxygenated venous blood to the lungs where gaseous exchange can occur and then to deliver the oxygenated blood to the tissues. Hemodynamic changes from cardiac lesions can alter the function of the lungs, as can the actual process of cardiac surgery. During the operation there are times when the lungs cannot be adequately expanded by the anesthesiologist, as this would block the operative field and slow the progress of the procedure.

The nurse should be most alert to pulmonary complications when the patient has cardiac lesions which pose these problems:

1. Overloading the lungs with excess blood:
   a. Patent ductus arteriosis.
   b. Left-to-right shunts from atrial or ventricular septal defects.
2. Underperfusion of the lungs with blood:
   a. Pulmonary stenosis.
   b. Tetralogy of Fallot.
   c. Triscupid stenosis or atresia.
3. Pulmonary hypertension due to back up of blood into the lungs:
   a. Mitral stenosis or insufficiency.
   b. Aortic stenosis with a failing left ventricle.

Respirations. CHEST EXPANSION. Whether or not the patient is breathing on his own or has artificial respiratory support, the first question is "Are respirations adequate enough to support the patient?" The nurse begins this evaluation by noting the chest expansion. If the patient is relaxed and has no respiratory difficulty, the nurse will observe (1) full and easy respirations, (2) symmetrical rise and fall of the chest, (3) an abdominal rise and fall with respirations, and (4) a normal respiratory rate.

If the patient is having respiratory distress, the nurse will observe certain clinical findings and should investigate the probable causes. Shallow, rapid respirations which may be caused by pain, restrictive chest dressings, hypoxia, or metabolic acidosis with the lungs compensating by blowing off CO_2. An asymmetrical rise and fall of the chest may indicate splinting (from pain) on the operative side, pneumothorax, flail chest, slippage of the endotracheal tube into either the right or left mainstem bronchus, or pleural effusion. Obstruction of air flow in the large air passages will cause problems of "forced" inspiration as noted with the use of the accessory muscles of the neck, shoulder girdles, and intercostal muscles, retraction of the intercostal and supraclavicular structures, flaring of the nares (especially in children), mouth breathing, and sitting upright and leaning forward with the arms supported and away from the chest. Obstruction of air flow in the small bronchi will cause problems of "forced" expiration as noted with conscious, forced tightening of the abdominal muscles on expiration, a prolonged expiratory phase with visible use of accessory muscles, and pursing of the lips. A tight abdomen that does not rise and fall with respirations usually indicates a tense patient who is not relaxed, a diaphragm which may not be functioning properly (phrenic nerve injury from surgery), or gastric dilation, especially if the abdomen is distended and tympanitic.

CHEST AUSCULTATION. Many pulmonary problems can be diagnosed and prevented from intensifying by frequent, knowledgeable auscultation of the chest. The more a nurse listens to a chest, the more accurate and comfortable she will be in detecting pulmonary changes in the patient. This evaluation goes back to an earlier statement—*the nurse must establish a baseline.*

A patient with healthy lungs will have normal vesicular breath sounds which have a louder sound on inspiration and a softer sound on expiration. They can be heard over most of the chest. Normal bronchial breath sounds will be heard only over the trachea and proximal bronchi.

The following are *abnormal* chest sounds.

Wheezes. Wheezes are high pitched piping or whistling sounds with a musical quality that occur either on inspiration or expiration, but are often louder and more persistent during expiration. In either case they indicate a partial blockage of air flow that can be caused by bronchospasm, edema, dried out mucus, or scarring of the different air passages. Wheezes will often be present in patients with chronic lung disease. When they are so gross as to cause dyspnea, treatment is indicated. Agents that relax bronchial smooth muscle, such as Isuprel, aminophylline and Adrenalin, will counteract the bronchospasm and alleviate the wheezing.

Rales. Fine, crackling rales that are delayed until the peak of inspiration are caused by fluid accumulation within the alveoli. This sound can be mimicked by bringing hair next to the ear and gently rubbing it together. To detect rales earlier when congestive heart failure is suspected, encourage the patient to take deep inspirations when you listen to his chest. Fine rales are heard when left ventricular failure causes a "back-up" of blood into the lungs, or when excessive fluid administration causes overloading of the lungs with fluids. Overloading of the lungs with fluids is sometimes so severe that gross pulmonary edema develops. The alveoli become so full of fluid that rales are present during inspiration and expiration and will be heard throughout the whole chest.

Rales will be heard first in dependent areas of the lungs, therefore the nurse should listen posteriorly and at the bases on a patient who is sitting up, and she should listen anywhere posteriorly on a patient who is lying flat. Whenever the nurse detects rales she should listen frequently to the patient's chest to determine how rapidly the lungs are filling with fluid and whether or not immediate treatment is needed. The patient usually will be more comfortable sitting upright in bed and will profit from oxygen administration. At this time, the nurse should check the neck veins, the central venous pressure, and the intake and output for evidence of fluid overload and, if present, should slow the intake until a physician has been summoned. If congestive heart failure is developing, diuretics and digitalis preparations will be needed. If the failure is severe enough to cause pulmonary edema, help should be summoned immediately, as this is an emergency. The nurse should immediately let the patient assume any position that is comfortable, begin oxygen administration, start IPPB, and give mild sedation if it is ordered.

A coarser type of rale that begins early in inspiration usually originates in the larger air passages and is caused by retained mucus or conditions like bronchiectasis. Usually, coughing and suctioning will lessen or eliminate this type of rale. Coarse rales are usually heard in the dependent portions of the lungs, reflecting the effects of gravity.

Rhonchi. Rhonchi are very coarse, loud rattling or snoring sounds, beginning very early in inspiration. They occur when foreign matter like mucus or aspirated material is present in the larger air passages, and will usually clear with good coughing or suctioning.

Bronchial or Tubular Breathing. Bronchial breathing is unlike normal vesicular breathing in that the expiratory sound is louder, longer, and of a higher pitch than the inspiratory sound. It sounds like air moving in and out of a large hollow tube, which is exactly what is happening. Bronchial breathing occurs when the alveoli in a segment or lobe of the lung are not ventilated and collapse, as in atelectasis. These collapsed areas must be reopened by effective coughing, suctioning of obstructing mucus, or by effective IPPB.

Decreased Breath Sounds. In a normal individual, vesicular breath sounds are heard over all areas of the chest. The breath tones may be somewhat "distant" if the person is obese, has an increased A-P diameter of the chest, or has long-standing pulmonary disease. When breath sounds are markedly decreased or totally absent, the nurse should suspect pneumothorax, pleural effusion, marked atelectasis or consolidation, and hemothorax.

Pleural Friction Rub. Both the inside of the chest cavity and the lungs are covered with a thin lining called the *pleura*, which is very smooth and slides easily when the lungs expand and contract. When the lung surface or the pleura becomes roughened, a pleural friction rub will develop. A pleural friction rub may be either low or high pitched, and sounds like leather squeaking. It is heard on inspiration or expiration, and is heard best at the bases and at the lower part of the axillary line where the underlying disease is usually present. A pleural friction rub is commonly associated with pulmonary embolus but may also be heard with lung consolidation.

RESPIRATORY RATE AND VOLUME. The respiratory rate is as important in maintaining adequate blood gases as the heart rate is in maintaining a cardiac output. The normal adult has a respiratory rate of 10 to 12 per minute, a tidal volume (the amount of air exchanged with each breath) of 600 to 800 cc, and a minute volume (the amount of air exchanged per minute) of 6 to 7 liters per minute. The formula for the minute volume is:

$$\text{Minute volume} = (\text{tidal volume}) \times (\text{respiratory rate})$$

The nurse should be alert to any changes in the respiratory rate and minute volume. These changes can lead to problems in maintaining a normal acid-base balance. Any time either the tidal volume or the respiratory rate decreases, hypoxia or carbon dioxide retention may be anticipated. Sometimes the respiratory rate will slow as a compensatory mechanism to retain carbon dioxide in order to form more carbonic acid, counterbalancing an excess of base, as is formed in metabolic alkalosis. With an increase in the tidal volume or the respiratory rate, respiratory alkalosis may be anticipated. An increase in rate may also indicate compensation by the lungs for hypoxia or for metabolic acidosis.

CO_2 NARCOSIS. When a patient is not able to ventilate adequately, excess carbon dioxide can be retained causing total anesthesia and death as an end result. As the arterial P_{CO_2} rises, there usually is an increase in the systolic blood pressure which the nurse should be alert to detect. When the P_{CO_2} reaches 80 mm Hg, the respiratory center in the brain becomes depressed, and when the P_{CO_2} is 100 mm Hg or above, death is imminent.

The symptoms of CO_2 narcosis in order of progression are a slight cyanosis with hyperventilation at rest, mental vagueness, twitching of the fingers occurring only at rest (a very important sign), sleepiness, deep cyanosis without dyspnea or increased respirations, headache, warm hands (due to the hyperemia from the high CO_2), and coma.

Whenever a patient cannot be awakened, the nurse should think of a cerebral insult, an overdosage of analgesics, or CO_2 narcosis. Since high levels of carbon dioxide cause peripheral vasodilatation, many times the patient will be pink and warm without signs of cyanosis. Therefore, the nurse should not be dependent upon evidence of cyanosis for a diagnosis of CO_2 narcosis, but will need blood gas determinations to make a definitive diagnosis.

HYPOXIA.   When oxygen levels are lower than normal, a patient is hypoxic. Hypoxia develops when a patient is unable to adequately oxygenate his blood and has arterial P_{O_2} of 60 mm Hg or less breathing room air. Hypoxia can be caused by either a low cardiac output or impaired lung function.

Since cyanosis is a late sign of hypoxia, the nurse should be alert to earlier signs, such as tachycardia and tachypnea, so earlier treatment can be instituted. This treatment usually involves oxygen administration and reversal of the underlying cause. Hypoxic patients may exhibit restlessness, mental vagueness or confusion, mild to profound cyanosis, tachycardia, and tachypnea.

Whenever a patient becomes hypoxic, sedatives and narcotics (which can depress respirations) should be used as little as possible, unless continuous respiratory support is provided at a set rate or with the apnea control on. Death can result if the depressed respirations cause any further progression of the hypoxia.

BLOOD GAS EVALUATION.   Alkalosis, acidosis, CO_2 narcosis, and hypoxia each merit a review. The body constantly strives to balance bases (or alkalis) and acids in order to maintain a pH that is compatible with life. The pH (reflecting the number of hydrogen ions in the body) is influenced primarily by the amount of carbon dioxide and bicarbonate that is available and the ratio they maintain.

In order to have a normal pH (7.38 to 7.42 or 7.35 to 7.45), there must be 20 parts bicarbonate to one part carbonic acid (which essentially is carbon dioxide).

$$\text{Normal pH} = \frac{20 \text{ parts bicarbonate } (HCO_3^-)}{1 \text{ part carbonic acid } (H_2CO_3)}$$

The body depends upon the kidneys and the lungs for keeping

this 20:1 ratio. The main function of the kidneys is the regulation of bicarbonate. If the body is short on bicarbonate or has an excess of acid that needs buffering, the kidneys reabsorb bicarbonate instead of excreting it. The reverse is true when the body has an excess of bicarbonate or a deficit of acid. The kidneys also regulate how much acid is saved or excreted in the urine.

The lungs, on the other hand, are responsible for regulating carbon dioxide (CO_2). In normal everyday living, carbon dioxide and water are formed as the end products of metabolism.

$$CHO + O_2 = CO_2 + H_2O$$
(carbohydrate) (oxygen) (carbon (water)
dioxide)

Since carbon dioxide readily binds with water to form carbonic acid (H_2CO_3), it is necessary to prevent excess acid build up by eliminating carbon dioxide through the lungs. It is the primary function of the lungs not only to provide oxygen but to eliminate carbon dioxide.

Therefore, in thinking of an acid-base balance and the maintenance of a normal pH, the following is important:

$$\frac{\text{Bicarbonate is regulated by the kidneys}}{\text{Carbon dioxide is regulated by the lungs}}$$

The body has a unique system of compensatory mechanisms to aid in maintaining a normal pH. There are various buffers in the blood but, for our purposes, we will be discussing the role of the lungs and the kidneys.

The lungs respond within minutes to changes in pH due to stimulation of receptors which relay information to the respiratory center in the brain. Although the lungs respond quickly, they cannot provide an effective, complete compensation. Therefore, they cannot be relied upon to provide adequate compensation when metabolic problems arise.

On the other hand, the kidneys can provide an effective, complete compensation for metabolic and respiratory problems as long as the arterial P_{CO_2} is not greater than 80 mm Hg. Although the kidneys begin compensating almost immediately, it may take 24 to 48 hours for their effects to be complete enough to be noted. As a rule of thumb, the kidneys usually rid the body of whatever excess it has. Therefore, if the patient has acidosis, the urine should become acid (urinary pH of 4 to 6), while the urine should become alkaline (urinary pH 6 to 8) when the patient has alkalosis.

The normal arterial blood gas values with a patient breathing room air are:

pH   7.38 to 7.42 or 7.35 to 7.45 (depending on the laboratory)

P_{O_2} 80 to 100 mm Hg
P_{CO_2} 40 mm Hg
HCO_3^- 24 to 28 mEq/L
BE   −3 to +3 (the base excess is usually the difference between
            the normal serum HCO_3 and the patient's HCO_3)

Alkalosis.   When the pH is above 7.42 (or 7.45), the patient is alkalotic from either too much base or too little acid. The cause of the alkalosis can be metabolic, respiratory, or both.

With *respiratory alkalosis,* the patient has breathed so rapidly or so deeply that he has "blown off" too much carbon dioxide and thus has lost carbonic acid.

$$H_2O \; + \; CO_2 \; = \; H_2CO_3$$
(water)   (carbon   (carbonic acid)
          dioxide)

Some of the potential causes of respiratory alkalosis are (1) emotion, (2) fever, (3) exercise, (4) salicylate poisoning (early stages), (5) central nervous system problems (encephalitis, tumors), (6) low oxygen tension in inspired air, (7) sudden correction of respiratory acidosis, (8) congestive heart failure, and (9) acute alcohol intoxication.

To reverse the respiratory alkalosis, the carbon dioxide levels must be returned to normal. The only way the carbon dioxide can be returned to normal is to prevent the patient from hyperventilating and in essence to hypoventilate or underbreathe him. Ways of doing this include breathing into a bag, adding dead space tubing to the ventilator or decreasing the respiratory rate or tidal volume in order to decrease the minute volume. Sometimes sedation or analgesics will lessen the anxiety or pain which has precipitated the elevated respiratory rate.

The blood gases for respiratory alkalosis have an elevated pH and a low carbon dioxide (P_{CO_2}). If metabolic compensation is taking place and the kidneys are excreting bicarbonate, then the bicarbonate level will be low.

UNCOMPENSATED RESPIRATORY ALKALOSIS	COMPENSATED RESPIRATORY ALKALOSIS
pH 7.5 ↑	pH 7.40
P_{CO_2} 30 ↓	P_{CO_2} 30 ↓
HCO_3^- 25	HCO_3^- 20 ↓
BE +1	BE −5 ↓

In the uncompensated respiratory alkalosis, the HCO_3 has remained normal and the patient has lost carbonic acid by dropping the P_{CO_2}, thus elevating the pH. With the compensated respiratory alkalosis, the pH has returned to normal since the HCO_3 has dropped (as is reflected in the BE of -5) counter-balancing the loss of carbonic acid.

With metabolic alkalosis, the patient either ingests too much base or loses too much acid through the gastrointestinal tract or kidneys.

Potential causes of metabolic alkalosis are:

1. Vomiting or nasogastric suctioning of acid stomach contents.
2. Excessive ingestion of alkali (antacids, sodium bicarbonate).
3. Adrenal cortical excess (Cushing's syndrome).
4. Hypokalemia.
5. Congenital infantile diarrhea.
6. Acute renal failure (diuretic stage).
7. Mercurial diuretics or chlorthiazide.
8. Hypercalcemia.

The treatment for the metabolic alkalosis is the correction of the underlying cause of either the low acid or the high alkali levels.

The blood gases for metabolic alkalosis have an elevated pH and a high bicarbonate level. If there is respiratory compensation, the P_{CO_2} will be elevated.

UNCOMPENSATED METABOLIC ALKALOSIS	COMPENSATED METABOLIC ALKALOSIS
pH 7.5 ↑	pH 7.42
P_{CO_2} 40	P_{CO_2} 52 ↑
HCO_3^- 31 ↑	HCO_3^- 31 ↑
BE +7 ↑	BE +7 ↑

In the uncompensated metabolic alkalosis, the pH is elevated owing to the high HCO_3^-, as is reflected in the elevated base excess. In the compensated metabolic alkalosis, the pH has been returned to normal owing to an elevation in the P_{CO_2} which counterbalances the excess base.

Alkalotic patients may exhibit tight, bandlike headaches, restlessness, tingling or pins-and-needles sensations around the mouth or in the extremities, tetany, convulsions, tachycardias, arrhythmias, hypocalcemia, and hypokalemia.

Acidosis.   Whenever the pH is less than 7.35 (or 7.38), the patient is acidotic from either too much acid or too little base. The cause of the acidosis can be respiratory, metabolic, or both. Although a patient can readily tolerate a moderate alkalosis, acidosis is poorly tolerated and should be corrected as soon as possible.

Respiratory acidosis occurs when ventilation has been inadequate to eliminate carbon dioxide. Potential causes of respiratory acidosis are:

1. Respiratory arrest.
2. Respiratory depression (narcotics, sedatives, anesthesia, or high O_2 flows in chronic lung disease).
3. Chest wall problems (chest trauma, poliomyelitis, obesity, kyphoscoliosis).
4. Primary pulmonary disease (severe emphysema, atelectasis, pneumonia, pulmonary fibrosis).
5. Airway obstruction.
6. Pulmonary problems (pneumothorax, mechanical hypoventilation, pleural effusion).
7. Congestive heart failure.

The only way to reverse respiratory acidosis is to adequately ventilate the patient and to correct the primary problem. By ventilating the patient, the excess carbon dioxide will be eliminated. If the respiratory acidosis is severe or persistent, intubation or a tracheostomy may be indicated.

The blood gases in respiratory acidosis have a low pH and a high carbon dioxide. The serum bicarbonate levels will be elevated if renal compensation is occurring.

UNCOMPENSATED RESPIRATORY ACIDOSIS	COMPENSATED RESPIRATORY ACIDOSIS
pH 7.30 ↓	pH 7.40
P_{CO_2} 56 ↑	P_{CO_2} 56 ↑
HCO_3^- 24	HCO_3^- 30 ↑
BE −1	BE +6 ↑

In the uncompensated respiratory acidosis, the pH has fallen owing to an elevated P_{CO_2} (forming carbonic acid). In the compensated respiratory acidosis, the pH has returned to normal owing to an elevation in the HCO_3^- which is buffering the excess carbonic acid.

Metabolic acidosis occurs when there is an excess of metabolic acids or a loss of bicarbonate. Potential causes of metabolic acidosis are:

1. Low cardiac output or cardiac arrest.
2. Uncontrolled diabetes mellitus.
3. Renal failure.
4. Congenital infantile diarrhea.
5. Hepatic failure.
6. Salicylate poisoning.
7. Generalized hypoxemia.

8. Ingestion of acidifying agents (ammonium chloride, calcium chloride, paraldehyde).

The underlying cause will need treatment, but in the meantime, if the patient is very acidotic, the low bicarbonate should be replaced. To determine the amount of bicarbonate a patient with metabolic acidosis needs, the following formula is used:

Patient weight in kg × 0.4 × BE = mEq of sodium bicarbonate to be given

Assuming that the patient weighs 70 kg and has a base deficit of −11:

$$70 \times 0.4 \times -11 = 308 \text{ mEq sodium bicarbonate}$$

The blood gases with metabolic acidosis have a low pH and a low bicarbonate. If pulmonary compensation is effective, the P_{CO_2} will be low:

UNCOMPENSATED METABOLIC ACIDOSIS	COMPENSATED METABOLIC ACIDOSIS
pH 7.23 ↓	pH 7.35
P_{CO_2} 40	P_{CO_2} 22 ↓
HCO_3^- 16 ↓	HCO_3^- 16 ↓
BE −11 ↓	BE −11 ↓

The pH is low in the uncompensated metabolic acidosis owing to excess acid or a loss of bicarbonate (as is reflected in the base excess). The pH has returned to normal in the compensated metabolic acidosis owing to a low P_{CO_2} with a consequent loss of carbonic acid.

Acidotic patients may exhibit lethargy and sluggishness, semi-coma to coma, impaired nervous tissue conduction (increased PR interval or widened QRS), heart block, ventricular fibrillation, or asystole, hypercalcemia, and hyperkalemia.

When the nurse is involved in drawing arterial blood gases, the following things are important. (1) Only rinse the syringe used for the blood gases with heparin, as the P_{O_2} of heparin that has been exposed to air is 150 mm Hg and this can distort the true P_{O_2}. (2) Remember to use firm, digital pressure over the site of the arterial puncture for five to 10 minutes if the patient is not anticoagulated. To determine if this pressure has been effective, palpate the artery to ascertain if any swelling has occurred. If swelling is present, the pressure should be continued.

Figure 11–3 and its legend will summarize these acid-base and blood gas considerations.

Clearing secretions. Secretions can be removed from the

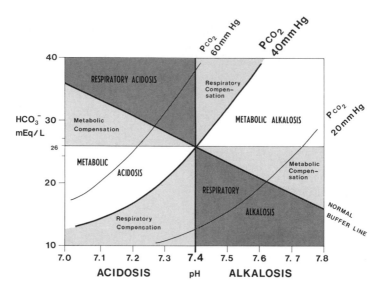

Figure 11–3. Diagram of acid-base relationships.

This acid-base diagram will enable the nurse to work more effectively with blood gas determinations. By plotting the blood gases, the nurse will learn the acid-base diagnosis and will be able to follow the patient's progress.

The pH values run horizontally, with the pH of 7.4 being the average normal value. The area to the right of pH 7.4 represents alkalosis, while the area to the left of pH 7.4 represents acidosis. The further the pH moves away from the center to the periphery of the diagram, the more the patient's condition is deteriorating.

The bicarbonate (HCO_3^-) values are listed on the left side of the diagram and increase in value as they move vertically upward. The average normal value for HCO_3^- is 26 mEq/L. A patient with metabolic acidosis will have a low bicarbonate, while a patient with metabolic alkalosis will have an elevated bicarbonate.

The P_{CO_2} values are represented by the sloping lines (isobars) that cut diagonally across the diagram. The normal average value for the P_{CO_2} is 40 mm Hg. If the P_{CO_2} falls to the left of the 40 mm Hg isobar, the patient has respiratory acidosis. If it falls to the right of the 40 mm Hg isobar, he has respiratory alkalosis.

The point at which the normal average values for the pH, HCO_3^-, and P_{CO_2} intersect represents the "absolutely normal" person. Whenever the patient deviates from this central area, he is developing an acid-base imbalance.

In order to plot the patient's blood gases, it is necessary to have values for the pH and either the P_{CO_2} or the HCO_3^-. It is possible to determine the third value from plotting two of the variables. For instance, if the pH is 7.3 and the P_{CO_2} is 30 mm Hg, the lines intersect at a HCO_3^- of 16 mEq/L and fall within the boundaries of metabolic acidosis with respiratory compensation. On the other hand, if the pH were 7.3 and the HCO_3^- was 30 mEq/L, these lines would intersect on the P_{CO_2} line of 59 mm Hg, giving a diagnosis of respiratory acidosis. (After Davenport, H.: The ABC of Acid-Base Chemistry. 5th ed. Chicago, Illinois, University of Chicago Press, 1969.)

lungs by having the patient cough deeply and productively or by suctioning. Nasotracheal and orotracheal suctioning are commonly used after thoracic surgery to remove copious secretions which are difficult for the patient to raise. Suctioning is a frightening, uncomfortable experience, during which the patient needs a great deal of support and understanding.

In order to effectively and safely remove secretions from a patient, the following will be useful.

1. Loosen secretions and bring them higher in the tracheobronchial tree before suctioning.
   a. Hyperventilate the patient on the respirator or with a ventilatory bag.
   b. Lavage through the endotracheal tube or tracheostomy, then hyperventilate the patient.
   c. Have the patient cough.
2. Place the catheter where suctioning is needed, by listening to the lungs to locate the mucus, then:
   a. Hyperextend the head and turn it to the left in order to suction the right lung.
   b. Hyperextend the head and turn it to the right in order to suction the left lung.
3. Suction intermittently only while coming out of the trachea, and for no longer than 30 seconds at a time. This precaution will lessen the chances of hypoxia and will cause less trauma to the respiratory mucosa.
4. Prolonged suctioning or the use of large catheters (especially in children) can cause:
   a. Vagal stimulation with resultant cardiac slowing and possible cardiac arrest.
   b. Severe hypoxia, especially in someone with a low P_{O_2}.
   c. Laryngospasm.
   d. Vomiting and possible aspiration.
5. If the suction catheter has holes along the sides, rotate it as you suction to pick up more mucus.
6. By pressing inward and downward on the trachea just above the sternoclavicular notch, it is possible to cause coughing. This process is more effective in children and young adults as their tracheas are more pliable.

If suctioning is necessary and a tracheostomy or endotracheal tube is not being utilized, then nasoendotracheal suctioning should be initiated. Nasoendotracheal suctioning involves the same principles and precautions as previously mentioned, but is different in that the patient must be positioned properly, and the insertion of the suction catheter must be done in coordination with the patient's breathing.

SUCTIONING

To apply nasotracheal suction properly to a patient follow these steps:

1. Sit the patient upright with the head back and the neck hyperextended.

2. Examine the nares to be sure there is no obstruction to passage of the catheter.

3. Prepare the suction catheter, lubricant, and gloves (as sterile as possible).

4. Have the patient stick out his tongue.

5. Hold the tongue forward with a piece of gauze.

6. Gently advance the suction catheter (with the suction off) until the patient coughs.

7. The catheter has passed into the trachea when the patient goes into spasms of coughing and has difficulty speaking.

TRACHEOSTOMIES AND ENDOTRACHEAL TUBES. These tubes have the advantage of making suctioning easier and making it possible to give a patient continuous support from a respirator; however, they present potential dangers if not cared for properly.

Endotracheal Tubes. Endotracheal tubes can be inserted through the mouth or nose. The latter is usually more comfortable for the patient. In either case, they should be secured to the patient to prevent them from coming out or from slipping inward and blocking one of the major bronchi.

If the tube is inserted through the nose (1) prevent pressure areas and possible ulceration of the nares by applying an ointment to the inside of the nose and (2) prevent excess tension on the tube and keep it positioned as comfortably as possible. If it is inserted through the mouth, (1) it is harder to provide good oral hygiene and to remove secretions from the mouth and nasal pharyngeal areas, and (2) there is danger that the patient may occlude the tube by biting down on it. To lessen this danger, an oral bite block can be made of a roll of gauze sponges, or an oral airway may be left in place. If the patient is exceptionally cooperative, these measures may not be necessary, as long as the patient is instructed properly.

Endotracheal tubes are not painful unless the patient suddenly moves his head. These tubes will temporarily prevent the patient from talking, cause a feeling of fullness in the throat, give the patient the desire to swallow, and may cause a gagging sensation. If the patient is informed of these things before surgery, he will be better able to tolerate the endotracheal tube postoperatively.

Tracheostomies. A tracheostomy is performed when a patient needs long-term respiratory support, while an endotracheal tube is usually a temporary measure and is generally left in place no longer than 72 hours. Tracheostomies also need good humidification. The nurse can suspect that humidification has been inadequate whenever the moistened suction catheter sticks to the sides of the tube or when dry secretions are obtained.

The nurse will need to frequently clean the inner cannula of tracheostomy tubes to keep the airway patent, and she should determine the frequency of cleaning depending upon the amount and the character of the secretions. Since most tracheostomy tubes are inserted with an obturator in place, it is wise to keep the obturator and another sterile tracheostomy tube taped onto or near the bed.

When a tracheostomy is "fresh," the nurse will need to observe for (1) excessive bleeding around the incision, (2) subcutaneous crepitus around the incision, and (3) fresh blood being suctioned from the lungs. If any of these occur, a physician should be notified.

Cuffs on endotracheal and tracheostomy tubes. Cuffs are necessary in order to provide a closed system between the patient and the respirator and to prevent aspiration of gastric contents into the lungs. Unless the cuff is properly inflated, air will leak around the tube and up into the mouth. If this leak is large enough, the patient will lose too much of his minute volume and will not be adequately ventilated.

If the cuffs are not released often enough, or are filled at greater than minimal pressures, necrosis of tracheal tissue can occur. In order to release the cuff properly, the following should be done:

1. Suction the nasopharynx and oropharynx before deflating the cuff in order to prevent mucus in the nasopharynx and oropharynx from dropping into the lungs. Even with thorough suctioning, mucus may remain; thus it is helpful to release the cuff just as inspiration occurs to let air from the respirator blow any remaining mucus up into the mouth where it can be suctioned.

2. Release the cuff slowly to lessen the coughing and spasm that can occur with abrupt deflation.

3. Observe the patient for evidence of dyspnea, tachycardia, or cyanosis which could necessitate stopping the suctioning, and returning the patient to the respirator.

4. If the patient cannot tolerate being off the respirator for long enough periods of time, teach him how to keep his mouth and nose shut while on the respirator with the cuff deflated. This process is similar to that of a patient using a respirator with a mouthpiece with his nose sealed. If the patient can do these things, his cuff can be released as often as needed while supplying him with the necessary respiratory support. If some air leak exists around the tracheostomy or endotracheal tube, larger volumes of inspired air can be given to compensate for the air leak.

5. When reinflating the cuff, it is not a good practice to predetermine the amount of air that will be needed to provide a good seal.

The amount of air will vary owing to stretchage of the cuff and the fit of the tube within the trachea. The nurse should slowly inflate the cuff with just enough air so that no leakage can be felt around the tube, the mouth, or the nose. Some physicians recommend leaving a small air leak around the tube to lessen pressure on the trachea by the cuff.

Some cuffs are secured permanently to the tube while others are just slipped into place. The latter have a tendency for the cuff to slip, which can occlude the end of the tube, causing asphyxiation. Occlusion of the tube by the cuff should be suspected when (1) the patient increases his respiratory rate or attempts to override a rate-controlled respirator by taking more inspirations than the respirator provides, (2) respirations become labored, (3) breathing becomes easier on inspiration with the cuff deflated, but expiration is difficult or impossible (owing to the cuff being sucked back into the tube), and (4) it becomes difficult to pass a suction catheter through the tube.

Ways to aid breathing. Other than clearing secretions by using respirators, endotracheal tubes, and tracheostomies, there are other ways the nurse can make breathing easier for the patient.

1. Give adequate analgesics to control pain, but not to the point of depressing respirations.

2. A semi-Fowler's or high-Fowler's position is good for increasing the tidal volume by allowing the diaphragm to descend more easily. This position aids patients with excess fluid in the alveoli by causing the fluid to pool in the lower portions of the lung and by decreasing venous return to the heart.

3. The chest will expand more easily with the arms away from the side of the body which can be done by supporting them with pillows.

4. If the patient has a pleuritic type of pain, lying him on the side of the pain will normally lessen it; however, this position will also limit the expansion of that side of the lung and this must be taken into consideration.

5. For aiding respirations in children, it is helpful to put a small rolled towel just under the shoulders to hyperextend the neck, allowing for better air exchange.

6. Relieving abdominal distention by nasogastric intubation or placement of a rectal tube will allow the diaphragm to descend without encountering resistance from a distended abdomen.

Cerebral Considerations

A generalized cerebral insult may result from hypotension, hypoxemia, or a low cardiac output, while a localized cerebral lesion can occur from a blood clot or an embolus of air, fat, or calcium. In either case, the patient should be carefully observed and evaluated, as immediate supportive or therapeutic treatment may be indicated.

If abnormal neurologic signs are present, the nurse should be particularly alert to clinical changes that may indicate an increase in intracranial pressure. In the early, compensated stages of increased intracranial pressure, the nurse will see the loss of consciousness, the pupils going from constriction with fixation to dilation with fixation on the involved side, the systolic blood pressure rising and the diastolic blood pressure falling (resulting in a wide pulse pressure), the heart rate falling and the pulse becoming full and bounding. If treatment is not initiated during this early stage, the patient is likely to die. In the later, decompensated stages of increased intracranial pressure, the nurse will see an unconscious, unresponsive patient, bilaterally dilated and fixed pupils, a decreasing systolic blood pressure with a rising diastolic blood pressure, a rising pulse with some irregularities, and the onset of Cheyne-Stokes respirations (cycles of gradually increasing tidal volumes followed by gradually decreasing tidal volumes) or Biot's breathing (respirations coming in couples, triples, quadruples, and so on rather than waxing and waning as with Cheyne-Stokes). At this point, death is imminent.

To determine if cerebral damage is present, especially in the immediate postoperative period, the nurse should observe and determine:

1. Are both pupils equal and do they briskly react to light?
2. Can the patient be easily aroused?
3. Can the patient move all extremities?
4. Is the patient hyperactive to any kind of stimulus?
5. Is decerebrate positioning present?
6. Are Cheyne-Stoke's or Biot's respirations present?

Temperature

Changes in body temperatures have important effects on the cardiovascular system and cellular metabolism. If the nurse is to effectively control fever and initiate hypothermia when indicated, she must have an understanding of heat production and heat loss within the body.

Temperature control mechanisms. Heat production is controlled in the posterior portion of the hypothalamus. This center uses several mechanisms to control heat production. Vasoconstriction prevents heat loss through the skin, thyroxin and epinephrine increase metabolism, and shivering increases the metabolic rate. This latter process is particularly important, as the increase in muscle tone in preparation for shivering can increase the metabolic rate 50 to 100 per cent, while the actual process of shivering can increase heat production by 200 or 300 per cent.

Heat loss is controlled in the anterior portion of the hypothalamus. This center can inhibit or counteract the heat production center by causing vasodilation, limiting the release of thyroxin and epinephrine, and decreasing muscle tone and shivering.

If there is a need to cool the patient, the nurse should utilize the principles of conduction or convection. With conduction, the body is in direct contact with an object that is cooler than the body, i.e., ice packs or a hypothermia blanket. With convection, heat is transferred from the body to the air. Therefore, the room temperature should be cooler than the body temperature, and the air should be circulating to displace the warm air next to the body with cooler air. Since one of the initial responses of the body to cold is vasoconstriction, convection and conduction will be of little value unless shivering and vasoconstriction are controlled.

Rewarming. When the cardiac surgical patient returns to the recovery room, he usually has a subnormal temperature that was created during surgery. Due to this low temperature, the patient will show signs of vasoconstriction, such as (1) cool, mottled, cyanotic skin; (2) weak, thready pulses; and (3) a blood pressure that is difficult to hear.

To aid the patient in attaining a normal temperature, the nurse can cover him with additional blankets, use warmed blankets, or use hot water bottles to accelerate the rewarming process. Care should be taken so that the patient does not get burned from the hot water bottles, as a patient's perception of heat is impaired when he is cold. Patients have a tendency to overshoot the desired temperature. Therefore, when the temperature is 2°F lower than the desired temperature, the extra blankets and warming devices should be removed. As the patient is being rewarmed, vasodilation can occur and the nurse should watch for increased chest drainage and a drop in the CVP, which could indicate a need to administer more blood and fluids.

Fever. Other than in the immediate period when the patient returns from the operating room and is cold, the nurse's main concern is controlling fever. Whether the etiology of the fever is dehydration, atelectasis, infection, "postpump fever," or brain damage, the goal of reducing the fever is the same—(1) decreasing the metabolic needs of the body, (2) lowering the body's oxygen consumption, and (3) lessening the work of the heart.

Some of the methods of controlling or reducing fever are:

1. Administration of aspirin or other antipyretics.
2. Ice packs to the axilla, groin, and back of the neck.

3. Sponging with tepid water or a mixture of water and alcohol.

4. Creating a cool environment (air conditioned room or cool oxygen tent).

5. Administration of corticosteroids.

6. Hypothermia via an ice blanket.

Hypothermia. The problems encountered in hypothermia and its proper use will be given special consideration, as hypothermia is one of the most effective, rapid methods of lowering temperatures. Hypothermia is most commonly used when there has been a neurologic insult and with fever when other methods fail to lower the temperature. A mild hypothermia of 87 to 95°F (30 to 35°C) is usually used when neurologic conditions develop.

Conduction by direct contact with a hypothermia blanket is best attained when the "insulating zone" is eliminated by keeping the patient's body in direct contact with a wet surface over the ice blanket. If the body is in contact with a dry sheet, the conduction of heat from the body to the trapped air between the sheet and ice blanket becomes equal and no more heat loss occurs. Therefore, if a hypothermia blanket is to be covered at all, it should be done initially with a wet sheet until the proper temperature has been reached. Obviously, more than one dry sheet should be avoided.

Any patient on a hypothermia blanket needs special skin care to prevent cold injury with frostbite and tissue necrosis. To avoid these problems, the hands and feet should be wrapped in cloth; the entire body should be rubbed down with a mixture of lanolin, mineral oil, or cold cream; the patient should be turned frequently; and bony prominences and pressure areas should be massaged.

To control shivering (which occurs primarily in the induction state), Demerol, Phenergan, or Thorazine may be administered as the muscle tone increases, preceding the actual process of shivering. When the muscle tone is increasing, the masseter, intercostal, and abdominal muscles will show a rippling motion. If the nurse waits until shivering has occurred before giving these medicines, the metabolic rate and oxygen consumption will have increased significantly by the time the medicine becomes effective. The nurse can also control shivering by applying covered hot water bottles to the feet of the patient. If the feet are kept warm, the brain will receive less stimulus that cold is occurring and thus there will be less vasoconstriction and muscle tensing to cause shivering.

When inducing or maintaining hypothermia, an accurate rectal temperature is needed to guide the course of therapy. The rectal probes that give a continuous reading via battery-operated meters have a tendency to be inaccurate and should be checked for accuracy against a regular glass thermometer at least every two hours. The nurse should also be aware that the cooling process should be stopped

2°F above the desired temperature, as there is a tendency for the body temperature to drift downward after the hypothermia has been stopped.

Some of the more important changes that occur with hypothermia are:

1. The decrease in circulation delays drug absorption from intramuscular sites and can cause drug accumulation. Intravenous drug administration is recommended as drug absorption and excretion will be more expedient and accurate.

2. Opiates may be potentiated by hypothermia; thus smaller doses are usually recommended.

3. Loss of blood preceding cooling (hemorrhage) causes a faster induction, which may bring the patient to dangerously low temperatures faster than normal.

4. Cooling may cause tissue breakdown and necrosis, thus careful observation of pressure areas, frequent turning, and good massages are necessary.

5. Respiratory embarrassment and cardiac arrhythmias may develop at temperatures below 86°F.

6. Shivering will occur during both cooling and on rewarming between 86 to 91°F.

7. The blood pressure will be harder to hear as the patient gets cooler, and palpation may be necessary to determine it.

Since different systems of measurement are used in hospitals, the following information on converting from one system to another will aid the nurse:

(1) To change from cm H_2O to mm Hg, divide the cm H_2O by 1.36.

(2) To change from mm Hg to cm H_2O, multiply the mm Hg by 1.36.

(3) To change from Centigrade to Fahrenheit, multiply the Centigrade value by 9/5, then add 32.

(4) To change from Fahrenheit to Centigrade, subtract 32 from the Fahrenheit value, then multiply by 5/9.

Fluids

Between 50 and 70 per cent of an adult's total body weight is composed of fluid, and anything that alters the fluid volume or composition can have a marked effect on homeostasis. For this reason it is important to accurately measure the intake and output, to use other clinical parameters in determining the level of hydration, and to understand the importance of certain electrolytes.

Intake. *Intravenous fluids* are used in the immediate postoperative period to keep the patient hydrated, the amount being determined by estimating the normal needs and probable losses of the patient. If an intravenous fluid is isotonic, the molecular concentration is comparable to the composition of our body fluids (i.e., 5 per cent dextrose and water and 0.9 per cent sodium chloride). If the solution is hypertonic, the composition of the solutes is higher than that of our body fluids (i.e., greater than 5 per cent dextrose and water or greater than 0.9 per cent sodium chloride). When a hypertonic solution is given rapidly, it draws fluid from the intracellular and interstitial compartments into the intravascular system. By suddenly increasing the intravascular volume it is possible to overburden the heart and cause cardiac failure. To avoid this complication, it is safest to administer a liter of hypertonic solution over a period of six hours or longer.

Care should be taken that all intravenous solutions, including special IVs (Lidocaine and Isuprel drips and so on) and flush solutions (for venous and arterial monitoring lines) are routinely included in the fluid intake for each shift.

Some useful hints when dealing with more than one intravenous infusion are the following. (1) Color code the intravenous solutions with methylene blue or IV vitamins, so potent medicines like Isuprel and Adrenalin can be easily recognized. (2) If the concentration of an IV solution containing a vasopressor or another potent drug is changed, tip the drip chamber to allow a small air bubble to enter the line. This air bubble will mark the place where the drug concentration has changed.

Nasogastric tubes can also provide a route for fluid intake. In the immediate postoperative period, antacids are commonly administered via the nasogastric tube to prevent the development of stress ulcers, particularly in patients with a previous ulcer history, during undue stress, or when corticosteroids are administered. Later, tube feedings may be indicated in order to provide additional nutritional intake that is rich in vitamins, calories, and proteins. For each gram of protein that is given, the body requires 50 ccs of fluid to handle the protein breakdown. If this additional fluid is not provided, the patient may become dehydrated.

Humidified air from respirators supplies a greater amount of water than is normally present in room air. This insensible fluid gain must be calculated by changes in the CVP and patient weight, as direct measurement of this fluid intake is impossible. Care should be taken when ultrasonic nebulizers are used with children, as they provide an extremely high water content in the inspired air. Also, when saline is used in the small nebulizers located near the airway, the saline will be readily absorbed by the lung and will bind with water in the body, resulting in more retention of water.

Lavaging the lungs to loosen tenacious secretions can become another source of fluid intake. Many times the solutions for lavaging are not recovered, and again, if this is a saline solution, it can cause more retention of water by the body.

Output. The *urinary output* depends upon the level of hydration, the condition of the kidneys, and the arterial pressure presented to the kidneys. Normally, an adult should have a minimum urinary output of at least 20 cc per hour, with a specific gravity of 1.010 to 1.025. If the patient is underhydrated, the urinary output will be low with a high specific gravity, while if the patient is overhydrated, the urinary output will be high with a low specific gravity.

If the patient's cardiac output is falling, and the arterial pressure is not sufficient to filter urine, the urinary output will decrease with little or no change in the specific gravity. If renal damage has occurred from prolonged hypotension, cardiac arrest, or an embolus to the kidney, there will be a decrease in the urinary output without a change in the specific gravity, or even anuria may result.

Measurement of the urinary pH will provide valuable information in evaluating the kidney's response to shifts in acid-base balance. The normal kidney can compensate fully for acid-base problems within 24 to 48 hours after the change has occurred. If the patient is alkalotic, the urine should become alkaline with a urinary pH as high as 8. With acidosis, the urine should be acidic with a urinary pH as low as 4.

Nasogastric tubes remove air and secretions that the stomach is incapable of moving through normal channels. Nasogastric drainage usually has high concentrations of acid, sodium, and potassium. These ions require accurate measurements so the amount and type of fluid and electrolyte replacement will be sufficient.

The nurse should closely observe the character, color, and amount of nasogastric drainage. If any blood (old or new) is present, the source of the bleeding should be investigated. The presence of bleeding may require additional blood administration, an evaluation of the clotting mechanisms, or the use of antacids.

Fluid losses through the skin occur normally, and are classified as a form of insensible fluid loss. While an average adult can lose 800 cc or more in a normal day's work, these fluid losses will increase greatly whenever fever, stress, or shock enter the patient's clinical course.

With *breathing*, fluid is lost from the body. This insensible fluid loss is accentuated whenever the patient is tachypneic or is breathing through his mouth. These fluid losses can run as high as 1000 to 2000 cc per day.

Diarrhea, especially in children, can cause considerable loss of fluids. Again, the pH and electrolyte concentrations are typically different and need to be calculated.

Blood loss through venipunctures can be surprisingly large when frequent blood samples are taken. This loss should be calculated in patients with small bodies, and more particularly, in infants and children.

The previous review of the pertinent variables in the measurement of a patient's intake and output, hopefully has shown that intake and output measurements alone are inaccurate in determining the patient's level of hydration. Other clinical observations invaluable in determining the amount and type of fluids that a patient needs will now be covered.

Evaluation of the hydration status. *Daily weights* can be a very reliable means of determining the patient's state of hydration. In order to make them as accurate as possible, they should be done at the same time of day, with the same scale, with the same amount of clothing, and by the same personnel.

The serum *electrolyte levels* and the *hematocrit* can reflect dehydration or overhydration, as their values are determined by the amount of blood in which they are contained. For example, if the patient is overhydrated, the electrolytes and hematocrit will have lower values owing to dilution. If the patient is dehydrated these values will be high, as the patient has lost water and the concentration of the elements in the blood has increased.

Observation of the patient will also help to determine the state of hydration. Since overhydration is more common than dehydration in the postoperative period, only the signs of overhydration will be reviewed here.

1. Tissue edema, especially in dependent areas (presacral, posterior thighs, ankles, and so forth).

2. Full neck veins that do not collapse when the patient is elevated to a 45 degree angle.

3. An enlarged liver (below the rib margin) that causes a visible reflux of blood into the neck veins when it is compressed (hepato-jugular reflux).

4. Fine crackling rales in the lungs.

5. Cardiac asthma or wheezing in the lungs.

A *central venous pressure* when correctly measured may be a good index of the circulating blood volume. The CVP will be accurate if the catheter is placed in the venae cava, innominate, subclavian, or iliac veins; if the patient is flat with the reference zero mark at the level of the right atrium or midaxillary line; if the patient is not straining; if the respirator is not delivering large volumes of air; and if the fluid level fluctuates with respirations.

The central venous pressure when correlated with other clinical observations and measurements can provide the following valuable information:

1. An increased blood volume with appropriate cardiovascular compensation will result in an increase in the CVP, stable or slightly elevated blood pressure, full pulses, and a warm dry skin.

2. Heart failure due to fluid overloading with backward failure from the left heart to the right heart will result in an elevated CVP, a decreased blood pressure, rales, and cool, dusky, moist skin.

3. Hypovolemia due to a loss of circulating blood volume will result in a decrease in the CVP, a low blood pressure with a narrow pulse pressure, and pallor.

4. Vasoconstriction due to cold or overactivity of the sympathetic nervous system causes a high CVP, a stable or slightly elevated blood pressure, and a cool, dry skin. Vasoconstriction can mask a fluid deficit, creating a smaller vascular bed by narrowing the lumen of the vessels, so the same amount of blood will occupy a smaller space. The fluid deficit may be uncovered by warming the patient (causing vasodilation) or by releasing the nervous system controls on the constricted arterioles (by administering phenothiazides or isoproterenol).

A *pulmonary artery* or *left atrial pressure catheter* may document signs of left ventricular failure before marked clinical changes occur in the patient, and usually before the left-sided failure progresses to right-sided failure. Pressures obtained by these catheters allow earlier intervention and preventive treatment. When either of these pressures rise above their normal values, the etiology may be due to fluid overloading or backward failure. The treatment is geared toward limiting fluids, diuresis, and giving inotropic agents such as digitalis which strengthen the myocardium.

Blood administration. Blood transfusions are a routine and necessary component in the postoperative care of the cardiac surgery patient. To minimize the possibility of a transfusion reaction, the patient's blood type and identification number and the serial number and type of the blood should be carefully checked by two people. The patient should be closely observed throughout the transfusion for signs of a transfusion reaction, and the blood should be discontinued after hanging at room temperature for six to eight hours. Closer observation for a transfusion reaction is indicated with infants, or patients who are heavily sedated or under anesthesia owing to their limited ability to perceive and to express symptoms. Infants usually need the closest observation as they seldom chill or shiver, and the only sign of a reaction may be pallor, slight cyanosis, or a drop in blood pressure with a rise in the pulse and temperature.

Reactions to blood transfusions may be manifested in one or more of the following ways:

1. Facial flushing or edema.
2. Throbbing headache.
3. Pain in the lumbar region.

4. Severe abdominal cramping.
5. Vomiting and diarrhea.
6. Bronchial spasm.
7. Urticaria (hives).
8. Fever.
9. Chills.
10. Elevated pulse.
11. Decreased blood pressure.

If a blood transfusion reaction has occurred, the nurse will need to closely monitor the patient's urinary output, since hemolytic reactions can cause deposition of damaged red blood cells in the renal tubules, producing oliguria or anuria. If the urinary output decreases, the physician should be notified; he may want to promote an osmotic diuresis and "flush the kidneys" by administering a hypertonic solution, such as 20 to 50 per cent glucose or mannitol.

Numerous blood transfusions of ACD-preserved blood over a short period of time can lower the body's ionized calcium enough to produce tetany. To maintain normal calcium blood levels, 10 cc of 10 per cent calcium gluconate is usually given after eight to 10 units of blood. This dosage can be repeated as often as every two units of blood thereafter, if indicated.

Electrolytes

Electrolytes are essential components of body fluids and are necessary to sustain life. The concentration of certain electrolytes is markedly different in the intracellular and extracellular compartments. Whenever these concentrations are changed, problems occur that an alert nurse can prevent by early detection.

Potassium. Extracellular potassium averages 4.0 mEq/L, while intracellular potassium averages 140 to 160 mEq/L. Since the extracellular potassium represents only 2 per cent of the total body potassium, it is important to obtain blood samples that do not distort the true value of the extracellular potassium by breakdown of the red blood cells. Red blood cell breakdown can be minimized by (1) leaving the tourniquet on for only a short period of time, (2) avoiding traumatic venipunctures in which blood does not return easily and air gets sucked into the syringe, and (3) not putting the blood into vacuum blood tubes through small needles. Whenever the lab report indicates that the blood sample has been hemolyzed (indicating red blood cell breakdown), another blood sample should be sent to assure an accurate potassium determination.

Hypokalemia, or a low serum potassium, can occur in the immediate postoperative period from various causes. Owing to the "stress" of the operation, the aldosterone levels may be elevated, resulting in a loss of potassium ion as sodium is saved by the body. If the patient is hyperventilated and develops a respiratory alkalosis, the serum potassium may drop. Hypokalemia can also result from an inadequate intake of potassium, diuretics, vomiting, diarrhea, and excessive nasogastric drainage.

Hypokalemia predisposes to digitalis toxicity, arrhythmias, a weakened myocardium, and metabolic alkalosis.

The nurse can suspect hypokalemia whenever the patient is lethargic, drowsy, irritable, or confused; whenever muscle tone lessens leading to paresthesia, flaccid paralysis, or abdominal distension. ECG changes of hypokalemia are a U wave more than 1 mm in height, AV block, low voltage, and flattened or inverted T waves.

The treatment for hypokalemia is potassium administration. Usually 40 to 120 mEq of potassium is diluted in 1000 cc of IV solution and not given faster than 15 to 20 mEq/hour.

Hyperkalemia, or a high serum potassium, can occur from (1) excessive potassium intake, (2) red blood cell breakdown, (3) tissue necrosis, (4) acidosis, (5) renal insufficiency, and (6) adrenal cortical insufficiency.

The patient with hyperkalemia may exhibit paresthesias of the extremities, weakness, mental confusion, listlessness, or nausea. The ECG will initially show a peaking and increase in the amplitude of the T wave, and then impaired electrical conduction with widening of the QRS and prolonged QT interval, which may eventually merge to form a sine wave pattern. Severe hypokalemia can result in cardiac arrest.

Immediate treatment to redistribute the high potassium includes the use of either IV sodium bicarbonate, or IV insulin and glucose to force the potassium back into the cells. Hyperventilation resulting in respiratory alkalosis can also lower the serum potassium. Definitive treatment to remove the potassium from the body includes giving ion-exchange resins like Kayexalate which binds the potassium, and the use of either peritoneal dialysis or hemodialysis. Hyperkalemia can be a life-threatening condition and deserves prompt treatment.

Sodium.   Hyponatremia, or low serum sodium, is more common than hypernatremia. Hyponatremia can occur when there is a "true" loss of sodium from the body, or when the sodium within the body is diluted from excessive water intake. There is a low total body sodium when a "true" loss has occurred. On the contrary, the total body sodium can be normal or elevated when hyponatremia is present owing to dilutional conditions. The patient will have peripheral edema with dilutional hyponatremia, and no edema with hyponatremia owing to a true loss of sodium.

Hyponatremia can occur from advanced congestive heart failure, advanced cirrhosis, or from overhydration. Since sodium is the main ion that binds with water, when the total body sodium is high, as with congestive heart failure, excess water is retained. When the total body sodium is low there is little to prevent large losses of water from the body. Whether the etiology of the low serum sodium is due to overhydration or lack of total body sodium, the consequences may be cardiovascular collapse from either too much or too little circulating blood volume. Also, cerebral edema from too much water entering the brain cells can result in swelling which can cause coma and death. Whenever the serum sodium value begins to fall below normal, treatment should be started.

The treatment of hyponatremia due to a "true" loss of sodium is the replacement of the sodium loss, which usually is given in hypertonic IV form. If the hyponatremia is dilutional, the treatment is aimed at restriction of sodium intake and ridding the body of the excess water through the use of diuretics.

A patient with dilutional hyponatremia can exhibit fatigue, weakness, anorexia, dry mouth, confusion, convulsions, seizures, coma, and vital sign changes similar to shock.

Calcium. Calcium has cardiac actions similar to digitalis and potentiates the action of digitalis. *Hypocalcemia,* or low serum calcium, is not uncommon in the postoperative cardiac patient. Serum calcium can be lowered from (1) multiple blood transfusions, since the ACD preservatives in the blood bind the calcium, and (2) from an alkalotic state, which drives calcium into the cell. Hypocalcemia can result in tetany and may necessitate additional doses of digitalis preparations. If the calcium levels suddenly return to normal, there is danger that the calcium will potentiate the excess digitalis to the point of causing digitalis toxicity.

Hypercalcemia produces changes similar to those of digitalis intoxication, i.e., sinus bradycardia, paroxysmal atrial tachycardia with block, AV block, and ventricular premature contractions. If the hypercalcemia is severe enough, cardiac rigor and asystole can occur, resulting in death.

Chest Drainage

Chest drainage tubes are inserted into the pleural cavity at the completion of the operation to provide a route for the evacuation of blood and air. If the blood is not adequately evacuated from the chest, pooling of blood and clot formation can occur, necessitating reoperation. The nurse is expected to understand the functioning of the chest drainage system and how to keep the chest tubes patent.

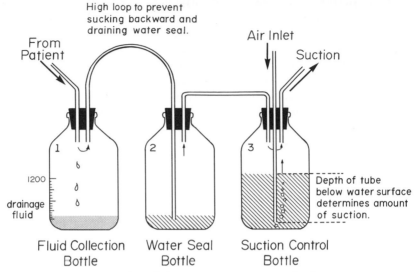

Figure 11-4. Pleural drainage system. See text for discussion.

Chest bottles. The chest tubes can be connected to either a one, two, or three bottle drainage system. Since a three bottle chest drainage system is more common, its major components will be discussed here (Fig 11-4).

A three bottle chest drainage system is composed of the following.

1 The bottle on the right controls the amount of suction. It has a water column of 15 to 20 cm which will provide the necessary suction of 15 to 20 cm of water, regardless of the force of the suction connected to this bottle. Therefore, the suction should be regulated to keep the water bubbling just slightly to indicate that the suction is connected and working. There is no need to cause excessive bubbling, as the height of the water column and not the amount of bubbling determines the amount of suction.

2. The middle bottle provides a seal of water over the end of the long tube, preventing air from being sucked back into the chest, thus avoiding a pneumothorax. No bubbling should be seen in this bottle unless the patient is coughing vigorously; a leak has occurred in the lungs or tubing; or the connections between the patient, the connecting tubing, or the bottles have loosened. Any bubbling in this container should be reported and the cause should be identified. If the bubbling is due to an air leak in the lungs, the nurse should be alert to the bubbling worsening, as other therapy may be indicated.

3. The drainage collection bottle (on the left) collects any fluid

that is drained from the chest. This bottle is usually marked in gradations to ensure accurate measurements of the chest drainage.

The chest drainage is usually copious and bloody immediately after surgery, and gradually decreases and becomes more serous until the drainage finally ceases. The nurse should be alert to a sudden cessation of bleeding or clot formation in the tubing which may indicate blockage of the chest tubes. She should also be aware that bleeding of over 200 cc per hour for a period of four to six hours in an adult indicates a need for evaluation of clotting mechanisms, and that reoperation for excessive bleeding may be necessary.

Chest tubes. The chest tubes are usually anchored to the skin with sutures, but as an extra precaution they should be taped securely to the patient and observed for slippage. If the chest tubes are patent, blood and fluid within the tube will fluctuate with either the respirations or the heart beat, depending upon the location of the tube within the chest. To ensure patency it is necessary to "strip" the tubes at least every half hour or more often in the period when bleeding is more profuse. To strip the chest tube correctly, the nurse secures the end of the tube that is next to the patient with one hand, and with the other hand (lubricated with lotion or oil to decrease resistance) she sequentially compresses the full length of the tubing from the patient to the chest bottle. If more than one chest tube is in place, she should clamp the tube that is not being stripped in order to create a better suction. If it appears that the chest tube is clotted, the nurse can either strip the tube toward the chest to push the clot off the end of the tube, use the rounded end of a large pair of forceps in order to compress the tube more completely, or insert a small needle into the tubing below a chest tube clamp to open a tube closed by negative pressure.

The patient with chest tubes. If the patient is properly instructed preoperatively, he will understand the purpose of the chest tubes and the sensations he will experience with them. Chest tubes are uncomfortable and usually cause pain when the patient inhales deeply, coughs, or when the tubes are being stripped. If the chest tubes are not sutured tightly in place, or if one of the drainage holes in the chest tube slips out of the thoracic cavity, subcutaneous emphysema or a pneumothorax can result.

Pooling of blood within the chest may occur even if the chest tubes are patent and draining well. To prevent pooling, the nurse should let the patient turn only toward the side of the chest tubes, or periodically change the patient's position (semi-Fowler's, completely flat, or sharply on the side of the chest tubes) to place the blood in a position in which it can be drained. If pooling occurs because of blockage of the chest tubes, it may be necessary for the physician to directly instill a solution into the chest tubes to loosen the blood clots and reopen the chest tubes.

When the chest drainage has ceased (usually within the first 48 hours), the chest tubes are removed. After the patient has taken a deep breath and has completely exhaled, the chest tube is quickly removed. The patient will experience a sharp burning pain at this time which will quickly disappear. If the patient has not been able to cooperate or the tube has been improperly removed, a pneumothorax may occur. After removal of the chest tubes, the nurse or physician should listen to the chest for an absence of breath sounds, indicating a pneumothorax. In some hospitals it is routine for chest x-ray films to be taken after the chest tubes are removed to make sure that a pneumothorax has not occurred.

Stomach Decompression

Following cardiac surgery, gastric dilatation is a very common occurrence. The stomach can become distended from air leaking around the endotracheal or tracheostomy tube, from the patient swallowing air, or from an accumulation of gastric fluid. Regardless of the cause it is necessary to decompress the stomach with a nasogastric tube to prevent vomiting, possible aspiration, and respiratory embarrassment.

Children are more prone to air swallowing and are more sensitive to respiratory embarrassment from abdominal distention. When the abdomen becomes distended it is difficult for the diaphragm to descend fully and to allow good tidal volumes. Eventually, if the distention is not corrected, respiratory embarrassment with tachypnea and hypoxia can result.

Pain

Different pain thresholds and abilities to tolerate pain are influenced by previous exposure to pain, cultural background, ego strength, and the amount of emotional support received at the time the pain occurs. Most of the patient's postoperative pain is caused by the physical trauma of surgery and surgical incisions (thoracotomies being more painful than sternotomies) and from the insertion of the chest tubes and other indwelling catheters.

Pain can cause physiologic changes in different organ systems overtaxing their function and lessening their performance. When pain occurs, there are certain responses that are particularly important in cardiac patients: (1) catecholamines (norepinephrine and epinephrine) are released, causing tachycardia, increasing the work load of the heart and the oxygen needs of the heart; (2) the acid level in the stomach may increase and eventually lead to stress ulcers; (3) the sympathetic discharge from pain may cause constriction of the afferent arterioles leading to the kidneys and may decrease glomerular filtration; and (4) the incisional pain can prevent deep breathing and coughing, often resulting in atelectasis and pneumonia.

It is only compassionate to alleviate pain and to prevent stress that pain inflicts on the patient. The following are some ways of lessening or alleviating pain:

1. Prepare the patient in advance for any painful experiences that he may encounter, and premedicate him if possible. Pain can be expected when the chest tubes are stripped or removed, from deep coughing, and from sighing on the respirator.

2. Control anxiety as much as possible, as anxiety and stress potentiate pain. The patient can be helped by providing emotional support and by explaining procedures, his progress, and the routine of the recovery room.

3. Enlist the patient's cooperation prior to moving or turning to decrease muscle resistance, which will only accentuate the pain.

4. Find positions which are most comfortable for the patient and splint incisions when the patient is coughing.

5. Since pain is harder to control and is intensified the longer it is untreated, frequent small doses of intravenous narcotics will be more effective than larger infrequent doses given intramuscularly.

6. If a patient is stoic or will not admit to having pain, knowing the signs that can accompany pain is important in interpreting when pain is really present. Some of the signs of pain are shallow respirations, tachycardia, restlessness, perspiration, increased blood pressure, and tense or grimacing facial expressions.

7. If the maximum dose of a narcotic is being used and is not effective, the addition of Phenergan may help to potentiate the narcotic and may also help the patient to relax.

8. If the patient is informed as to how often he can receive the narcotic and is encouraged to ask for it within these time intervals, he will be more active in decisions and may thus be able to tolerate his pain better.

9. Some patients have a fear of being "hooked" on drugs and may elect not to ask for their pain medication. The nurse should explain that some patients feel this way and that there is little danger of this happening.

Complications

Although some of the complications that will be covered in this section have previously been mentioned, they are of such importance in determining the patient's clinical course that it is worthwhile consolidating them here as to their etiology, signs, and treatment.

Shock.   Shock in cardiac surgical patients is most likely to occur from inadequate circulating blood volume or from myocardial failure. In either case, the patient can exhibit restlessness, thirst, a fast pulse, low blood pressure, narrow pulse pressure, slow capillary filling, cold, cyanotic, moist skin with weak, intermittent and thready pulses. Inadequate circulating blood volumes can occur from hemorrhage, vasodilatation, or inadequate blood replacement. Myocardial contractility will decrease with acidosis, hypoxia, electrolyte imbalance, or myocardial infarction. Myocardial infarctions developing after cardiac surgery may have the following etiology: (1) inadequate coronary artery perfusion during the operation; (2) tachycardias or severe hypotension causing poor coronary artery perfusion; and (3) air, blood clots, or calcium debris lodging in the coronary arteries.

Treating shock usually involves treating the underlying cause. For instance, if the shock is due to an inadequate circulating blood volume additional blood is administered. If the shock is due to myocardial failure the acidosis, electrolyte imbalance, and hypoxia are corrected and inotropic drugs like digitalis or Isuprel are given to strengthen the heart

Cardiac arrest.   Cardiac arrest should be anticipated in all cases, and can be diagnosed by the absence of pulses and respirations and later by dilated pupils. The initial treatment of a cardiac arrest is closed chest massage, mouth-to-mouth respiration, correction of the metabolic acidosis, and treatment of the underlying cause. The different major causes of cardiac arrest are respiratory arrest, massive hemorrhage, an irritable myocardium (ventricular tachycardia and ventricular fibrillation), a weakened myocardium (myocardial ischemia or hypoxia), and a depressed conducting system (marked bradycardia, complete heart block, and asystole). (Refer to Chapter 9 for more detailed information.)

To help the nurse move more efficiently when a cardiac arrest occurs, the following will be useful: (1) attach a three way stopcock at the IV site so medicines can be administered quickly; (2) keep a crayon or grease pencil handy so that the time, dosage, medicine, and treatment can be written on a window or panel by the bed, (3) use a No. 15 blunt needle to draw up solutions like sodium bicarbonate, and (4) if emergency drugs are used frequently in your unit, have the pharmacy check to see which drugs can be left drawn up in labeled syringes in the emergency cart.

Tamponade.   When blood or fluid collects between the lining of the heart (pericardium) and the myocardium, tamponade can develop. This collection of fluid can produce such pressure that the heart is compressed and is not able to adequately fill with blood during diastole and thus has less blood to pump out during systole. As this process continues, the patient will eventually go into profound shock. An early sign of tamponade is a rise in the CVP that is not attributed to excess fluid administration. The pulse will rise as the blood pressure falls and the pulse pressure narrows. The heart sounds will become distant, and the classic description of a "quiet, small heart" may be present. A pulsus paradoxicus of 10 mm Hg or more may be heard Kussmaul's sign or a rise in the jugular veins on inspiration can also indicate tamponade.

Tamponade in postoperative cardiac patients often will not result in an elevated CVP, as the mediastinal clots may only press upon the ventricles and not the atria. The only clue to the diagnosis may be signs of the low output syndrome associated with a falling urinary output. Usually a portable chest x-ray film will reveal a widening of the mediastinal shadow, giving strong evidence to the presence of tamponade.

Occasionally the tamponade can be treated by inserting a long needle through the chest wall to evacuate the blood between the pericardium and the heart. Usually, however, it is necessary to return the patient to the operating room, as large clots can form in this space and cannot be removed by a pericardial tap.

Pneumothorax.   A pneumothorax can occur when the lungs are punctured or when a connection between atmospheric air and the chest cavity exists, as with stab wounds or with the removal of chest tubes. The patient may experience a sudden, severe respiratory embarrassment when a large pneumothorax suddenly develops. There will be cyanosis, labored respirations, tachypnea, tachycardia, and either a decrease or absence of breath sounds on the side of the pneumothorax. A pneumothorax not only limits the amount of lung that is available for gaseous exchange, but can cause movement of structures within the chest toward the opposite side of the chest (mediastinal shift), especially if a tension pneumothorax develops. With a tension pneumothorax, tracheal and cardiac displacement are common; this usually is an emergency situation.

The treatment for a pneumothorax consists of the insertion of a chest tube into the upper portion of the thoracic cavity to evacuate air and re-expand the collapsed lung.

Pulmonary edema.   When the left ventricle fails to such an extent that blood backs up through the left atrium into the lungs, pulmonary edema may result. With acute, fulminating pulmonary edema there is a sudden onset of tachypnea, cyanosis, frothy pink sputum, a desire to sit erect, and symptoms of shock. The treatment is geared toward impeding venous return to the heart—(1) tourniquets on the extremities; (2) sitting the patient upright; (3) giving IV morphine to sedate the patient and vasodilate vessels, causing pooling of blood; (4) performing a phlebotomy to lessen the circulating blood volume; and (5) giving diuretics to decrease the total body fluid. The treatment is also geared toward removing the excess fluid in the alveoli by (1) using IPPB to increase the pressure in the alveoli and cause transudation of fluid back into the capillaries and (2) using agents that decrease surface tension (50 per cent alcohol) so the frothy fluid can be removed more easily.

After the initial emergency treatment is started, inotropic agents may be used to improve the cardiac performance to prevent backward failure from recurring.

Pulmonary embolus.   Blood clots that form in the venous system or in the right side of the heart can travel to the lungs and result in a pulmonary embolus. If the clot is large enough to completely occlude the pulmonary artery, the patient will suddenly collapse and death can shortly follow. If the clots come in small showers and do not completely block the pulmonary artery or one of its major branches, the patient has a good chance of surviving.

A patient with a pulmonary embolus will have respiratory difficulty, cyanosis, and hemoptysis and may have pleuritic pain or asthmalike symptoms. If the embolus causes infarction of lung tissue near the lung surface, a pleural friction rub, which sounds like squeaking leather varying with respirations, will be heard. Otherwise, the diagnosis can be made from blood gases, angiography, lung scans, or a chest x-ray film.

Patients who are most prone to having pulmonary emboli are those who (1) are on bedrest and do not have elastic leg stockings or who do not do leg exercises; (2) have diuresed large volumes of urine within a short period of time and have increased blood viscosity; (3) have atrial fibrillation which predisposes to clot formation in the atria, and (4) have such poor myocardial contractility that there is stasis of blood in the atria.

Pulmonary emboli are usually treated by anticoagulation or by inferior vena cava ligation if emboli recur. If the pulmonary function has been significantly impaired and respiratory support is indicated, the patient may need an endotracheal tube or tracheostomy. A pulmonary embolectomy may be needed if cardiovascular collapse occurs from a large pulmonary embolus.

Cerebral embolus.   A cerebral embolus can be caused by emboli of air, fat, calcium, or blood clots that are released into the arterial system and lodge within the brain. Cerebral emboli are more likely to occur following surgery on the left side of the heart, with right-to-left shunts in either the atria or ventricles, or if air or clots enter the left atrial monitoring line.

The nurse should suspect a cerebral embolism when the patient cannot move all extremities, does not awaken, or is hyperactive to any type of stimulus. The treatment is aimed at preventing or controlling cerebral edema by administration of corticosteroids, hypothermia, elevation of the head of the bed, and use of hypertonic solutions like urea or mannitol. The reversibility of this condition will depend upon the extent of the insult and the effectiveness of the treatment. The nurse can be most helpful at this time by being alert to signs that cerebral edema is developing.

Cerebral vascular accident (CVA). A cerebral vascular accident (or stroke) can be caused by blockage of local arterial blood flow to a portion of the brain, by hemorrhage within the brain, or by a generalized lack of cerebral blood flow due to profound systemic hypotension. If the stroke occurs on the dominant side of the brain, the patient will have speech difficulties or complete aphasia. The patient often shows weakness or total paralysis of one side of the body.

The treatment may include anticoagulation if the etiology was not due to hemorrhage, utilization of air mixtures high in carbon dioxide to elicit cerebral vasodilatation, cooling, steroids, and hypertonic IV solutions to prevent cerebral edema and supportive measures, such as physical therapy. The patient will be more comfortable if he is given injections on the paralyzed side which has less feeling; he should be touched for meaningful stimuli on the uninvolved side.

Renal failure. Cardiac surgical patients may develop renal failure during their postoperative course. Circulatory insufficiency is a common factor contributing to renal failure and may be caused by:

1. Hypovolemia, owing to a loss of blood, plasma, or fluids (dehydration).

2. Ineffective pumping action of the myocardium from congestive heart failure, myocardial infarction, tamponade, or pulmonary embolus.

3. Low circulatory resistance (associated with vasodilatation and hypotension) from toxins, drug-induced anaphylactic reactions, adrenal insufficiency, hyponatremia, or acidosis.

These preceding conditions contributing to circulatory insufficiency may lead to acute oliguric renal failure, which is characterized by (1) an oliguric-anuric stage; (2) an early diuretic stage, and (3) a late diuretic or recovery stage.

The oliguric-anuric stage begins when the urinary output is less than 400 cc per day in an adult and less than 50 cc per day in a child. Although this stage usually lasts from eight to 15 days, the greater the renal damage, the longer the oliguric-anuric stage. The patient's urinary output will be low or absent, and the serum creatinine, serum potassium, and BUN will rise.

The early diuretic stage follows the oliguric-anuric stage. As the kidneys recover, the urinary output increases with a fall in the specific gravity, the serum creatinine, and BUN. During this stage, death may occur from water or electrolyte depletion if treatment is not instituted.

During the late diuretic stage, the urinary output is good and the BUN and serum creatinine approach normal ranges.

The management of acute oliguric renal failure is aimed at maintenance of fluid and electrolyte balance, and the prevention of metabolic acidosis and infection.

1. The fluid intake is sharply restricted, especially during the oliguric-anuric stage, owing to the endogenous water production by the metabolism of food and body tissues. A fluid limit of 500 cc per day is not uncommon. When properly managed, the patient is expected to lose 0.3 to 0.7 kg of weight per day during the oliguric stage.

2. The potassium intake is limited owing to the high serum potassium levels from the loss of intracellular potassium (acidosis and catabolism of protein and tissues). If the potassium levels are too elevated, the use of IV sodium bicarbonate, IV glucose and insulin, kayexalate, or dialysis may be indicated. High serum potassium is more pronounced in the oliguric-anuric stage.

3. Dilutional hyponatremia resulting from endogenous water formation from metabolism may occur. If the patient gains weight during the oliguric-anuric stage, this problem should be suspected and confirmed by a low serum sodium. The treatment is to limit water intake and if necessary, give a hypertonic IV solution of sodium.

4. Metabolic acidosis due to an increase in organic acids or a loss of bicarbonate can be treated by buffering the excess acid with sodium bicarbonate or TRIS buffer (which is stronger than sodium bicarbonate and contains no sodium).

5. A diet high in carbohydrates and low in protein is given to prevent more protein breakdown. With less protein breakdown there will be less nitrogenous wastes, which can only be excreted by the kidneys. The patient is usually given a 100 gm carbohydrate diet with little or no protein (20 to 40 gm protein), limited sodium (500 mg), and little or no potassium

6. The dosage of drugs such as digoxin, which are primarily excreted through the kidneys, will have to be reduced or they may reach toxic levels.

7. Infections, especially pulmonary, are common with renal failure and cause a greater breakdown of protein. These patients develop pulmonary infections as they often have tenacious, copious pulmonary secretions as well as inadequate respiratory excursions. Antibiotic therapy is instituted when the organism has been isolated. The dosage of some of the antibiotics (especially streptomycin, colistin, and kanamycin) will need to be greatly reduced when oliguria or anuria are present, as they are excreted primarily through the kidneys.

In order to evaluate the patient's response to therapy, the nurse should look for signs of improvement in the patient—an increase in mental alertness, absence of a metabolic hand flap (previously called *liver flap*), and increase in the urinary creatinine clearance (usually 80 to 100 cc per minute in an adult).

Postoperative psychosis. Postoperative psychosis is more likely to occur in patients who have had psychologic and stressful unresolved problems preoperatively, who have been very sick before surgery, and who have experienced sensory deprivation postoperatively. The term *sensory deprivation* can be related to any unmeaningful stimuli, such as noise from monitors, respirators, and oxygen tents, frequent vital signs, lack of uninterrupted sleep, and painful treatments and procedures.

Meaningful stimuli evolve around close relationships with people who show concern of deep caring, and give the patient a feeling of being wanted, needed, and loved. Unfortunately, in most intensive care units, it is difficult to provide enough meaningful stimuli because of the multiple chores, heavy patient load, desire of some staff to protect themselves from close involvement with patients who run a high mortality rate, and the strict control of visiting hours.

Patient changes resulting from sensory deprivation usually begin after a lucid period of three to five days. They last from one to two days and are best treated by removing the patient from the intensive care unit and by sedating with Thorazine, Stelazine, or Trilafon.

The patient's symptoms usually begin with auditory and visual hallucinations leading to paranoia. Usually the patient will recover when he is removed from the intensive care unit and allowed to have uninterrupted sleep and resume a normal day and night schedule.

Besides allowing the patient to spend more time with loved ones, promoting closer staff-patient relationships and longer uninterrupted periods of sleep, the following changes in the ICU environment will be helpful:

1. Decrease the monotonous noise created by monitors, oxygen tents, and traffic through the ICU.

2. Allow the patient more mobility by removing catheters and monitoring devices as soon as possible, or placing them in positions that will not hinder his movement.

3. When the patient is more alert, allow him to have a radio or television set.

4. Provide calendars and clocks to help orient him to time.

5. Structure the unit so the patient is protected from the noises of emergencies around him, yet provide for the extra stimuli that a window facing a pleasant view can give.

6. Make the patient feel that he is important in promoting good care by including him in his health care plan, in determining his

needs, and by giving him choices in determining his own care, as it is geared toward the time of discharge.

The Convalescent Phase

The convalescent period begins after the patient has overcome the acute problems that usually occur within the first three to five days following surgery. During this time, healing and rest begin restoring the patient to a stronger state that leads to discharge from the hospital.

The patient is moved from the recovery room back to a general ward usually on the third to fifth postoperative day. He does not have special nurses unless he requests them or the patient load on the ward is so great that the regular staff can not provide his care. The recovery room had a smaller patient-nurse ratio which enabled the nurses to be more attentive to the patient's needs. Thus, when the patient is returned to the floor without a special nurse, he may experience a sensation of being "dumped." He feels neglected and forgotten. To avoid this feeling, there is a need for the nurses to provide a continuity of care between the recovery room and the general ward. This continuity can be accomplished in the following ways:

1. Prepare the patient for the feelings of "dumping" that he might encounter.

2. Encourage independence as soon as the patient is ready for it in the acute postoperative period.

3. Attempt to transfer the patient back to the ward and room from which he came before surgery.

4. Encourage the nursing personnel from the floor to visit the patient while he is in the recovery room.

5. Nursing personnel from the recovery room and particularly the nurse who has been with the patient in the preoperative and acute postoperative period need to continue interest and follow through on his care once he leaves the recovery room.

6. If the floor nurses have been briefed on pertinent preoperative and postoperative data, it will be easier for them to have a fuller understanding of the total picture, so continuity of care can be provided.

EMOTIONAL PROBLEMS

Isolation

Upon discharge from the recovery room, the patient is pleased that the worst is over, and is anxious to return to an environment in which he can get more sleep and spend more time with his family and friends. Later, he may develop feelings of isolation that can evolve from the larger physical design of the ward that does not allow direct visualization of the personnel. Isolation can also occur if the nursing personnel feel that the patient is demanding and know that they cannot provide the special attention he received while in the recovery room. Unless the patient understands that he is clinically better and does not require as much care, and unless the nursing personnel understand the patient's dependent state and his fear of being left alone, the gap will widen and the feelings of isolation will increase.

Dependence to Independence

During the convalescent period, independence should be encouraged in the patient. As the patient gains more strength, he needs to be encouraged to do more for himself so he will develop a sense of pride and a better self-image. Some patients will need to be watched for overexertion before they are physically ready, as this can cause setbacks. Patients who have used their cardiac disease as a "crutch" will fight to remain dependent upon the staff and the family. It is possible that the family of this dependent patient will continue to foster this type of dependency as they also have a need to maintain this type of relationship.

The patient will again need orientation so he can learn the role he will play in the convalescent period. The most obvious thing the patient will experience is a continual feeling of being tired and having little strength, especially upon exertion. His appetite will be poor at first and he will continue to experience incisional pain. Narcotics usually are not required at this time, unless the pains are sharp or intense If narcotics are still needed, the patient should be encouraged to take them so he can rest better, move more easily and participate more fully in his treatments.

The course of healing is not always a smooth one with a steady upward trend. Many times it is one of "hills and valleys" that may depress the patient and discourage him. If he is prepared for this type of course and is given encouragement when he hits the "valleys," he will not lose hope and will strive for the next "hill."

PHYSIOLOGIC PROBLEMS

Fluid Balance

To maintain a proper fluid balance it may be necessary for the patient to have a fluid limit, low salt diet, accurate recording of intakes and outputs, and daily weights. If the patient has been in congestive heart failure before surgery, the total body sodium will still be elevated and the tendency to retain fluids will prevail. If the patient has not adjusted to a low salt diet and finds it unpalatable, lemon juice, herbs, and salt substitutes can be utilized. Since salt substitutes contain calcium or potassium in place of sodium, it is wise to consult with the physician to determine which type of salt substitute would be best for the patient.

When the patient is under stress or is depressed, the body has a tendency to hold sodium and water. If the patient is in borderline failure, this emotional tone may be enough to cause frank cardiac failure. Thus, anything the nurse can do to help alleviate the depression or help the patient deal effectively with his feelings of depression might indirectly prevent him from retaining additional sodium and water.

Potassium-losing diuretics may be given daily or used intermittently when indicated. In either case, especially if digitalis preparations are being used, a potassium supplement is indicated. If the patient cannot tolerate the potassium supplements, he can benefit from learning which foods are high in potassium, so he can balance his diet in such a way that a potassium supplement may not be necessary.

Pulmonary Consolidations

A certain degree of atelectasis is present in all patients who undergo major cardiac surgery. It takes a great deal of effort and time to remedy this complication and to prevent the patient from developing further atelectasis or pneumonia. The need for pulmonary support is still indicated during the convalescent period, since the patient has a tendency to slack off on his pulmonary regimen (coughing and use of the IPPB). He needs to be encouraged to continue his pulmonary therapy until he is up and walking around a good portion of the day. While he is still weak and spends most of the day in bed, changing positions every couple of hours during the day will keep the lungs better aerated and enable the patient to raise mucus more effectively. Pain medications may still be indicated at this time to aid the patient in being more active in his pulmonary regimen and his daily exercises.

Pleural Effusions

A certain percentage of patients will develop pleural effusions in which fluid collects between the lungs and the lining of the chest cavity. This fluid will eventually create such pressure on the lungs that they will not be able to expand fully, and the removal of this fluid may be necessary. This problem is most prone to develop after the chest tubes have been removed.

A thoracentesis is performed to evacuate the fluid by inserting a needle through anesthetized tissue into the side of the chest where the pleural effusion has developed. Evacuating the fluid may cause sharp pains, which usually do not persist. The patient feels relief immediately after the procedure, and states that he can breathe more easily. After this procedure, the nurse or physician should auscultate the lungs to ascertain if the needle has punctured the lung, causing a pneumothorax.

Anticoagulation

Patients who receive prosthetic valves are routinely anticoagulated to prevent clot formation on the valve which could either impair its performance or release a clot into the circulatory system. Anticoagulation is started after the chest tubes have been removed and will often continue throughout the rest of the patient's life. The initial anticoagulation may be started with heparin in order to maintain the clotting time at two to two and one half times the normal clotting time of the patient. With a normal clotting time of 10 to 15 minutes, the therapeutic range of the Lee and White clotting time would be 25 to 40 minutes. When therapeutic clotting levels have been reached and the patient is able to take oral fluids, he is changed to an oral form of anticoagulation like Dicumarol or Coumadin. Many cardiac centers begin anticoagulation not with heparin but with Dicumarol or Coumadin.

It takes oral anticoagulants three to five days to reach therapeutic levels, so they are given in combination with the heparin until good prothrombin levels are attained. The therapeutic range for a prothrombin time usually is between 15 and 25 per cent. The prothrombin time will vary somewhat from lab to lab and from patient to patient. Therefore, special consideration should be given to the medications the patient is receiving that can alter the prothrombin time. Some of the more commonly used drugs in cardiac patients that alter the prothrombin time will be mentioned. Drugs increasing the prothrombin time are quinidine, salicylates, adrenocorticosteroids, dilantin, and sulfonamides. Drugs lessening the prothrombin time are barbiturates, chloral hydrate, meprobamate, and antihistamines.

The patient should be observed for any evidence of overanticoagulation, such as excessive bruising, bleeding, or blood in the urine. The patient and the family should be instructed to look for these things and to be alert to cuts that require more pressure for longer periods than normal in order to stop the bleeding. These patients should carry medical emergency cards in their wallets stating that they are taking anticoagulants.

Digitalization

Routinely, digitalis is stopped at least 24 hours prior to surgery and is usually resumed postoperatively within the first 24 to 48 hours. When the patient begins oral feedings, the digitalis preparations are changed from the intravenous to the oral route. Changing to an oral route may require further regulation of the dosages depending upon the state of the gastrointestinal tract and the kidneys. The patient should be observed and instructed as to the symptoms of digitalis toxicity. He may experience nausea, vomiting, "yellow vision," and anorexia. With monitored patients, the nurse may observe bradycardia, ventricular premature beats, an increased PR interval, first degree heart block, or paroxysmal atrial tachycardia with block. If these occur, the digitalis dosages may need to be decreased or stopped temporarily, and potassium may be given.

Cardioversion

Some cardiac patients will continue to have arrhythmias after surgery, i.e., atrial fibrillation. Since these arrhythmias can markedly decrease the cardiac output, it is advantageous to revert the patient to sinus rhythm by administering antiarrhythmic drugs or by doing a cardioversion. At present, cardioversion is favored more than drug therapy which takes more time and can result in drug toxicities.

In a cardioversion, an electrical current (usually direct current) is synchronized to discharge on the R wave of the ECG. This synchronization avoids the "vulnerable zone" (during the T wave) which could result in ventricular fibrillation. When this electrical energy is passed through the body by means of external paddles, the heart is instantaneously depolarized, hopefully allowing the sinus node to take over as the pacemaker of the heart. If the cardioversion is successful, maintenance of antiarrhythmic agents may be needed to keep the patient in sinus rhythm.

The patient may be given either general anesthesia or may receive an IV sedative such as Valium. When the patient does not receive general anesthesia, he will experience a "shocking" sensation throughout his body which may cause fear and pain at the time it occurs. A prepared patient will know that this shocking sensation is only instantaneous, and thus will experience less apprehension.

DISCHARGE FROM THE HOSPITAL

If there have been no major complications, the patient will be discharged from the hospital within two to three weeks after surgery. Plans are made with the physician, dietician, and visiting nurse to guide the patient and his family in understanding his medications, diet, and exercise tolerance. The family is taught how to prepare his diet and what they might do to temporarily rearrange things at home to cause less exertion for the patient. The planning for discharge actually begins with teaching in the preoperative period and is continued throughout the entire hospitalization. The patient and family need to understand how the disease has affected the physical abilities of the patient, how much he can do now, what limits to set for physical activity, diet, rest, and medicines, and how to observe for fluid retention.

This chapter has been developed to provide the nurse with a deeper, fuller understanding of the physiologic and emotional factors involved in caring for the cardiac surgical patient. Hopefully, this comprehensive view will prepare the nurse more effectively for establishing a *baseline*—the most essential component in determining patient care.

Bibliography

Abbey, J.: Nursing observations of fluid imbalance. Nurs. Clin. N. Amer. 3:77–86, 1968.
Abbey, J.: Temperature considerations. Unpublished paper. U.S.P.H.S., Grant #1147, 1967.
Banyai, A., and Levine, E.: Dyspnea: Diagnosis and Treatment. Philadelphia, F. A. Davis Company, 1963.
Betson, C., and Ude, L.: Central venous pressure. Amer. J. Nurs. 69:1466–1469, 1969.
Christman, L.: Patient role. J. Nurs. Ed. 6:17–21, 1967.
Chronic obstructive emphysema. Ciba Pharmaceutical Company, p. 51–54, 1968.
Crowley, D.: Pain and Its Alleviation. U.C.L.A. School of Nursing, 1962.
Delp, M. H., and Manning, R. T. (eds.): Major's Physical Diagnosis. 7th ed. Philadelphia, W. B. Saunders Company, 1968.
Guyton, A. C.: Function of the Human Body. 3rd ed. Philadelphia, W. B. Saunders Company, 1969.
Guyton, A. C.: Textbook of Medical Physiology. 4th ed. Philadelphia, W. B. Saunders Company, 1971.
Hazan, S. J.: Psychiatric complications following cardiac surgery. J. Thorac. Cardiovasc. Surg. 51:307–318, 1966.
Hickey, M.: Hypothermia. Amer. J. Nurs. 65:116–122, 1965.
Jourard, S.: The Transparent Self. Princeton, New Jersey, D. Van Nostrand Company, Inc., 1970.
Knowles, J.: Respiratory Physiology and Its Clinical Application. Cambridge, Massachusetts, Harvard University Press, 1959.
Kornfeld, D.: Psychiatric view of the intensive care unit. Brit. Med. J., p. 108–110, 1969.
Kornfeld, D. S., Maxwell, T., and Momrow, D.: Psychological hazards of the intensive care unit. Nurs. Clin. N. Amer. 3:41–51, 1968.

Kurihara, M.: Assessment and maintenance of adequate respiration. Nurs. Clin. N. Amer. 3:65–76, 1968.

Langendorf, R., and Pick, A.: Atrioventricular block, Type II (Mobitz) — Its nature and clinical significance. Circulation 38:819–821, 1968.

Meyer, J. H.: Effects of hypothermia on local blood flow and metabolism during cerebral ischemia and hypoxia. J. Neurosurg. 14:210–227, 1957.

Morrelli, H., and Melmon, K.: Pharmacologic basis for the use of antiarrhythmic drugs. Pharmacol. Physicians 1:1–7, 1967.

Muehecke, R.: Acute Renal Failure: Diagnosis and Management. Saint Louis, Missouri, C. V. Mosby Company, 1969.

Papper, S.: Hyperkalemia and hypokalemia. Disease of the Month, June 1964.

Rogers, C.: A counseling approach to human problems. Amer. J. Nurs. 56:994–998, 1956.

Rushmer, R.: Cardiovascular Dynamics. 3rd ed. Philadelphia, W. B. Saunders Company, 1970.

Scheinman, M., and Hutchinson, J.: Cavitary left atrial electrograms after open-heart surgery. J. Thorac. Cardiovasc. Surg. 57:400–407, 1969.

Young, J. F.: Recognition, significance, and recording of the signs of increased intracranial pressure. Nurs. Clin. N. Amer. 4:223–236, 1969.

Index

Page numbers in *italics* refer to illustrations.